Understanding the Electrocardiogram:
by Derek J Rowlands
Section 2: Morphological abnormalities

D J Rowlands
Consultant Cardiologist
Manchester Area Health Authority
Hon. Lecturer in Cardiology
University of Manchester

Illustrations and ECG art-work
Denis Gidion, Creative Workshop,
Macclesfield.

Typesetting and art-work
Gask and Hawley Limited, Manchester.

Acknowledgements

My debt to those who have helped, directly or indirectly, in the production of this volume is no less than it was in Section 1. The influence of all those whose contribution was acknowledged in that Section has, of course, continued undiluted in this Section.

It is true with regard to Section 2 as it was with regard to Section 1 that my greatest direct debt is to ICI Pharmaceuticals Division. Their collective commitment to this project has sustained me through periods of self-doubt and has given me unfettered freedom, in moments of self-confidence, to proceed with the work as I saw fit. The faith displayed by Bob Tomlinson and Ivor Townshend at a time when the whole project was no more than a concept would be easy to forget at this stage when the production of Section I has been extended to 30,000 copies – but I recall it with gratitude. More recently that faith has been supported and extended by Mike Asbury. The prime importance of design and of the quality of illustrations was acknowledged in Section 1. Responsibility for this aspect of production in Section 2 has been taken over by Steve Jackson. That he has so clearly maintained the previously set standards and added improvements where appropriate without producing inconsistencies speaks volumes for his expertise.

Each of the persons mentioned above was responsible in his own area for aspects of production. The needs of one area might, and often did, conflict with those of another. One person permanently occupied the centre of all ensuing struggles – Roger Tittensor. On his broad shoulders fell the greatest individual burden. He contributed to the production of this volume to an extent over and beyond the call of duty. Problems and brickbats from whatever source were automatically referred to him. Whether at work or at home he made himself available. He has my gratitude. I trust he has his wife's forgiveness.

The above acknowledgements refer to **direct** help in the production of this book. **Indirect** help from those who guided my approach to cardiology played no small part in my attitude to learning, to understanding and to teaching (a natural progression). I wish particularly to acknowledge Dr Morgan Jones, from Manchester, whose reasonable, balanced approach taught me so much during my first attachment in clinical cardiology, and Dr Howard Burchell, under whose clinical guidance I spent a year at the Mayo Clinic. Even the depth of his modesty and his self-effacing style could not disguise from me his true greatness.

D J ROWLANDS

How to use this book

As indicated in the advice on how to use Section 1 of this trilogy, there are, in general, three recognisable approaches used by students attempting to learn from a book:—

Approach 1. The student wishes to have rapid access to information enabling him to discriminate among normal appearances, specific abnormalities and non-specific abnormalities without being committed to "background reading". Whilst this approach can never give true understanding it may, occasionally, be expedient. To fulfil such a requirement the student should be sure that he has mastered those pages specified for this approach in Section 1, together with the data contained in the blue

"diagnostic boxes"

contained on pages 118, 124, 133, 137, 139, 141, 148, 155, 162, 165, 196, 215 and 219. Pages containing such boxes are indicated by a blue triangle in the top outer corner – as on this page. He should also pay particular attention to pages 265 to 269.

Approach 2. The student wishes to understand the basis of the normal electrocardiogram and the more important principles underlying the commoner morphological abnormalities of the ECG, but does not wish to concern himself with aspects which are conceptually difficult, contentious, less important or rare or with any combination of these three. Such a student should read through the text sequentially, omitting parts marked with a coloured paragraph edge as shown here.

Approach 3. The student wishes to follow each step in the full understanding of the electrocardiogram. This student must follow the whole text through sequentially.

Whatever the approach, the student should follow the advice, given in Section 1, to study as much of the book as possible within the first few weeks of obtaining it. However, unlike the situation which obtains when one sets out to understand the normal electro-cardiogram – where the understanding of each part is dependent upon the understanding of those parts preceding and following the part in question, it is possible to understand each section in its own right. It is, therefore, possible to study a chapter at a time in this section. However, it should be realised that the **sequence** of the chapter has been chosen to minimise conceptual difficulties and to reduce the likelihood of diagnostic error (thus, for example, left bundle branch block must be understood before myocardial infarction is covered and ventricular pre-excitation must be **referred to** before bundle branch block, even though it will not be covered until later).

Introduction

Inter-relationships between Morphological and Rhythm Information

The electrocardiogram provides greater or lesser degrees of information about the structure, shape, orientation, size and state of health of the atrial and ventricular myocardium (**"morphological" information**) and on the direction, timing and sequence of the depolarisation of myocardium and the relationship between atrial and ventricular depolarisation (**"rhythm" information**). In the majority of electrocardiograms the morphological information and the rhythm information are mutually discrete. Occasionally, however, a disturbance of the cardiac rhythm may interfere with morphological analysis (as when ventricular tachycardia precludes the recognition of ventricular hypertrophy, bundle branch block or myocardial infarction) and sometimes a morphological abnormality may interfere with the determination of cardiac rhythm (as when bundle branch block occurring in association with a supraventricular tachycardia may lead to an incorrect diagnosis of ventricular tachycardia). In most electrocardiograms it is possible both to determine the cardiac rhythm and to assess the morphological state. Reports of electrocardiograms should always give both items of information, wherever possible.

Simple electrocardiographic reports therefore often take one of the general forms illustrated below:-

1. "Sinus rhythm. The record is within normal limits."

2. "Sinus rhythm. Left bundle branch block."

3. "Sinus bradycardia. Acute myocardial infarction."

4. "Ventricular tachycardia. This precludes morphological evaluation of the electrocardiogram."

This whole section (Section 2) will be concerned entirely with morphological abnormalities of the electrocardiograms. **Unless otherwise stated, normal sinus rhythm will be assumed.** The criteria for normality of the QRS complexes, S-T segments and T waves given in Section 1 depend upon the normal sequence of depolarisation and of repolarisation of the ventricular myocardium. This normal sequence is only possible if the activation (depolarisation) wave reaches the ventricles via the normal route, i.e. through the A-V node from a more proximal, primary initiating site. The criteria for QRS complexes, S-T segments and T waves (i.e. the ventricular part of the ECG) therefore apply to all rhythms initiated from a **supraventricular** site, i.e. sinus rhythm, sinus arrhythmia, sinus tachycardia, sinus bradycardia, atrial ectopic beats, atrial tachycardia, atrial flutter, atrial fibrillation, nodal ectopic beats, nodal rhythm and nodal tachycardia.

The only exception to this rule arises from the fact that the right and left bundle branches have different refractory periods (normally the refractory period of the right bundle is longer than that of the left bundle). Because of this, when the supraventricular rate is rapid it is possible for the depolarisation wave to emerge from the distal end of the atrio-ventricular node at a time when one bundle (usually the left) has recovered and the other has not. In this event the depolarisation wave spreads through the ventricular myocardium by pathways preferentially served by that bundle which has recovered and the QRS complexes, S-T segments and T waves are all altered. This rate-dependent conduction down one bundle only is known as **functional bundle branch block** or as **aberrant intraventricular conduction.** If the bundle which, in these circumstances, fails to conduct is the right bundle no disease of the bundle is implied. If the bundle which fails to conduct is the left bundle it is likely that the left bundle is abnormal (simply because in normal circumstances its refractory period is less than that of the right bundle).

Rate-related (functional) bundle branch block most commonly occurs in association with atrial tachycardia in which case usually each QRS complex, S-T segment and T wave is affected. It also occurs intermittently in atrial fibrillation – usually only being present in those cardiac cycles which follow closely on the preceding cycle (i.e. where the ventricular rate is transiently rapid). Sinus tachycardia is never rapid enough to give rise to "normal" functional bundle branch block, though it may give rise to bundle branch block on a rate-dependent basis by unmasking disease in one or other bundles, i.e. the occurrence of bundle branch block in association with sinus tachycardia implies disease in the appropriate bundle.

Beats which are initiated within the ventricle (ventricular ectopic beats, ventricular tachycardia) cannot possibly follow the normal pathway since they actually start in the wrong place! Such beats therefore necessarily produce abnormal QRS complexes and this primary abnormality of the QRS complex inevitably gives rise to secondary abnormalities of the S-T segments and T waves.

Sensitivity and Specificity

Electrocardiographic interpretation is an empirical process. An abnormality of the electrocardiogram is **defined** as such only because the "abnormal" feature is not generally (if ever) found in electrocardiograms taken from normal, healthy subjects. The **recognition** of any given electrocardiographic abnormality depends upon the satisfaction of the appropriate criteria. Most electrocardiographic abnormalities depend upon the presence of more than one criterion. The criteria themselves are the result of the accumulated experience of empirical interpretation of electrocardiograms and each criterion will have a greater or lesser degree of **sensitivity** and **specificity.**

A 100% sensitive criterion for any abnormality is one which guarantees that whenever it is applied to a community, every case of that abnormality within the community will be detected.

Sensitivity is defined as follows:-

$$\text{Sensitivity} = \frac{\text{Number of true positive detections}}{\text{Number of positives in the group tested}}$$

Sensitivity thus gives an index of the capability of a test to detect an abnormality.

A 100% specific criterion for any abnormality is one which guarantees that whenever it is applied to a community every case in which the test indicates that the given abnormality is present will actually have that abnormality.

Specificity is defined as follows:-

$$\text{Specificity} = \frac{\text{Number of true normals detected}}{\text{Total number of normals in the group tested}}$$

Specificity thus indicates the ability of a test to recognise a normal subject.

In practice no electrocardiographic criterion is 100% specific or 100% sensitive and when several different criteria are applicable to a given diagnosis the greater the number of criteria fulfilled the more confident can one be of the diagnosis.

Diagnostic Criteria and Associated Findings

Most electrocardiographic diagnoses require the presence of certain minimal, essential criteria. These are the *sine qua non* of the diagnosis. In addition, it may be possible to recognise certain changes which are frequently found in association with the condition in question, but which are not **essential** to the diagnosis. The presence or absence of these associated findings may be the result of matters independent of the condition in question (e.g. may depend upon the degree of cardiac rotation or the overall body build). Whenever possible, criteria subsequently given will be divided into **"diagnostic criteria"** and **"associated findings".** Unless otherwise indicated, **all** the diagnostic criteria must be fulfilled for the ECG diagnosis to be made.

In addition, it is sometimes important to note certain **negative** points in the diagnostic process, i.e. that certain features are not actually part of the diagnostic process (are neither "diagnostic criteria" nor "associated findings") and their presence indicates some additional abnormality. Such features (of which there are a very large number of possibilities) will only be mentioned if they are frequently but wrongly considered to be part of the primary diagnosis.

There is general but not absolute agreement among cardiologists on the criteria of normal and most abnormal electrocardiographic appearances. However, since agreement is not absolute, some variation in criteria amongst authors is to be expected. Wherever possible, in this presentation, reasonable criteria are given with which most would agree.

Primary and Secondary Interpretation of the Electrocardiogram

The view is widely held and frequently expressed that the electrocardiogram should never be interpreted without prior knowledge of the relevant clinical data. In fact, this viewpoint is virtually unchallenged. It is a view with which the author completely disagrees. In the author's view the electrocardiogram should be "read" and interpreted in the **absence** of clinical data ("primary interpretation"). Both this primary interpretation and the electrocardiogram on which it is based should then be re-appraised in the light of relevant clinical data ("secondary interpretation"). It is a fallacy to believe that the two processes can take place concurrently. The danger when primary and secondary interpretation are not undertaken **consecutively** is that the criteria for making a given electrocardiographic diagnosis may be modified by clinical knowledge and the modified criteria used to support the clinical conclusion. This is scientifically indefensible. When a blood sample is sent to the biochemistry laboratory with a request for estimation of the blood urea level, the chemist makes the assessment independently of the clinical data. The urea level is, or is not, raised as the case may be, irrespective of whether there is clinical evidence of renal damage ("primary interpretation" of the urea level). The clinician must then use secondary interpretation of the chemist's result in the light of the clinical data. If the chemist finds that the urea level is at the upper extreme of the normal range he says just that. He does not say it is abnormal if he knows that there is previous clinical evidence of renal damage nor does he say that it is normal if there is no such evidence. If the interpretation of an independent test is modified by prior clinical judgement, the test cannot subsequently be said to support or prove the clinical judgement. For example, if an ECG shows non-specific S-T, T changes in the left precordial leads, the report should state that fact. The clinical knowledge that the patient takes digitalis clearly means that digitalis is a possible cause of the S-T, T changes. However, it is not certain that digitalis is the cause, it could be ischaemia, electrolyte disturbances, inflammation, injury, etc. If the patient has never taken digitalis, clearly that cannot be the cause.

Primary interpretation is a definitive statement of the electrocardiographic diagnosis – an indication of whether the record is within normal limits or whether specific or non-specific abnormalities are recognisable. Secondary interpretation is an assessment of the significance of normal or abnormal appearances in the light of the full clinical picture. The author absolutely agrees that the latter process must **always** take place but it should not be allowed to interfere with a very disciplined approach to the former. A few examples may help to clarify this concept.

Example 1

A man of 45 presents with chest pain. The electrocardiogram is entirely normal.

Primary interpretation

The ECG is within normal limits.

Secondary interpretation

The electrocardiogram could still be that of a patient with myocardial ischaemia.

Secondary interpretation is essential for primary interpretation alone might result in inappropriate management.

Example 2

A fit 25-year-old man who plays squash regularly has a routine ECG for insurance purposes. The record shows abnormally tall R waves in V_5 and V_6 and abnormally deep S waves in V_1 and V_2. In other respects the record is normal.

Primary interpretation

The voltage criteria for left ventricular hypertrophy are fulfilled.

Secondary interpretation

This man is thin and athletic. The voltage criteria have high sensitivity and low specificity in the diagnosis of left ventricular hypertrophy. Although the electrocardiographic appearances suggest the possibility of left ventricular hypertrophy, in this situation they do not prove it and it is perfectly possible that the heart is completely normal.

Example 3

A grossly overweight man of 50 has a systolic murmur suggestive of aortic stenosis. His electrocardiogram is identical with that of the man in Example 2.

Primary interpretation

The voltage criteria for left ventricular hypertrophy are fulfilled.

Secondary interpretation

Obesity reduces the QRS voltages of surface electrocardiographic recordings. In the light of this fact, the abnormal R wave in V_5 and V_6 and the abnormal S waves in V_1 and V_2 more strongly point to true left ventricular hypertrophy. The presence of systolic murmur of aortic stenosis provides a possible explanation for the left ventricular hypertrophy but does not itself add to the evidence that left ventricular hypertrophy is actually present.

Perhaps a final illustration outside electrocardiography might help to highlight the pitfalls associated with interpreting a clinical test initially in full conjunction with clinical data. A clinician suspects that a patient has a mitral diastolic murmur but is not sure of this. He requests a chest X-ray. If he provides no clinical information about his suspicion on the X-ray request card and the radiologist thinks that the left atrium is slightly enlarged, the radiological opinion legitimately re-enforces the possibility of mitral stenosis. If, however, the clinician writes "? mitral stenosis" on the X-ray request card, there is the danger that the radiologist might, despite seeing appearances which he would otherwise regard as normal, be tempted by the clinical information on the card to write some such report as "Normal appearances. There is perhaps minimal left atrial enlargement". Should this happen the clinician might then, quite unjustifiably, use this dubious information as supportive evidence of his own doubtful opinion. The radiologist should just have said "Normal appearances" if the criteria for abnormality were not fulfilled. In that situation, the clinician would still be able to entertain his initial diagnosis but this would no longer be falsely reinforced via an interpretation of a test distorted by the initial clinical suspicion.

Intraventricular Conduction Disturbances

The Pacemaker and Conducting Tissue

The three waves most easily recognisable in the normal electrocardiogram are the result of electrical activity in **myocardium,** i.e. not in the cardiac conducting tissue. The P wave, QRS complex and T wave are the surface electrocardiographic manifestations of atrial myocardial depolarisation, ventricular myocardial depolarisation and ventricular myocardial repolarisation respectively. (Atrial myocardial repolarisation gives rise to the Ta wave on the surface ECG, but this is completely obscured in most records by the QRS complex which is much larger and which occurs at about the same time). Myocardium cannot **initiate** depolarisation but it has the ability to **conduct** a depolarisation wave once it has been initiated and myocardial depolarisation is followed by **myocardial contraction.**

The pacemaker and conducting tissue of the heart is histologically different from myocardium and can be seen to consist of modified myocardium with very few contractile elements. It, too, has the ability to **conduct** any depolarisation process already initiated, but it differs from myocardium in that (a) **it can initiate such depolarisation,** and (b) **depolarisation** (whether conducted or initiated) **does not result in contraction** (Table 1).

Table 1

	Properties		
Tissue	Conduction of depolarisation	Contraction in response to depolarisation	Initiation of depolarisation
Myocardium	+	+	−
Pacemaker and conducting tissue	+	−	+

The pacemaker and conducting tissue of the heart are arranged as shown in Figure 74. It consists of the sino-atrial node, the atrio-ventricular node, the common bundle (bundle of His) the right bundle branch, the left bundle branch (which has antero-superior and postero-inferior divisions) and the Purkinje network emanating from the bundle branches.

The **sinus node** (sino-atrial node, SA node) is located in the right atrium at the mouth of the superior vena cava. It is approximately 15mm in length, 5 to 7mm wide and 1.5 to 2mm thick. It is the primary cardiac pacemaker. The **atrio-ventricular node** (AV node) lies on the right side of the lower part of the interatrial septum. It is about 5-6mm long, 2-3mm wide and 0.5 to 1mm thick. The **common bundle** (bundle of His, AV Bundle) is continuous with the AV node. It penetrates the central fibrous body of

the heart to reach the crest of the interventricular septum. It is 10-20mm in length and 1-4mm in diameter. The **right bundle branch** runs directly down from the common bundle, on the subendocardial surface of the right ventricle. After a "bare" initial portion, fine branches of the **Purkinje tissue** (Purkinje network, Purkinje arborisation) arise from the remainder of its length to spread over the endocardial surface of the right ventricle. The **left bundle branch** is a less discrete structure than the right bundle. It has two major subdivisions, the antero-superior and the postero-inferior divisions. Each division forms a fan, rather than a fasciculus, of fibres, spreads on the endocardial surface of the left ventricle and gives rise to Purkinje tissue in the same way as the right bundle. Purkinje branches arise earlier (i.e. more proximally) from the left than from the right bundle.

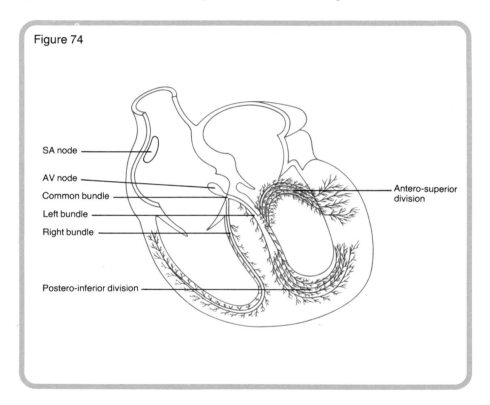

Figure 74

Normal Atrio-ventricular and Intraventricular Conduction

The sino-atrial node, all parts of the right and left atrial myocardium and the AV node are in electrical continuity (i.e. a depolarisation arising in any part is normally conducted to all other parts). This whole supraventricular system maintains electrical continuity with the ventricular system only via the common atrio-ventricular bundle (bundle of His). In normal circumstances, no electrical conduction is possible directly from atrial myocardium to ventricular myocardium, because of the interposition of the non-conducting, fibrous atrio-ventricular ring (which is electrically bridged by the His bundle). It follows that the depolarisation wave (which, if the rhythm is sinus, originates from the sino-atrial node) reaches ventricular myocardium only after its passage through the bundle of His and the beginnings of the right and left bundle branch systems. Thus the first part of the intraventricular myocardium to be depolarised is the superior part of the

interventricular septum adjacent to the mitral and tricuspid valves. The main stem of the left branch (before it bifurcates into its two divisions), is very short and the left bundle branch gives off fine Purkinje fibres more proximally than the right bundle branch. Because of this **the first (superior) part of the interventricular septum is depolarised from left to right.** Sequential depolarisation of the left and right ventricles then occurs, the sequence being dependent upon (a) the site of initiation of septal depolarisation and (b) the distribution of the fast conducting pacemaker tissue. The rate of conduction through the common bundle, bundle branches and Purkinje system is rapid (4000mm/sec) compared with that through the ventricular myocardium (400mm/sec). The AV node ("AV" junction) conducts most slowly of all at 200mm/sec.

The excitation wave arising at the AV node (having been conducted through atrial myocardium after initiation at the SA node) thus passes down the common bundle and simultaneously down both bundle branches. Because of the earlier origin of Purkinje fibres on the left, the superior part of the interventricular septum is depolarised from left to right. Lower down, the septum is depolarised simultaneously from both sides and subsequently the free walls of the ventricles are depolarised from endocardium to epicardium. Because of the relatively great speed of conduction down the bundle branches and Purkinje cells, the entire endocardial surface of both ventricles becomes depolarised at about the same time. Conduction then spreads more slowly transmurally from endocardium to epicardium.

It is therefore possible to simplify the sequence of depolarisation of the ventricular myocardium into three phases (as discussed on page 29). Phase 1 (Figure 75) represents depolarisation of the superior portion of the interventricular septum. This occurs initially and on its own. Phase 2 represents depolarisation of the free wall of the right ventricle and Phase 3 that of the free wall of the left ventricle – in both cases from endocardium to epicardium. Phases 2 and 3 are effectively simultaneous.

Figure 75

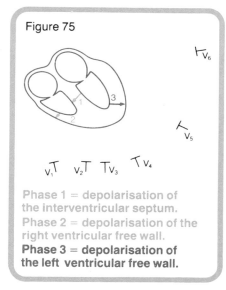

Phase 1 = depolarisation of the interventricular septum.
Phase 2 = depolarisation of the right ventricular free wall.
Phase 3 = depolarisation of the left ventricular free wall.

This sequence of ventricular myocardial depolarisation gives rise to the typical normal QRS wave forms in V_1 and V_6 (Figures 76, 77).

Figure 76

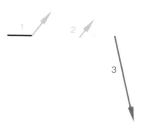

(a) V_1 sees these 3 waves

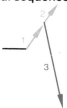

Three phases of depolarisation are shown. Phases 1 and 2 give positive and Phase 3 negative deflections in V_1. The relative magnitudes of their resulting deflections are represented by the length of the arrows. Phase 3 produces the largest effect because of the dominance of the left ventricle in terms of mass and therefore, of electrical activation.

(b) V_1 sees the waves in this temporal sequence

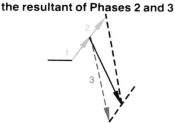

Phase 1 occurs initially alone. Phases 2 and 3 follow, together.

(c) V_1 records Phase 1 followed by the resultant of Phases 2 and 3

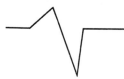

The resultant of Phases 2 and 3 acting simultaneously is determined by constructing the parallelogram of vectors.

(d) V_1 shows the following deflection:-

When the recorded deflection is over, the pen returns to the baseline.

(e) The QRS deflection in V_1 typically appears as follows:-

The magnitude of the Phase 1 wave was exaggerated in (a) to (d) for clarity. The deflections were also spread out for the same reason. **The typical QRS deflection in V_1 has a small initial positive wave followed by a larger negative wave.**

Figure 77

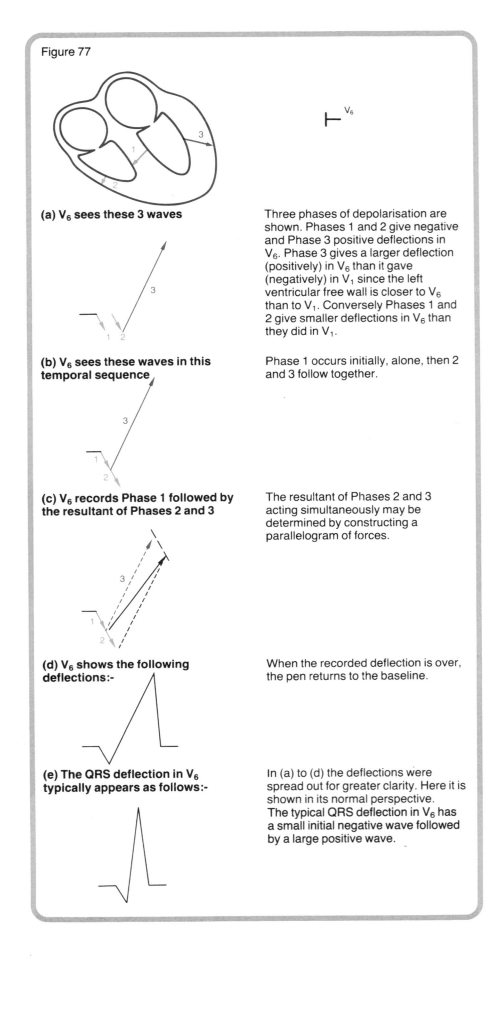

(a) V₆ sees these 3 waves

Three phases of depolarisation are shown. Phases 1 and 2 give negative and Phase 3 positive deflections in V_6. Phase 3 gives a larger deflection (positively) in V_6 than it gave (negatively) in V_1 since the left ventricular free wall is closer to V_6 than to V_1. Conversely Phases 1 and 2 give smaller deflections in V_6 than they did in V_1.

(b) V₆ sees these waves in this temporal sequence

Phase 1 occurs initially, alone, then 2 and 3 follow together.

(c) V₆ records Phase 1 followed by the resultant of Phases 2 and 3

The resultant of Phases 2 and 3 acting simultaneously may be determined by constructing a parallelogram of forces.

(d) V₆ shows the following deflections:-

When the recorded deflection is over, the pen returns to the baseline.

(e) The QRS deflection in V₆ typically appears as follows:-

In (a) to (d) the deflections were spread out for greater clarity. Here it is shown in its normal perspective. The typical QRS deflection in V_6 has a small initial negative wave followed by a large positive wave.

Ventricular Pre-excitation

Ventricular pre-excitation is a relatively rare condition in which an abnormal (additional or "accessory") atrio-ventricular conduction pathway exists between the atrial and ventricular myocardium. The accessory pathway usually conducts the depolarisation wave more quickly than does the normal atrio-ventricular conducting tissue. The accessory pathway makes electrical contact with the ventricular myocardium at a location other than that which is the usual starting point for ventricular myocardial depolarisation. It follows that, in the presence of ventricular pre-excitation, myocardial depolarisation commences at an "abnormal" location and the whole sequence of ventricular myocardial depolarisation must therefore follow an abnormal pathway. This results

in the development of an abnormal QRS complex in association with the short P-R interval which is indicative of the accelerated atrio-ventricular conduction.

The concept of ventricular pre-excitation and the changes induced by it on the electrocardiogram are fully discussed in the section on "Miscellaneous Abnormalities" (pages 212 to 249). However, it is necessary at this stage to be aware of its existence for the discussion which follows and the scheme for analysis of normal and abnormal electrocardiograms will both subsequently require modification in the light of the possibility of ventricular pre-excitation. All discussion prior to the formal consideration of pre-excitation will involve the assumption that atrio-ventricular conduction is normal.

Abnormal Intraventricular Conduction

When the normal sequence of conduction of a depolarisation wave is disturbed after it has descended through the AV node an intraventricular conduction disturbance is said to have occurred. The following intraventricular conduction disturbances are recognisable (with greater or lesser degrees of facility) on the 12-lead ECG:

Right bundle branch block (RBBB – partial or complete, permanent or intermittent)

Left bundle branch block (LBBB – partial or complete, permanent or intermittent)

Left anterior hemiblock (LAH – also known as left superior intraventricular block)

Left posterior hemiblock (LPH – also known as left inferior intraventricular block)

RBBB+LAH
RBBB+LPH
Diffuse intraventricular block

Right Bundle Branch Block (RBBB)

When there is total failure of conduction in the right bundle branch system (Figure 78), there is no change in the direction of depolarisation of the interventricular septum (Phase 1) and no change in the timing or direction of depolarisation of the free wall of the left ventricle (Phase 3), but depolarisation of the free wall of the right ventricle (Phase

2) is delayed and prolonged since the depolarisation wave reaches the right ventricular myocardium after slow conduction through the myocardium of the septum. Phase 2 depolarisation starts later than normal and takes longer to reach its peak and these features give rise to typical changes in the precordial electrocardiogram (Figures 79 and 80).

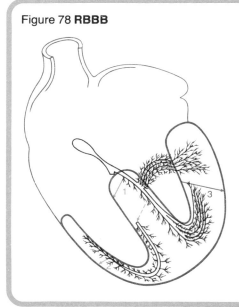

Figure 78 **RBBB**

There is failure of conduction in the right bundle branch proximally. Septal depolarisation (Phase 1) is unaffected since it is initiated via Purkinje fibres which arise proximally from the left bundle before its division into two fasciculi. Left ventricular depolarisation takes place at the normal time and at normal rate. Right ventricular depolarisation is delayed because of the slow conduction through myocardium which forms the only electrical continuity between the nearest Purkinje fibres arising from the left bundle and the distal, functioning part of the right bundle (interrupted arrow). The extent of the defect in the right bundle determines the extent of the delay in initiating and in completing right ventricular depolarisation.

Both in V_1 and V_6 the QRS complex differs from normal in its terminal portion only. The overall QRS duration is prolonged (since Phase 2 depolarisation starts late and takes longer than normal), a secondary slurred R wave occurs in V_1 and a secondary slurred S wave occurs in V_6.

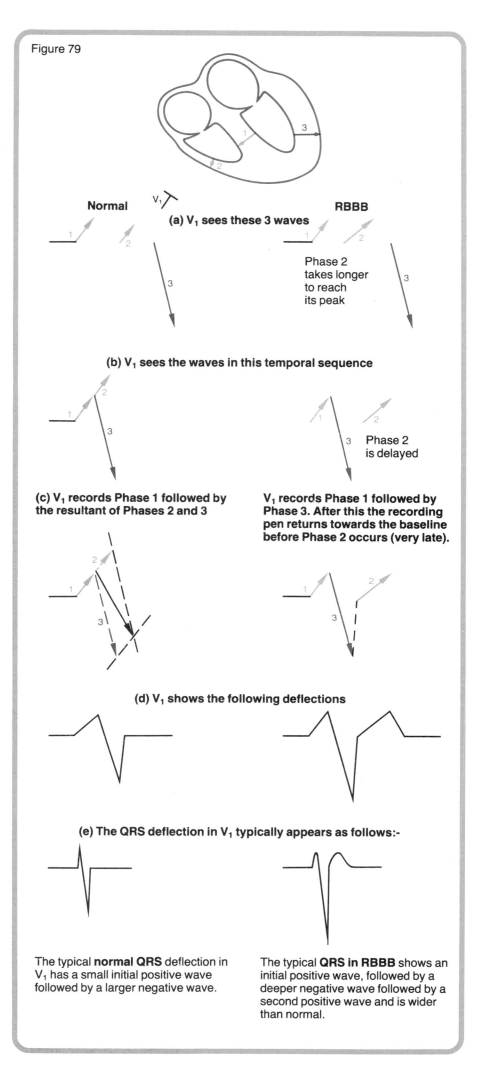

Figure 79

Normal V_1 **RBBB**

(a) V_1 sees these 3 waves

Phase 2 takes longer to reach its peak

(b) V_1 sees the waves in this temporal sequence

Phase 2 is delayed

(c) V_1 records Phase 1 followed by the resultant of Phases 2 and 3

V_1 **records Phase 1 followed by Phase 3. After this the recording pen returns towards the baseline before Phase 2 occurs (very late).**

(d) V_1 shows the following deflections

(e) The QRS deflection in V_1 typically appears as follows:-

The typical **normal QRS** deflection in V_1 has a small initial positive wave followed by a larger negative wave.

The typical **QRS in RBBB** shows an initial positive wave, followed by a deeper negative wave followed by a second positive wave and is wider than normal.

Figure 80

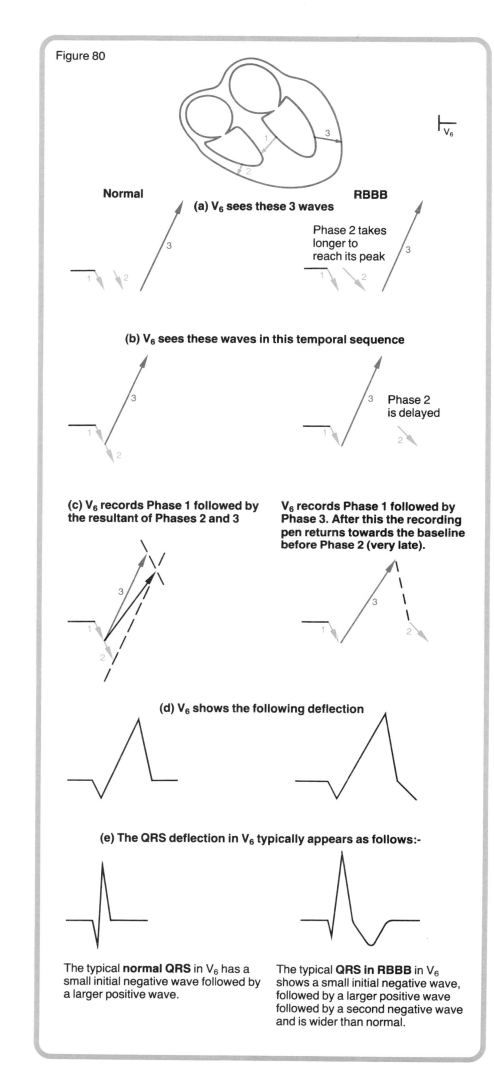

Normal   **(a) V₆ sees these 3 waves**   **RBBB**

Phase 2 takes longer to reach its peak

(b) V₆ sees these waves in this temporal sequence

Phase 2 is delayed

(c) V₆ records Phase 1 followed by the resultant of Phases 2 and 3

V₆ records Phase 1 followed by Phase 3. After this the recording pen returns towards the baseline before Phase 2 (very late).

(d) V₆ shows the following deflection

(e) The QRS deflection in V₆ typically appears as follows:-

The typical **normal QRS** in V₆ has a small initial negative wave followed by a larger positive wave.

The typical **QRS in RBBB** in V₆ shows a small initial negative wave, followed by a larger positive wave followed by a second negative wave and is wider than normal.

The changes in ventricular depolarisation (which are represented by the QRS changes) inevitably give rise to secondary changes in ventricular repolarisation (i.e. changes in the S-T segment and T waves). In consequence, there is often S-T segment depression and T wave inversion in the right precordial leads. Leads I and aVL tend to show appearances similar to those in V_6. The mean frontal plane QRS axis is not abnormal in uncomplicated right bundle branch block, although it may not infrequently be indeterminate. These features are all illustrated in Figure 81. This ECG would be reported as follows: "Sinus rhythm. The mean frontal plane QRS axis is indeterminate. There is complete right bundle branch block."

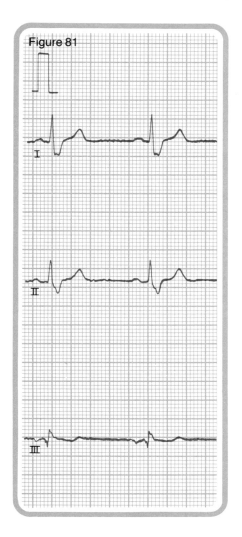

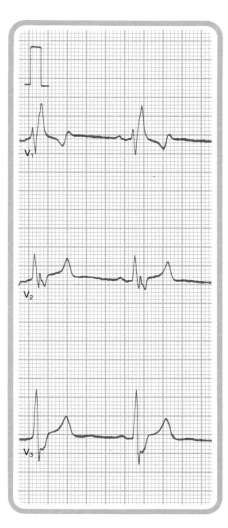

Figure 81

The rhythm is sinus. The total QRS duration is abnormally long (0.16 sec – most easily seen in the first QRS in V_1 or the second QRS in I). V_1 has a large secondary R wave (i.e. it has an rSR′ complex). The combination of prolongation of the total QRS duration with a secondary R wave in V_1 is diagnostic of right bundle branch block. As is usually the case there is a broad, slurred S wave in V_6 (the equivalent of the broad, slurred R wave in V_1). The mean frontal plane QRS axis is indeterminate but, as is often the case, the QRS appearances in V_6 are transmitted to I and aVL. There is secondary S-T segment depression in V_1 (often is present in V_2 and V_3 as well).

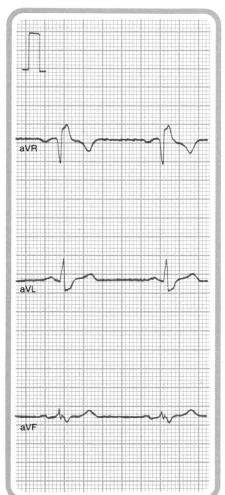

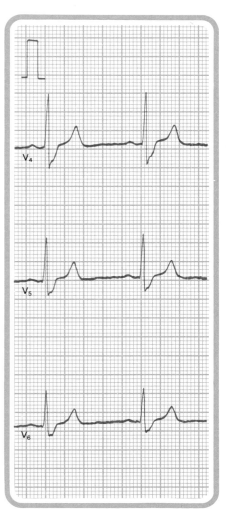

Diagnostic criteria for right bundle branch block

(Assuming the rhythm to be supraventricular)

1. Total QRS duration is 0.12 sec or greater.
2. A secondary R wave is seen in V_1. The secondary wave is usually broad and slurred, (the complex in V_1 may be rsr', rSr', RSr', RSR', or M-shaped).

Additional features frequently present in right bundle branch block

1. Deep, slurred S waves are seen in the left precordial leads (typically V_4, V_5 and V_6, though they may also be seen in V_3 and even V_2 if there is counterclockwise rotation, or they may be seen only in V_6 if there is clockwise rotation).
2. Deep slurred S waves are usually seen also in I and aVL.
3. S-T segment depression and T wave inversion are seen in the right precordial leads (typically $V_1 - V_3$, but only in V_1 in counterclockwise rotation and possibly from $V_1 - V_5$ in clockwise rotation).

Important negative points in right bundle branch block

1. The mean frontal plane QRS axis is usually within the normal range in uncomplicated complete right bundle branch block. The axis may move 15–30° towards the right when right bundle branch block develops but **abnormal** right axis deviation is **not** a routine feature of right bundle branch block. The axis is often indeterminate (page 48). This is not in itself an abnormality. When right bundle branch block is combined with a clearly abnormal axis, bifascicular block (i.e. RBBB+LAH if there is abnormal left axis deviation or RBBB+LPH if there is abnormal right axis deviation) is considered to be present (pages 139 to 142).
2. The initial part of the QRS complex is normal in every lead. In fact, each lead only differs from the normal QRS because of the presence of a late, slurred "addition" to the basic waveform (Figure 82).

Figure 82

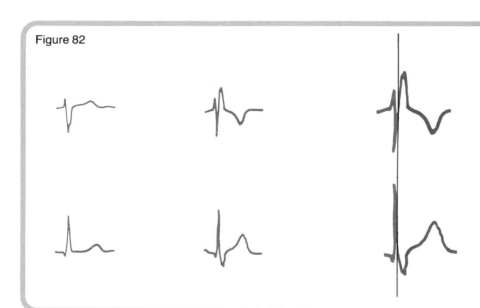

The left-hand column shows typical normal QRS configurations, S-T segments and T waves in V_1 and V_6. The central column shows typical appearances in right bundle branch block. The right-hand column shows the same appearances as the central column, enlarged by a factor of 2 to emphasise that in both these leads (and in fact in all 12 leads) both the initial and the dominant deflections of the QRS complexes in right bundle branch block are almost identical with those in the presence of normal intraventricular conduction. (The parts of the QRS deflections to the left of the vertical line are virtually the same as those in the normal QRS complexes).

The main reasons that all but the terminal part of the QRS is normal are because:
1. The direction of septal depolarisation (the earliest part of ventricular depolarisation) is normal and therefore the initial direction of the QRS in every lead remains unchanged, and
2. The depolarisation of the left ventricular free wall (which is the influence dominating QRS deflections in all leads in most circumstances) is unaltered.

Because the most important diagnostic parts of the QRS complexes are unaltered in right bundle branch block, the criteria for normality or abnormality of voltage, R wave progression and q waves can be applied (e.g. it is still possible to diagnose left ventricular hypertrophy or myocardial infarction).

Incomplete Right Bundle Branch Block

Incomplete right bundle branch block is diagnosed when:

1. A secondary R wave is seen in V_1 (which therefore has an rsr′, rSr′, rSR′, Rsr′, RSr′, RSR′ or M-shaped complex), and

2. The total QRS duration is 0.11 sec or less. An example is shown in Figure 83.

The ECG in Figure 83 would be reported as follows: "Sinus tachycardia. The mean frontal plane QRS axis is +45°. There is incomplete right bundle branch block".

When the term "right bundle branch block" is used without qualification, it is deemed to refer to complete right bundle branch block.

Although incomplete right bundle branch block can occur in disease states (listed below) it is usually of no clinical significance, being found in 2–3% normals.

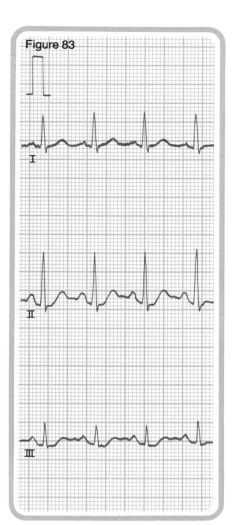

Figure 83

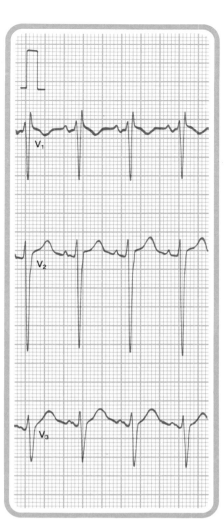

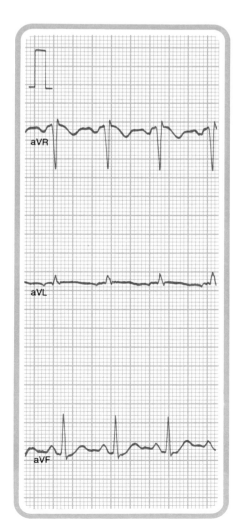

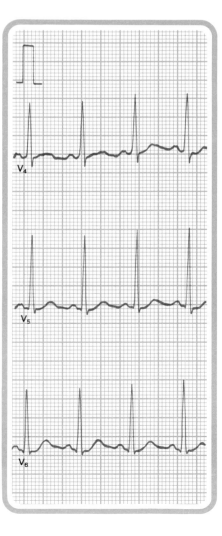

Figure 83

The rhythm is sinus. There is an rSr′ configuration to the QRS complex in V_1. However, the total QRS duration is within normal limits at 0.09 sec (best seen in V_1). There is therefore incomplete right bundle branch block.

Intermittent Right Bundle Branch Block

Right bundle branch block may develop secondary to myocardial infarction or ischaemia, may develop in the pulmonary embolism and may appear as a functional disturbance whenever the supraventricular rate exceeds a critical value. In all of these situations, the right bundle branch block may disappear and normal intraventricular conduction may return when the underlying abnormality improves. Rarely, right bundle branch block, unassociated with any overt cardiac abnormality may be present intermittently.

Clinical Significance

Complete right bundle branch block may occur congenitally in hearts which are in all respects completely normal. When it is the sole "abnormal" finding it must not be taken to be conclusive of the presence of cardiac disease.

It can, however, develop in a variety of cardiac diseases including ischaemic heart disease, hypertension, pulmonary embolism, cardiomyopathy, myocarditis, rheumatic heart disease, pericarditis, Chagas disease, and can be found congenitally in atrial septal defect (in which condition it is always found – complete or incomplete) and Fallot's Tetralogy.

Left Bundle Branch Block (LBBB)

When there is total failure of conduction in the left bundle branch system (Figure 84) there is delay in the initiation and in the velocity of depolarisation of the free wall of the left ventricle – Phase 3. (This is the precise corollary of the delay in depolarisation of the free wall of the right ventricle in the right bundle branch block). However, in LBBB there is a very important additional change – complete reversal of the direction of depolarisation of the interventricular septum (Phase 1). This latter feature produces dramatic changes in the electrocardiogram for it alters the initial direction of the QRS complex in every lead – all those leads which formerly showed an initial r wave will now have an initial q wave, and the leads with initial q waves will now have initial r waves.

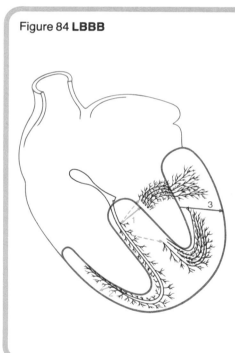

Figure 84 **LBBB**

There is failure of conduction in the left bundle branch system. Septal depolarisation arrow (1) is reversed (since it must take place from the earliest Purkinje fibres arising from the right bundle). In addition to this reversal of the direction of septal depolarisation, the depolarisation of the myocardium of the left ventricle starts later than normal and takes longer than normal because of the slow conduction through myocardium which forms the only electrical continuity between the nearest Purkinje fibres arising from the right bundle and the distal, functioning parts of the left bundle. Each of the two major divisions of the left bundle will receive the depolarisation wave (2 interrupted arrows) in the same way. The extent of the defect in the left bundle determines the extent of the delay in initiating and in completing left ventricular depolarisation.

The two changes from normal produce typical changes in the precordial QRS complexes (Figures 85 and 86). Both in V_1 and V_6 the QRS complex differs radically from normal in its configuration. The overall QRS duration is prolonged (since Phase 3 starts late and takes longer than usual). The cardinal features are absence of the (normal) septal q wave in V_6 and prolongation of the total QRS duration.

Figure 85

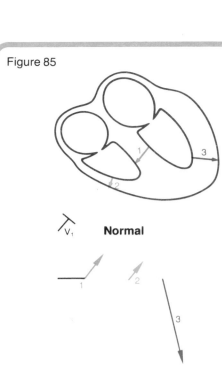

Normal   V₁   LBBB

(a) V₁ sees these 3 waves

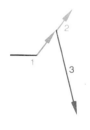 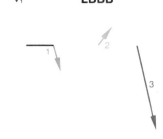

(b) V₁ sees these waves in this temporal sequence

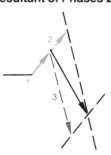 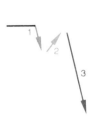

(c) V₁ records Phase 1 followed by resultant of Phases 2 and 3

(c) V₁ records Phase 1 (reversed) followed by Phase 2 followed by Phase 3.

 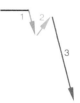

(d) V₁ shows the following deflections

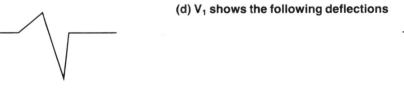 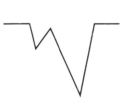

(e) The QRS deflection in V₁ typically appears as follows:-

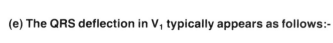 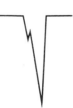

The typical **normal QRS** deflection in V₁ has a small initial positive wave followed by a larger negative wave

The typical **QRS in LBBB** in V₁ shows no initial positive wave, a deep negative wave and is wider than normal.

Figure 86

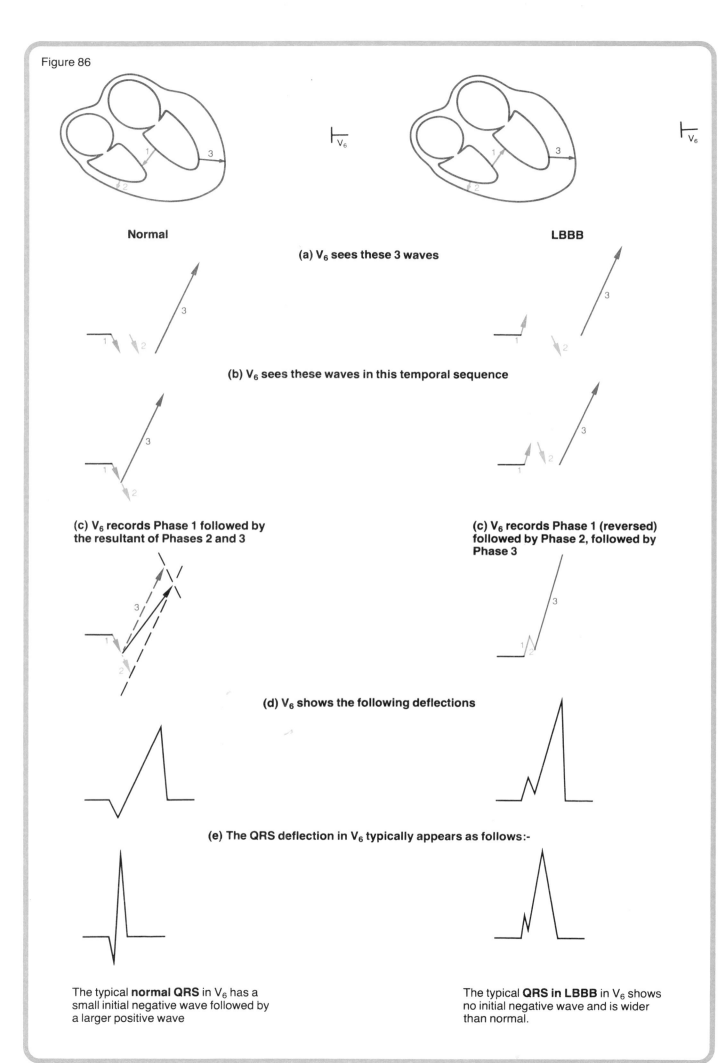

Normal   **LBBB**

(a) V₆ sees these 3 waves

(b) V₆ sees these waves in this temporal sequence

(c) V₆ records Phase 1 followed by the resultant of Phases 2 and 3

(c) V₆ records Phase 1 (reversed) followed by Phase 2, followed by Phase 3

(d) V₆ shows the following deflections

(e) The QRS deflection in V₆ typically appears as follows:-

The typical **normal QRS** in V₆ has a small initial negative wave followed by a larger positive wave

The typical **QRS in LBBB** in V₆ shows no initial negative wave and is wider than normal.

The changes in ventricular depolarisation (which are represented by the QRS changes) inevitably give rise to secondary changes in ventricular repolarisation (i.e. changes in the S-T segment and T waves). There is therefore often S-T segment depression and T wave inversion in the left precordial leads and S-T segment elevation with tall T waves in the right precordial leads. Leads I and aVL tend to show appearances similar to those in V_6. The mean frontal plane QRS axis is not abnormal in uncomplicated left bundle branch block, although it may be indeterminate. These features are illustrated in Figure 87. This ECG would be reported as follows: "Sinus rhythm. The mean frontal plane QRS axis is +15°. There is complete left bundle branch block".

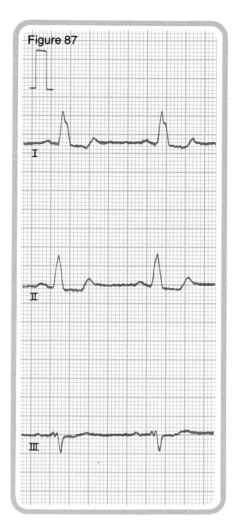

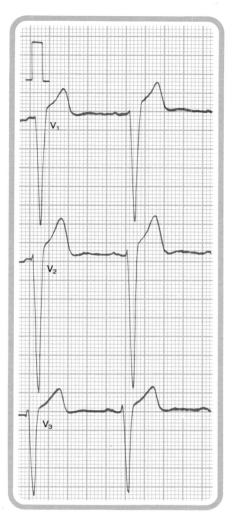

Figure 87

The rhythm is sinus. The total QRS duration is abnormally long (0.14 sec – most easily seen in the first QRS complex in V_6). Deep S waves (in this case with a small initial r wave) are seen in V_1. There is no secondary R wave in V_1 to indicate right bundle branch block. There is no initial (septal) q wave in V_6 or in leads further to the left than V_6 (i.e. I and aVL). In the absence of right bundle branch block this combination of absent left-sided q waves and abnormally long total QRS duration is indicative of left bundle branch block. S-T segment depression (which is secondary to the QRS abnormality) is seen in V_6, I, II and aVL. The frontal plane QRS axis is within the normal range of +15°. The heart is horizontal (page 53) and because of this the appearances in left ventricular leads (typically V_6) are transmitted to Leads I and aVL (i.e. to those frontal plane leads which lie closest to the direction of the frontal plane axis).

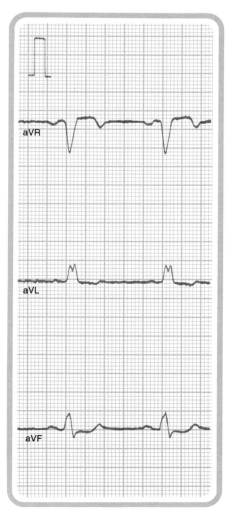

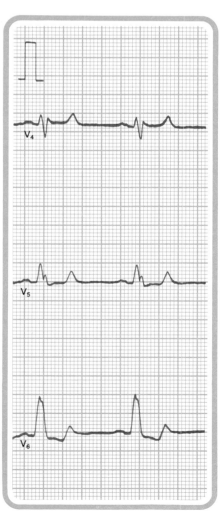

123

Diagnostic criteria for left bundle branch block

(Assuming that the rhythm is supraventricular and that there is no ventricular pre-excitation[†]).

1. Total QRS duration is 0.12 sec or greater.
2. There is no secondary R wave in V_1, to indicate RBBB[*].
3. There is no septal q wave in V_5, V_6 or in leads further to the left (in the case of horizontal hearts, I and aVL).

Additional features frequently present in left bundle branch block

1. The QRS complexes in some leads may be notched (e.g. Leads I, aVL, V_5 and V_6 in Figure 87).
2. The QRS complexes in V_5, V_6, I and aVL tend to have rsR', "M" pattern or broad monophasic R waves. If the heart is clockwise-rotated V_5, V_6, I and aVL tend to show RS complexes.
3. Secondary S-T segment depression and possibly T wave inversion may be present in left precordial leads and also in I and aVL.
4. The S-T segments are often elevated and the T waves abnormally tall in the right precordial leads.
5. The S waves in the right precordial leads are often abnormally deep.
6. The initial r waves in the right precordial leads may be very small or absent. If absent the QRS complexes, by definition, have deep Q waves not deep S waves.
7. In the precordial leads the dominant direction of the T waves and the S-T segments tends to be opposite to the dominant direction of the QRS complexes in any given lead.
8. In the limb leads there is an abnormal angle between the mean frontal plane QRS and T wave axes – or the QRS axis is highly determinate and the T wave axis indeterminate (which is equally abnormal (page 58)).

Note
[*] It is necessary to include this criterion since it is possible for no initial q wave to be visible in V_6 normally (page 67). If right bundle branch block develops on top of this normal variation the combination of (1) prolongation of the total QRS duration, and (2) absence of septal q waves in V_6 would lead to an incorrect diagnosis of LBBB. (The criteria for the recognition of RBBB would not be affected by this possibility (Figure 88)).
[†]See pages 212 to 220 and 266.

Important negative points in left bundle branch block

1. The mean frontal plane QRS axis is usually within the normal range in uncomplicated cases. The axis may move 15–30° towards the left (Figures 90 and 91) when left bundle branch block develops but **abnormal left axis deviation is not a routine feature of left bundle branch block.** Sometimes the axis may be indeterminate. This is not in itself an abnormality (page 48). When LBBB is combined with abnormal left axis deviation, extensive disease of the left ventricular conducting tissue is likely to be present involving the peripheral part of the antero-superior division of the left bundle branch system as well as the proximal part of the main left bundle. When LBBB is combined with right axis deviation, the possibility of co-existing right ventricular hypertrophy should be considered.

2. The initial part of the QRS complex in every lead takes place in a direction opposite from normal. Therefore, **once the diagnosis of left bundle branch block has been established, no further diagnostic processes utilising criteria for QRS complexes, S-T segments or T waves should be used - except for the measurement of the frontal plane QRS axis.**

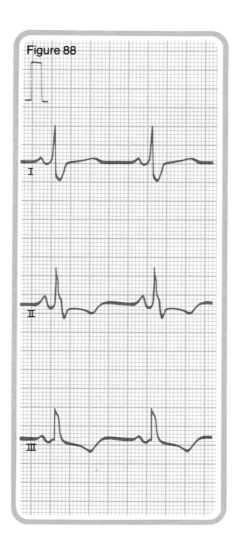

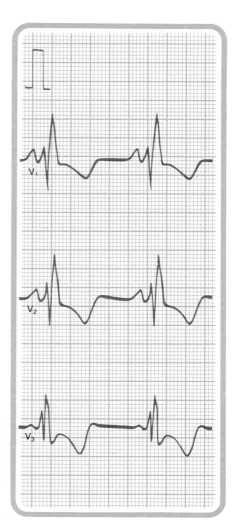

Figure 88

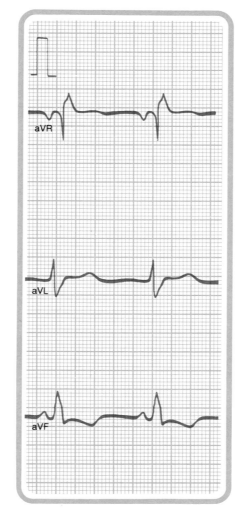

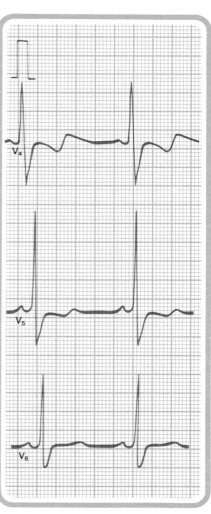

Figure 88

The rhythm is sinus. There is an rSR′ configuration of the QRS complex in V_1 and the total QRS duration is prolonged to 0.12 sec (best seen in V_1). There is therefore complete right bundle branch block. (No septal q wave is seen in V_6 or I. This is not in itself, abnormal. Had there been no septal q wave in V_6 and a prolongation of the total QRS duration **without a secondary r wave in V_1,** there would have been **left** bundle branch block. In that event one would have expected deep S (or Q) waves in V_1). There is S-T segment depression with T wave inversion from V_1 to V_4. These are changes commonly associated with right bundle branch block and no additional abnormality need be invoked.

Incomplete Left Bundle Branch Block

Incomplete left bundle branch block is diagnosed when there is no septal q wave in left-sided precordial leads or in Lead I or aVL and when the total QRS duration is 0.10 or 0.11 sec. Thus the only difference between complete and incomplete LBBB is the duration of the QRS complex. An example is shown in Figure 89. This record would be reported as follows:

"Sinus tachycardia. Incomplete left bundle branch block. There are non-specific S-T, T changes throughout the limb leads and in the left precordial leads. These may well be secondary to the intraventricular conduction disturbance. Left atrial hypertrophy."

When the term "left bundle branch block" is used without qualification, it is deemed to refer to complete left bundle branch block. When the total QRS duration is 0.10 sec (i.e. still acceptable as "normal") and there is no septal q wave in V_5, V_6, I or aVL it does not necessarily indicate disease* (even though it is technically incomplete left bundle branch block) since the q wave can sometimes be absent in these leads under normal circumstances (page 67).

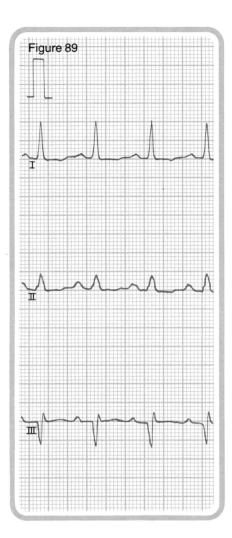

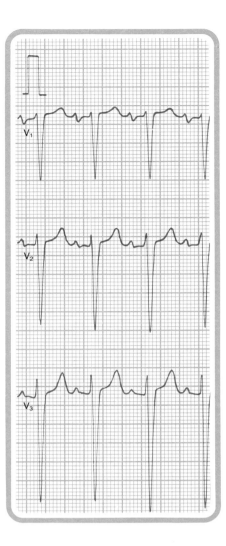

Figure 89

The rhythm is sinus but the rate is more rapid than 100 per minute, therefore the rhythm is actually sinus tachycardia. The S waves in the right precordial leads are deeper than normal, the R waves in the left precordial leads are taller than normal, but the important point to note is that there is no evidence of any normal septal q wave in V_5, V_6, Lead I or aVL. The septum is therefore depolarising from right to left and not from left to right as is the normal situation.

This suggests* a defect of conduction in the left bundle branch system. Total QRS duration is only 0.11 sec (best seen in the first QRS complex in V_2) and there is therefore incomplete left bundle branch block. The T waves are of low voltage throughout the limb leads and there is T wave inversion and S-T segment depression in the left precordial leads. These are non-specific changes which may well be secondary to the intraventricular conduction disturbance. The P waves are also abnormal (page 163).

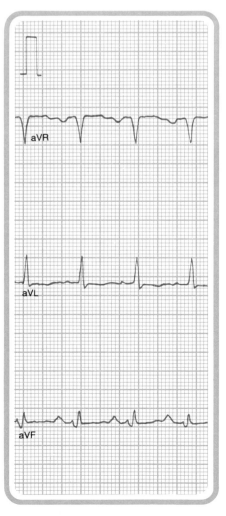

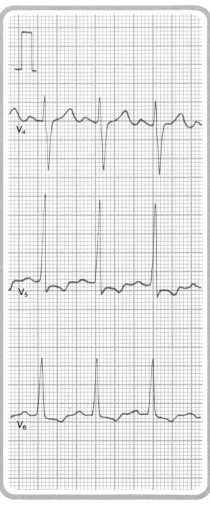

126

Intermittent Left Bundle Branch Block

Left bundle branch block may be intermittently present in relation to varying pathology, such as myocardial ischaemia. It can sometimes appear as a functional disturbance when the ventricular rate exceeds a certain value, but is less likely to do so than is right bundle branch block. In all of these situations, the left bundle branch block may disappear and normal intraventricular conduction may return when the underlying abnormality improves.

Figures 90 and 91 are taken from a patient with intermittent left bundle branch block.

Figure 90 shows the electrocardiogram of a patient with hypertrophic cardiomyopathy. The rhythm is sinus, there is normal intraventricular conduction. The record is within normal limits. Note that the frontal plane QRS axis is +15°.

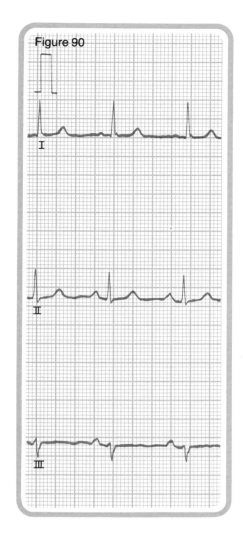

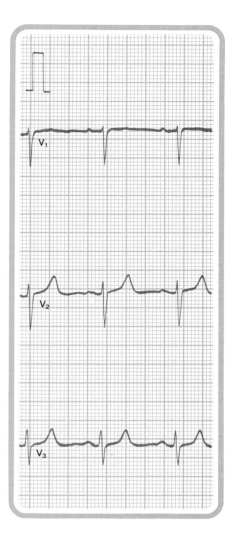

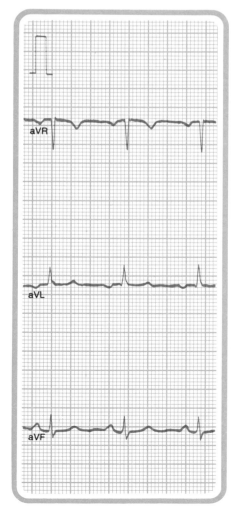

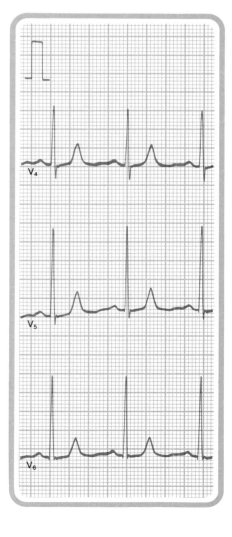

Figure 90

A normal ECG from a patient with hypertrophic cardiomyopathy.

Figure 91 shows an ECG taken from the same patient as that in Figure 90 and about 2 weeks later. Complete LBBB has developed. (The record is recognisably that of the same patient as Figure 90 since the P wave configuration in each lead is identical in the two records). Note that with the development of LBBB the frontal plane QRS axis has moved from +15° (Figure 90) to −15°. This degree of left-axis shift on developing LBBB is typical.

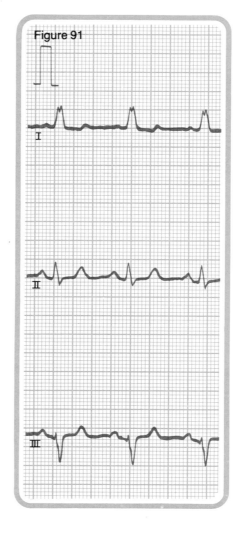

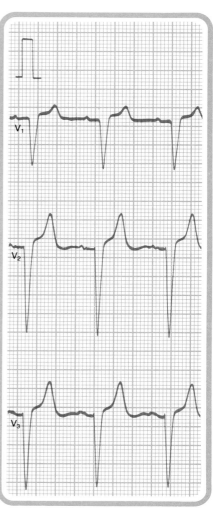

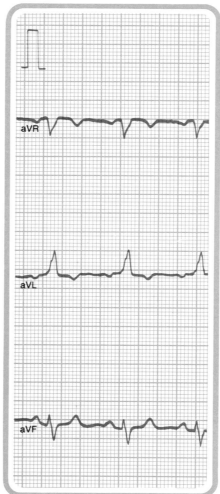

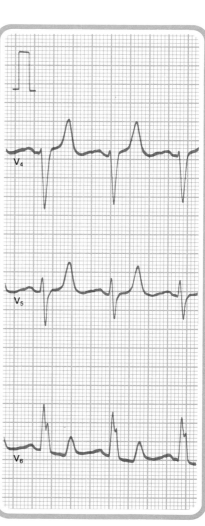

Figure 91

A record taken from the same patient as that in Figure 90, about 2 weeks later. Left bundle branch block has developed. The axis has moved minimally to the left but is still within the normal range. This patient developed and lost LBBB intermittently over many months. Cardiac catheterisation confirmed the (clinical) diagnosis of hypertrophic cardiomyopathy and coronary angiography showed normal coronary vessels.

Clinical Significance

Left bundle branch block always indicates the presence of significant cardiac disease. It occurs most commonly in ischaemic heart disease, hypertension, aortic stenosis and fibrous degeneration within the conducting tissue. It may also occur in congestive and in hypertrophic cardiomyopathy, myocarditis, acute rheumatic fever, syphilis, cardiac tumours, following cardiac surgery and in congenital heart disease.

Fascicular Blocks

The concept of "fascicular blocks" has caused much confusion, partly because there is some genuine disagreement about the meaning of the terms used, but mainly because of loose application of the terms. According to this concept there are three fascicles of conduction, those of the right bundle branch, the anterior division of the left bundle and the posterior division of the left bundle.

Unifascicular block thus includes (1) RBBB, (2) LAH and (3) LPH,

Bifascicular block includes (1) LBBB (2) LAH+RBBB and (3) LPH+RBBB

Trifascicular block corresponds to complete AV block where uni- or bifascicular block has been known to be present previously. Complete heart block can, of course, also arise because of complete failure of conduction through the AV node or through the common bundle.
(It should be noted that LBBB can arise either from a discrete lesion proximally in the left bundle branch or from simultaneous LAH and LPH).

The Hemiblocks

It is possible to recognise blocks which involve either of the two divisions of the left bundle branch system.

When we first considered a simplified system describing the sequence of depolarisation of the ventricular myocardium, we divided myocardium depolarisation up into three phases (page 29). These were:

Phase 1 – Depolarisation of the interventricular septum.

Phase 2 – Depolarisation of the free wall of the right ventricle, and

Phase 3 – Depolarisation of the free wall of the left ventricle.

As long as the two divisions of the left bundle branch system are either both conducting normally or are both failing to conduct, this simplified scheme still explains the basic form of the QRS complex in the various leads. However, when we come to consider the hemiblocks it is necessary to consider Phase 3 depolarisation as having two separate parts (Figure 92).

Figure 92

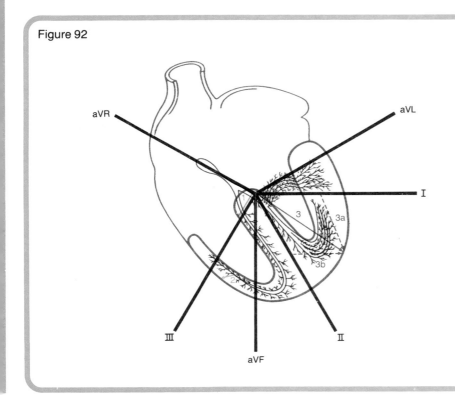

Phases 1, 2 and 3 represent depolarisation **(in the frontal plane)** of the interventricular septum, of the free wall of the right ventricle and of the free wall of the left ventricle respectively. Phase 3 is a result of depolarisation of the left ventricle simultaneously from two directions – a depolarisation wave spreading from below upwards and to the left as a result of transmission through the posterior (inferior) division (3b) and a depolarisation wave spreading from above downwards and to the left as a result of transmission down the anterior (superior) division (3a). In both cases the depolarisation wave also spreads from endocardium to epicardium. The phases of depolarisation can then be simplified as in Figure 93. Phase 1 occurs first, then Phases 2, 3a and 3b occur simultaneously, 3a and 3b add together to give 3 and Phases 3 and 2 add together to produce a resultant deflection which follows Phase I (Figure 93).

Normally the two parts of Phase 3 occur simultaneously with each other and with Phase 2 and they both follow Phase 1. The sequence of ventricular depolarisation in the frontal plane is therefore as outlined in Figure 93, with initial (septal) depolarisation downwards and to the right of the heart (towards Lead III) and subsequently a greater voltage depolarisation downwards and to the left of the heart. It is in this way that the normal counterclockwise direction of the vector loop in the frontal plane is inscribed and the resultant normal frontal plane axis (in the case shown in Figure 93 approximately +45°) is achieved.

The hemiblocks refer to failure of normal Phase 3a (anterior hemiblock) or of Phase 3b (posterior hemiblock) conduction.

The important functional disturbance produced by a hemiblock is a dramatic shift in the mean frontal plane QRS axis without any change in the initial direction of ventricular (septal) depolarisation.

Figure 93

Phase 1 occurs initially, alone. This is followed by Phases 2, 3a and 3b, all occurring simultaneously. Phases 2, 3a and 3b can be considered as acting from the point in time and in space at which Phase 1 ends.

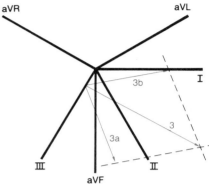

Starting from this point, Phases 3a and 3b can be seen to give rise to Phase 3:-

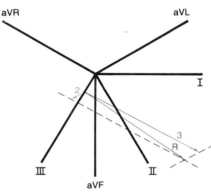

Phases 2 and 3 acting from this same point in time and space can be seen to give rise to R (which is the resultant of 2, 3a and 3b, all acting simultaneously).

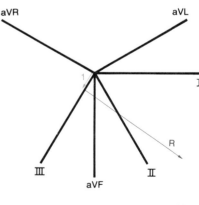

Thus the frontal plane representation of ventricular depolarisation has two sequential phases (1 and R).

This gives rise to the normal frontal plane loop (in this case with an axis of 45°). (The axis is the direction in which the frontal plane loop "points").

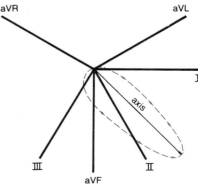

Left Anterior Hemiblock (LAH)

In left anterior hemiblock the antero-superior part of the left ventricle is not activated through the fast-conducting antero-superior division of the left bundle branch. Instead, it is activated only by the transmission of the depolarisation wave after it emerges from the postero-inferior part of the left ventricular myocardium which receives the depolarisation wave in normal manner through the postero-inferior division of the left bundle (Figure 94).

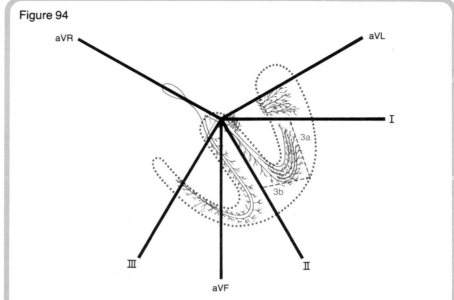

Figure 94

The antero-superior division of the left bundle totally fails to conduct. Septal depolarisation (Phase 1) and depolarisation of the free wall of the right ventricle (Phase 2) take place normally. Depolarisation of the inferior portion of the left ventricle (Phase 3b) also takes place normally. As usual Phase 1 occurs first, alone. Phases 2 and 3b then occur simultaneously. Depolarisation of the superior part of the left ventricle can only occur when a depolarisation wave reaches it from the postero-inferior division (i.e. after Phase 3b). However, since the impulse travels rapidly down the fast-conducting posterior division, Phase 3a is only minimally delayed. Since depolarisation of the superior part of the ventricle starts from the lower end rather than (as normal) from the upper end, the direction of Phase 3a is reversed.

The two basic changes, therefore, are:-
1. **Delay in the initiation of, and**
2. **Reversal of the direction of Phase 3a**

The depolarisation delay is much less than that in bundle branch block since there is rapid travel down the inferior bundle to the mid-portion of the left ventricle. The total QRS duration is therefore not abnormal, though it does tend to be at the upper end of the normal range.

The effects of these changes are shown in Figure 95.

Figure 95

Left anterior hemiblock.
The antero-superior division of the left
bundle totally fails to conduct.

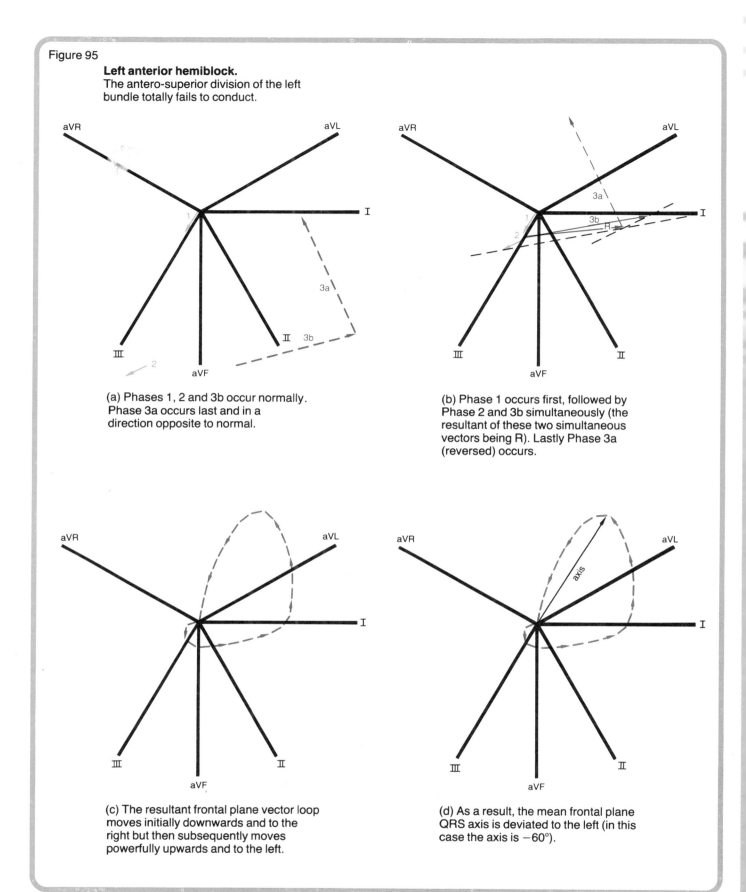

(a) Phases 1, 2 and 3b occur normally.
Phase 3a occurs last and in a
direction opposite to normal.

(b) Phase 1 occurs first, followed by
Phase 2 and 3b simultaneously (the
resultant of these two simultaneous
vectors being R). Lastly Phase 3a
(reversed) occurs.

(c) The resultant frontal plane vector loop
moves initially downwards and to the
right but then subsequently moves
powerfully upwards and to the left.

(d) As a result, the mean frontal plane
QRS axis is deviated to the left (in this
case the axis is −60°).

The cardinal features of left anterior
hemiblock are thus an abnormal degree
of left axis deviation with an initial
movement of depolarisation directed
inferiorly (i.e. left axis deviation but with
initial r waves in II, III and aVF).

Diagnostic criteria for left anterior hemiblock

1. A mean frontal plane QRS axis more negative than −30°.
2. Initial r waves in all inferior limb leads (II, III, aVF).
3. Other recognised causes of left axis deviation must be absent.

Other causes of abnormal left axis deviation

Other recognised causes of left axis deviation include some types of ventricular pre-excitation (the electrocardiographic features of the Wolff-Parkinson-White Syndrome), hyperkalaemia, tricuspid atresia, ostium primum atrial-septal defect. The only one of these easily missed is the Wolff-Parkinson-White Syndrome (see page 212). Artificial cardiac pacing from the apex of the right or left ventricle and injection of contrast in the left coronary artery are even more obviously recognisable alternative causes of left axis deviation.

Inferior myocardial infarction is an important, common cause of abnormal left axis deviation but does not come into the differential diagnosis if the diagnostic criteria (above) are fulfilled, since there is loss of the initial r waves in the inferior limb leads (II, III and aVF) in inferior infarction (see page 197).

Associated feature frequently present in left anterior hemiblock

The total QRS duration is usually at the upper end of the normal range (0.09 or 0.10 sec).

Important negative point in left anterior hemiblock

The total QRS duration is not prolonged beyond normal limits.

An example of left anterior hemiblock is shown in Figure 96.

This record would be reported as follows:-
"Sinus rhythm. The mean frontal plane QRS axis is −45°.
Left anterior hemiblock. Clockwise cardiac rotation".

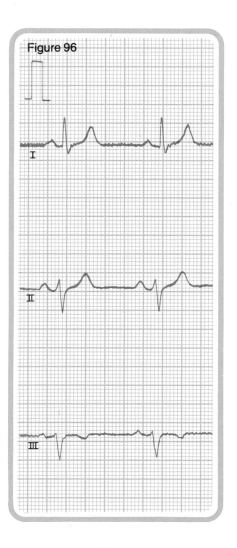

Figure 96

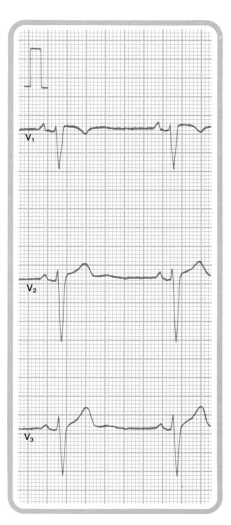

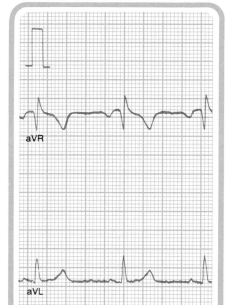

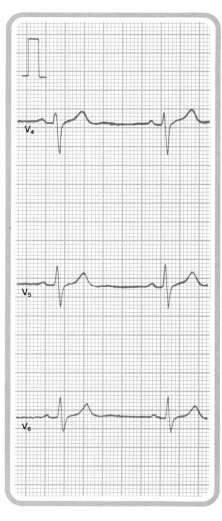

Figure 96

The rhythm is sinus. The mean frontal plane QRS axis is −45°. Normal initial r waves are seen in the inferior leads (II, III and aVF) and the abnormal degree of left axis deviation therefore indicates the presence of left anterior hemiblock (also known as left superior intraventricular block). The total QRS duration is 0.10 sec (best seen in the first QRS complex in Lead II). There is pronounced clockwise cardiac rotation (see pages 34–37). This accounts for the fact that no septal q waves are seen in the V_6. They are absent also from Lead 1 but are present in aVL and because of the latter, incomplete left bundle branch block cannot be said to be present.

Intermittent Left Anterior Hemiblock

Just as left and right bundle branch block can be intermittent if the pathological condition giving rise to the conduction problem varies, so left anterior hemiblock can be intermittent.

Clinical Significance

Chronic left anterior hemiblock is most commonly found in elderly people without other evidence of heart disease. In this situation it probably reflects fibrous degeneration in the anterior division of the left bundle branch. It may also be present in chronic ischaemic heart disease (e.g. in patients with chronic stable angina) in acute ischaemic heart disease (e.g. after acute ischaemia or infarction involving the appropriate division of the left bundle), in hypertension, in congestive cardiomyopathy, in hypertrophic cardiomyopathy, in calcific aortic stenosis (the calcium may extend into the conducting tissue), in myocarditis and as a result of surgical trauma (e.g. after aortic valve replacement).

Important differential diagnoses of left anterior hemiblock

The most striking feature of left anterior hemiblock is abnormal left axis deviation. The second commonest cause of abnormal left axis deviation is inferior myocardial infarction. The vital difference in the electrocardiogram between left anterior hemiblock and left axis deviation due to inferior myocardial infarction is the presence of initial r waves in the inferior leads (II, III and aVF) in left anterior hemiblock, compared with the abnormal Q wave in the inferior leads in inferior infarction (page 205). The third most common cause of left axis deviation is Wolff-Parkinson-White syndrome. This is easily missed unless looked for early in the assessment of the ECG (page 266). Other causes of left axis deviation are usually obvious and are listed on page 133.

Left Posterior Hemiblock (LPH)

Left posterior hemiblock occurs less frequently than left anterior hemiblock but as in anterior hemiblock the most dramatic change it produces is in the frontal plane QRS axis.

In left posterior hemiblock the postero-inferior part of the left ventricle is not activated through the fast-conducting postero-inferior division of the left bundle branch. Instead it is activated only by the transmission of the depolarisation wave after it emerges from the antero-superior part of the left ventricular myocardium which receives the depolarisation wave in the normal manner through the antero-superior division of the left bundle (Figure 97).

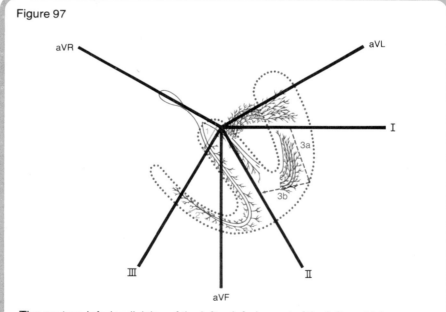

Figure 97

The postero-inferior division of the left bundle totally fails to conduct. Septal depolarisation (Phase 1) and depolarisation of the free wall of the right ventricle (Phase 2) take place normally. Depolarisation of the superior portion of the left ventricle (Phase 3a) also takes place normally. As usual, Phase 1 occurs first, alone. Phases 2 and 3a then occur simultaneously. Depolarisation of the inferior part of the left ventricle can only occur when the depolarisation wave reaches it from the antero-superior division. However, since the impulse travels rapidly down the fast-conducting anterior division, Phase 3b is only minimally delayed. Since depolarisation of the inferior part of the ventricle starts from the upper end, the direction of Phase 3b is reversed.

The two basic changes, therefore, are:-
1. **Delay in the initiation of, and**
2. **Reversal in the direction of, Phase 3b**

The depolarisation delay is much less than that in bundle branch block since there is rapid travel down the superior bundle to the mid-portion of the left ventricle. The total QRS duration is therefore not abnormal, though it does tend to be at the upper end of the normal range.

The effect of these changes is seen in Figure 98.

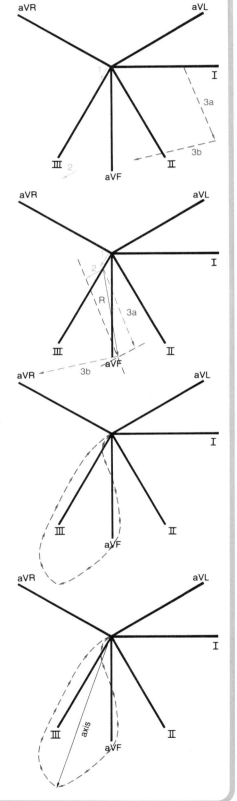

Figure 98

Left posterior hemiblock.
The postero-inferior division of the left bundle totally fails to conduct.

Phases 1, 2 and 3a occur normally. Phase 3b occurs last and in a direction opposite to normal.

Phase 1 occurs first, followed by Phase 2 and 3a simultaneously (the resultant of these two simultaneous vectors being R). Lastly Phase 3b (reversed) occurs.

The resultant frontal plane vector loop moves initially downwards and to the right. It then moves more definitively downwards. Finally it moves markedly to the right before returning to the origin.

As a result, the mean frontal plane QRS axis is deviated to the right (in this case the axis is +110°).

Cardinal feature of left posterior hemiblock

Unfortunately, it is not possible to be totally dogmatic about the presence of this lesion. One cannot, therefore, legitimately talk of "diagnostic criteria" but only of the "cardinal feature".

Its only electrocardiographic feature is a mild degree of right axis deviation (between $+90°$ and $+120°$). The total QRS duration is usually at the upper end of the normal range at 0.09 to 0.10 sec.

Such relatively subtle alterations as slight right axis deviation and a total QRS duration at the upper end of the normal range make it impossible to be totally confident of the diagnosis from the electrocardiogram alone. Other possible causes of right axis deviation must be excluded (on clinical or investigative grounds), before it can reasonably be concluded that left posterior hemiblock is present. These alternative causes include:- a vertical heart in a tall thin subject, emphysema, right ventricular hypertrophy, atrial-septal defect and extensive antero-lateral myocardial infarction.

An example of left posterior hemiblock is shown in Figure 99.

The ECG of Figure 99 would be reported as follows:- "Sinus rhythm. The mean frontal plane QRS axis is $+105°$. This is an abnormal degree of right axis deviation. There is no evidence of right ventricular hypertrophy and the appearance could be indicative of left posterior hemiblock. The frontal plane T waves are minimally abnormal".

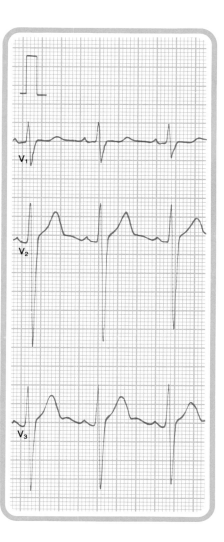

Figure 99

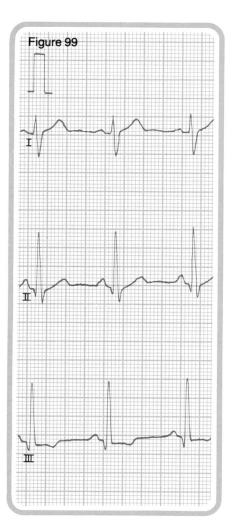

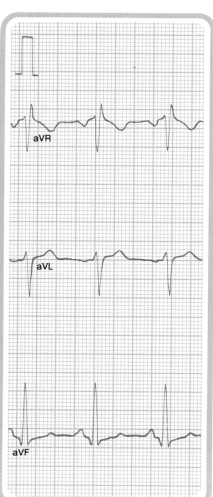

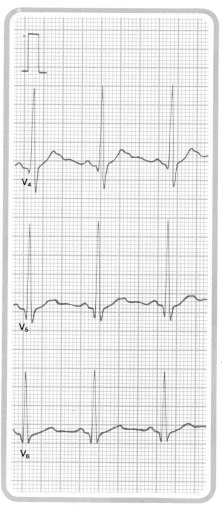

Figure 99

The rhythm is sinus, the mean frontal plane QRS axis is slightly deviated towards the right at +105°. The mean frontal plane T wave axis is +30°. The angle between this and the mean frontal plane QRS axis (75°) is thus abnormal (pages 56 and 57).
The T waves in the frontal plane are therefore minimally abnormal. There is no evidence in the precordial leads of right ventricular hypertrophy to account for the right axis deviation. There is no clockwise cardiac rotation such as might be found in the presence of chronic lung disease. Left posterior hemiblock is therefore a real possibility, but one cannot be totally dogmatic about this. If one had been able to see an earlier electro-cardiogram in the same subject which was similar in all respects but showed an axis within the normal range, then it would have been reasonable to conclude that left posterior hemiblock had developed.

Bifascicular Blocks

The term "Bifascicular block" is used when two fascicles are blocked simultaneously. The more common combination is right bundle branch block and left anterior hemiblock, and the less common combination is right bundle branch block and left posterior hemiblock. (The combination of left anterior hemiblock and left posterior hemiblock is indistinguishable from left bundle branch block).

Right Bundle Branch Block with Left Anterior Hemiblock

This combination is relatively easy to recognize. The criteria for right bundle branch block are fulfilled and there is an abnormal degree of left axis deviation (i.e. more negative than −30°).

Criteria for right bundle branch block with left anterior hemiblock

1. Total QRS duration is 0.12 sec or greater.
2. A secondary R wave is seen in V_1 (see page 118).
3. The mean frontal plane QRS axis is more negative than −30°.
4. An initial r wave is seen in the inferior limb leads (II, III and aVF).

An example is shown in Figure 100. The ECG in Figure 100 would be reported as follows:- "Sinus rhythm. There is complete right bundle branch block. There is left anterior hemiblock giving rise to a mean frontal plane QRS axis of −75°. There is left atrial hypertrophy and pronounced clockwise cardiac rotation and the r waves are of abnormally low voltage in the left precordial leads".

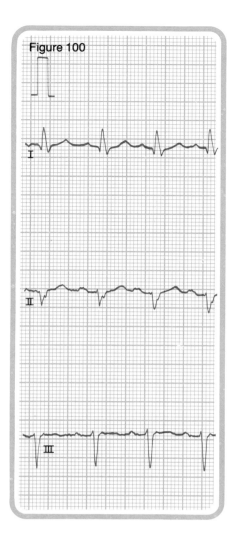

Figure 100

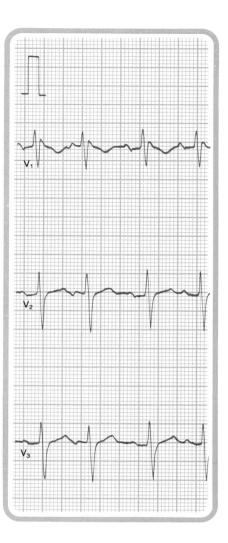

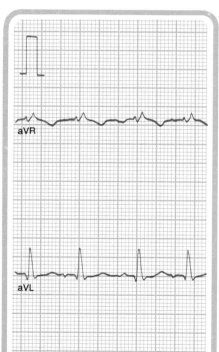

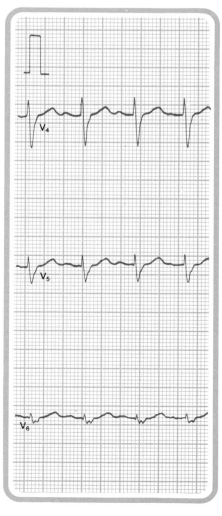

Figure 100

The rhythm is sinus. There is a secondary r wave in V_1. The total QRS duration is 0.13 sec (best seen in the first QRS complex in I). There is therefore right bundle branch block. The mean frontal plane QRS axis is $-75°$ and there are small initial r waves in II, III and aVF. There is therefore also left anterior hemiblock. (The bifid P waves in II and biphasic P waves in V_1 suggest left atrial hypertrophy – see later). There is clockwise cardiac rotation with very poor R wave progression across the precordial leads (such changes can occur in obesity and in anterolateral infarction – see later).

Right Bundle Branch Block with Left Posterior Hemiblock

Just as it is impossible from the ECG alone to be certain that there is left posterior hemiblock, so it is impossible to be **certain** of the combination of right bundle branch block and left posterior hemiblock. The criteria required are those for right bundle branch block and, in addition, an abnormal degree of right axis deviation. However, as is also true with regard to the diagnosis of right posterior hemiblock alone, other recognisable causes of right axis deviation must be included before the diagnosis of the combination can be made.

Cardinal features of right bundle branch block with left posterior hemiblock

1. Total QRS duration of 0.12 sec or greater.
2. A secondary R wave in V_1.
3. A mean frontal plane QRS axis more positive than $+90°$.

The first two criteria are those for right bundle branch block. The third criterion is that for left posterior hemiblock but is not specific, therefore other causes of right axis deviation need to be eliminated before the diagnosis can be made with confidence.

An example of the combination is shown in Figure 101. The ECG in Figure 101 would be reported as follows:- "Sinus rhythm. Complete right bundle branch block. Abnormal right axis deviation ($+120°$) consistent with right posterior hemiblock. Clockwise cardiac rotation."

Figure 101

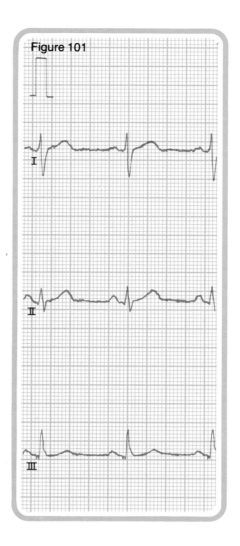

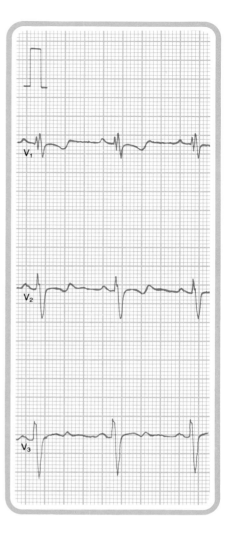

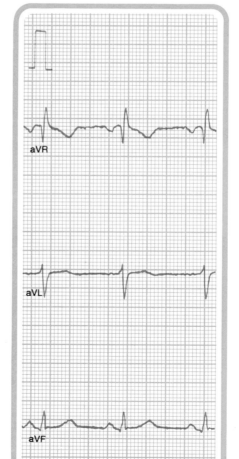

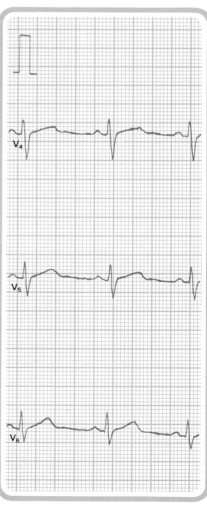

Figure 101

The rhythm is sinus. There is an rsR′S′ pattern in V₁. The total QRS duration is prolonged, at 0.12 sec (best seen in the first QRS complex in V₁). There is therefore complete right bundle branch block. There is an abnormal degree of right axis deviation (+120°). Since no other clinical or investigative cause for right axis deviation was apparent, right posterior hemiblock is a possible explanation. There is also clockwise cardiac rotation.

Clinical Significance of Bifascicular Blocks

The combination of right bundle branch block and left anterior hemiblock is relatively common. It is most frequently found in asymptomatic elderly patients with fibrotic degeneration in the conducting tissues, and only rarely does it proceed to complete heart block. It may also be seen in atherosclerotic heart disease, calcific aortic stenosis, hypertrophic cardiomyopathy, congestive cardiomyopathy and congenital endocardial cushion defects. When it occurs in the context of acute myocardial infarction some 25–50% may progress to complete heart block, but when found in other situations only 5–15% of the patients progressed to complete block.

Right bundle branch block with left posterior hemiblock is a much less frequent combination, but may occur in any of the conditions listed for combination of right bundle branch block and left anterior hemiblock (above). However, when it does occur it is much more likely to progress to complete heart block and this happens in 60–70% of the patients in whom the combination is found.

The main reason that left posterior hemiblock is much less common than left anterior hemiblock is because the posterior division is thicker and shorter and has a much better blood supply than the anterior division. Higher vulnerability of the anterior division explains why right bundle branch block and left anterior hemiblock is more common than right bundle branch block and left posterior hemiblock and also why the combination of right bundle branch block and left posterior hemiblock is more likely to progress to complete heart block.

Other Forms of Intraventricular Block

The terms "parietal block" and "peri-infarction block" have been used for many years, but are poorly defined and are often used by different authorities to mean different things. These terms are therefore best abandoned and will not be discussed further.

The term "diffuse intraventricular block" refers to a rare but defined condition in which the delay occurs in the myofibrils rather than in the conducting tissue. The **diagnostic criteria** are the presence of abnormally wide (0.11 sec or longer) QRS complexes with a normal frontal plane QRS axis and with a QRS configuration which is either similar to normal or to that of left bundle branch block. This rare condition is most commonly seen in severe cardiomyopathy or myocarditis. It may also occur in infiltrative myocardial disease, occasionally in severe rheumatic disease, in ischaemic heart disease (especially in the presence of ventricular aneurysms), in hyperkalaemia, severe hypoxia, hypothermia and sometimes following over-dosage with quinidine or procainamide.

Ventricular Hypertrophy

Appreciable hypertrophy of the right or left ventricle produces characteristic changes in the electrocardiogram. Lesser degrees of hypertrophy may be present without ECG changes or with only non-specific changes. This is more often true in the case of right than of left ventricular hypertrophy. In general, the limb leads are of less diagnostic value than the precordial leads in detecting these conditions. Once again, this is particularly true with respect to right ventricular hypertrophy and, indeed, there is no certain way of diagnosing right ventricular hypertrophy from the limb leads alone – however severe the changes.

In normal circumstances the thickness of the left ventricular free wall is about three times greater than that of the right ventricular free wall. The mass of the left ventricular myocardium is therefore many times greater than that of the right ventricle (page 22). The voltages generated by left ventricular depolarisation are of the order of ten times greater than those generated by right ventricular depolarisation and, for this reason, in normal circumstances (and in most abnormal circumstances) left ventricular depolarisation is the dominant influence in determining the appearances of the QRS complexes and the resultant S–T segment and T waves. As would be expected, therefore, left ventricular hypertrophy produces, in effect, an exaggeration of the normal QRS pattern whereas right ventricular hypertrophy alters the QRS pattern in the various leads. In both cases secondary S–T segment and T wave changes follow the primary changes in QRS complexes.

Left Ventricular Hypertrophy (LVH)

The increased myocardial bulk associated with hypertrophy of the left ventricle results in an increase in the voltage contribution of Phase 3 depolarisation (Figure 102 and 103). This gives **taller R waves in the left precordial leads** and **deeper S waves in the right precordial leads**. The increased bulk also gives rise to prolongation in the time taken to travel from endocardium to the (now more distant) epicardium. This time, known as the "ventricular activation time" or the "intrinsicoid deflection time" is measured from the onset of the QRS complex to the peak of the R wave (page 39). It is measured only in left precordial leads showing a qR complex.

With the development of LVH the total QRS duration may increase minimally compared with its volume before the development of LVH. It usually still remains within the normal range but may sometimes reach 0.10 or 0.11 sec. It does not reach 0.12 sec. The primary depolarisation (QRS) abnormality gives rise to secondary repolarisation changes in the form of S–T segment depression and T wave inversion in leads facing the left ventricle. The precordial leads which face the left ventricle are, of course, the left precordial leads. The limb leads which face the left ventricle are Leads I and aVL (when the heart is horizontal) or II and aVF (when the heart is vertical). In the presence of left ventricular hypertrophy, the heart is usually but not always horizontal.

Figure 102

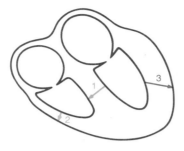

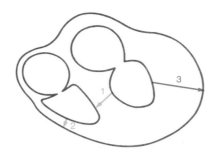

Normal

(a) The timing, sequence and relative voltages of the three phases of ventricular depolarisation are as shown:-

Left Ventricular Hypertrophy

(a) The timing and sequence of the three phases of ventricular depolarisation are normal. The voltage resulting from Phase 3 is substantially increased. That resulting from Phase 1 may also be slightly increased.

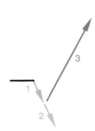

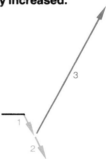

(b) The normal QRS complex in V₆ is of the qR pattern:-

(b) The qR configuration of the QRS complex in V₆ is unchanged, but the R wave height and the ventricular activation time are increased.

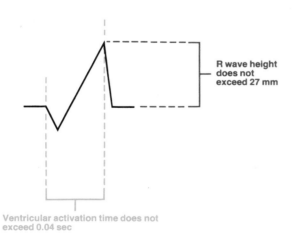

R wave height does not exceed 27 mm

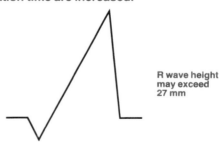

R wave height may exceed 27 mm

Ventricular activation time may exceed 0.04 sec

Ventricular activation time does not exceed 0.04 sec

(c) The normal qR complex is followed by an iso-electric S-T segment and upright T wave

(c) The abnormal QRS complex is followed by a depressed S-T segment and an inverted T wave.

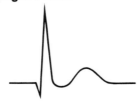

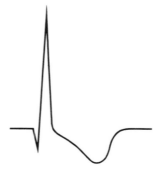

Figure 103

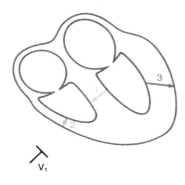

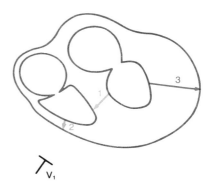

Normal

Left Ventricular Hypertrophy

(a) The timing, sequence and relative voltages of the three phases of ventricular depolarisation are as shown:-

(a) The timing and sequence of the three phases of ventricular depolarisation are normal. The voltage resulting from Phase 3 is substantially increased. That resulting from Phase 1 may also be slightly increased.

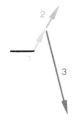

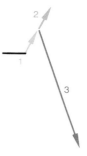

(b) The normal QRS complex in V₁ is of the rS pattern:-

(b) The normal rS configuration of the QRS complex in V₁ is unchanged but the S wave depth is increased.

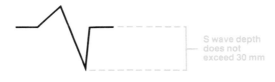

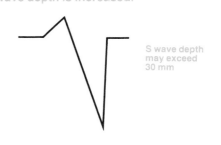

(c) The normal rS complex is followed by an iso-electric S-T segment. The T waves may be upright, flat or inverted.

(c) No definitive changes in the S-T segment or T wave occur in this lead.

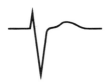

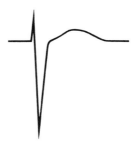

146

An example of severe left ventricular hypertrophy is shown in Figure 104. This ECG would be reported as follows:- "Sinus rhythm. The mean frontal plane QRS axis is −15°. There are pronounced changes of left ventricular hypertrophy. There is evidence of left atrial hypertrophy". (Left atrial hypertrophy is described in the next chapter. It is usually present when there is left ventricular hypertrophy).

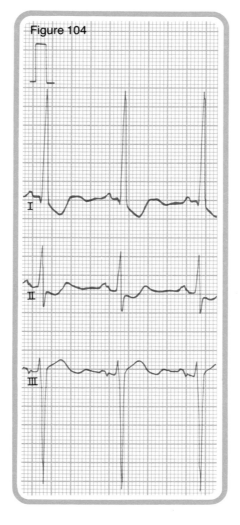

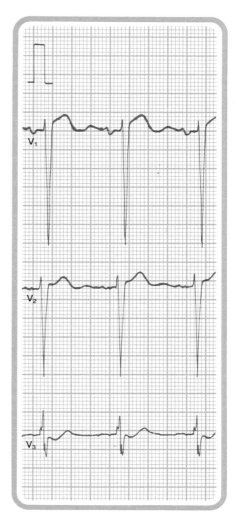

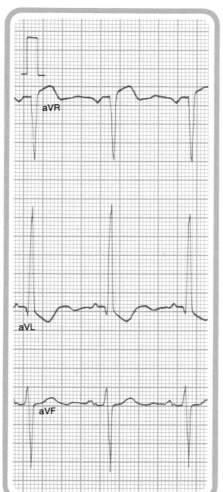

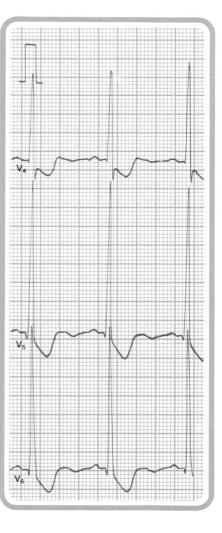

Figure 104

The rhythm is sinus. The axis is towards the left end of the normal range (−15°) i.e. the heart is horizontal. R wave height in V_5 and V_6 is abnormal (the peak R wave height in V_5 is 41mm). The S wave depth in V_1 is abnormal (31mm). The ventricular activation time in V_5 and V_6 is prolonged (0.06 sec). There is S–T segment depression and T wave inversion in the left precordial leads. Since the heart is horizontal the changes seen in the left precordial leads are also shown in I and aVL. There is also evidence of left atrial hypertrophy (page 165).

Criteria for left ventricular hypertrophy*

(Normal calibration assumed (pages 64 and 65))

1. The R waves in any one or more of the Leads, V_4, V_5 or V_6 exceeds 27mm.
2. The tallest R waves in any of the Leads V_4, V_5 or V_6 plus the deepest S waves in any of the Leads V_1, V_2 or V_3 exceeds 40mm.
3. The S waves in one or more of the Leads V_1, V_2 or V_3 exceeds 30mm.
4. R wave in aVL exceeds 13mm.
5. R in aVL exceeds 20mm.
6. The ventricular activation time (intrinsicoid deflection time) exceeds 0.04 sec (i.e. equals or exceeds 0.05 sec) **.
7. Abnormal S-T segment depression (i.e. more than 1mm below the iso-electric line (page 42)) in any lead facing the left ventricle (i.e. in V_4, V_5 or V_6, and in Lead I and aVL when heart is horizontal or in II and aVF when the heart is vertical).
8. T wave inversion in leads facing the left ventricle (as outlined in (7) above).

Unfortunately, there are no internationally agreed criteria for left ventricular hypertrophy. The above criteria would meet general but not universal acceptance. The voltage criteria (1–5 above) are generally sensitive criteria. As such they are frequently fulfilled in the absence of definitive, clinical or pathological evidence of left ventricular hypertrophy. **R waves beyond the normally accepted height or S waves beyond the normally accepted depth are often found in thin-chested persons (especially if they indulge in regular physical activity which may induce "physiological" hypertrophy). If the voltage criteria only are fulfilled it is better to report the ECG as "the voltage criteria for left ventricular hypertrophy are fulfilled" rather than "left ventricular hypertrophy" for the former can be normal in thin-chested persons.** This is a good example of "secondary" interpretation of the electrocardiogram in the light of clinical data (page 109).

Prolongation of the ventricular activation time is a more specific criterion but is considerably less sensitive than the voltage criteria.

Note

* Left ventricular hypertrophy is a **graded** abnormality (not an all-or-none abnormality like complete bundle branch block). Because of this there are no "diagnostic" criteria. A whole range of criteria may point towards left ventricular hypertrophy. Some are more sensitive than specific (page 108) and some more specific and sensitive. In general the greater the number of criteria fulfilled, the more likely the diagnosis becomes.

** The small squares on the ECG graticule indicate 0.04 sec and it is not considered possible to distinguish differences less than 0.01 sec. If this is accepted, "exceeds 0.04 sec" is the same as "equals or exceeds 0.05 sec".

Systolic overload, diastolic overload, "strain"

Hypertrophy of the left ventricle can be produced by conditions giving rise to additional load in the ventricle during systole (e.g. aortic stenosis) or during diastole (e.g. aortic incompetence). The so-called "Systolic overload pattern" is one in which the S–T segment and T wave changes are **relatively** more prominent than the QRS changes. The so-called "Diastolic overload pattern", conversely, is one in which the QRS changes are **relatively** more pronounced than the S–T segment and T wave changes. However, it should be stressed that these are "soft" (i.e. ill-defined) concepts and are not reliable indicators of the cause of the hypertrophy.

The term "strain" is even less well-defined (and carries physical, physiological and prognostic overtones which it cannot possibly justify). Like "systolic overload" it refers to the pronounced S–T segment and T wave changes **thought to have arisen on the basis of ventricular hypertrophy**. The term is not significantly different in concept from "systolic overload". For this reason (and also because the terms imply pathophysiological consequences which cannot possibly be predicted from the ECG) the terms "strain" and "strain pattern" are best avoided. The terms "systolic overload pattern" and "diastolic overload pattern" do have some minor discriminatory power but are not of major usefulness.

Associated features in left ventricular hypertrophy

1. Since the physical size of the left ventricle is increased in left ventricular hypertrophy, there is more left ventricle underlying the chest leads. Because of this, left ventricular (i.e. qR) complexes may appear further to the right in the precordial leads than the usual V_4 to V_6 – i.e. **there is often counterclockwise cardiac rotation** (pages 34 to 37).
2. Usually the development of left ventricular hypertrophy results in a **slight** shift of the mean frontal plane QRS axis towards the left. However, the axis usually remains within the normal range and typically it is between $+30°$ and $-30°$. This means that the heart is **horizontal** (page 53). In this event the changes in QRS complexes, S–T segments and T waves induced in the left precordial leads will be seen also in I and aVL.

Occasionally, left ventricular hypertrophy can occur with a mean frontal plane QRS axis of $+60°$ to $+90°$ – i.e. the heart is vertical (page 53). In this situation the changes in the QRS complexes, S–T segments and T waves induced in the left precordial leads are seen also in II and aVF.

Figure 104 shows a typical example of left ventricular hypertrophy in a horizontal heart. Leads I and aVL show appearances similar to those found in V_5 and V_6. Figure 105 shows an example of left ventricular hypertrophy in a vertical heart (the mean frontal plane QRS axis is $+60°$). Leads II and aVF show appearances similar to those found in V_5 and V_6.

The ECG of Figure 105 would be reported as follows:–
"Sinus rhythm. The mean frontal plane QRS axis is $+60°$. The precordial QRS complexes satisfy the voltage criteria for left ventricular hypertrophy".

3. Electrocardiographic evidence of left atrial hypertrophy usually accompanies that of left ventricular hypertrophy. Electrocardiographic evidence of atrial hypertrophy can only be recognised if the rhythm is sinus.
4. Prominent U waves are often seen in the right and mid-precordial leads of patients with left ventricular hypertrophy.

The U Wave

The U wave is a small, rounded, upright wave occurring immediately at the end of the T wave. It is part of the repolarisation process. It is visible in many normal electrocardiograms. It becomes more prominent in left ventricular hypertrophy, myocardial ischaemia, hypokalaemia and following exercise. It is thus a non-specific change. A U wave is deemed to be definitively abnormal if it is taller than the T wave preceding it (in the same lead). Prominent, but not abnormal, U waves are seen in V_1–V_3 of Figure 105. In this figure small U waves are also visible in V_4.

The normal U wave is described in more detail on page 195. Conditions giving rise to abnormally tall U waves are listed on page 263.

Important negative points in left ventricular hypertrophy

Left ventricular hypertrophy does not give rise to an abnormal degree of left axis deviation. The presence of an axis more negative than −30° in an electrocardiogram showing left ventricular hypertrophy suggests the presence of left anterior hemiblock (provided initial r waves are visible in the inferior limb leads).

Clinical Significance

The main causes of recognisable left ventricular hypertrophy on the electrocardiogram are systemic hypertension, aortic stenosis, coarctation of the aorta, mitral incompetence, aortic incompetence and hypertrophic cardiomyopathy. Of these, systemic hypertension almost certainly represents the commonest cause. Aortic and mitral incompetence both cause diastolic loads on the left ventricle and patent ductus arteriosus may do the same if the shunt is very large. The other causes listed result in systolic overload of the ventricle.

It is partly because left ventricular hypertrophy is associated with a **slight** shift of the frontal plane axis towards the left (though usually still within the normal range) and partly because those conditions most commonly giving rise to left ventricular hypertrophy tend to present in the middle and later age groups (when the axis normally lies towards the left end of the normal range) that left ventricular hypertrophy is usually associated with a horizontal heart. If appreciable left ventricular hypertrophy develops in a child, the heart may well be vertical, for the normal frontal plane QRS axis is at the extreme right hand end of the normal range in infancy and progresses gradually towards the left hand end of the range with increasing age. Left ventricular hypertrophy with a vertical heart is thus most commonly seen in childhood in association with valvar or subvalvar aortic stenosis or coarctation of the aorta.

Figure 105

The rhythm is sinus. The frontal plane QRS axis is +60° and the heart is therefore vertical. The precordial QRS complexes satisfy the voltage criteria for left ventricular hypertrophy. In other respects the record is within normal limits. Since the heart is vertical, the form of the QRS complexes in II and aVF is similar to that in V_6. Contrast this with Figure 104, where the heart is horizontal (frontal plane axis −15°). In this situation, Leads aVL and I show QRS appearances similar to those in V_6.

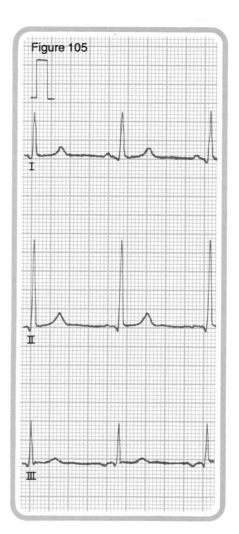

Figure 105

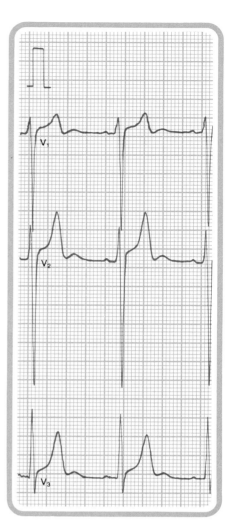

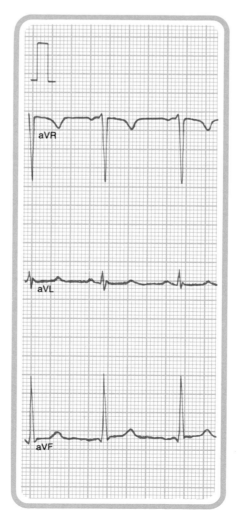

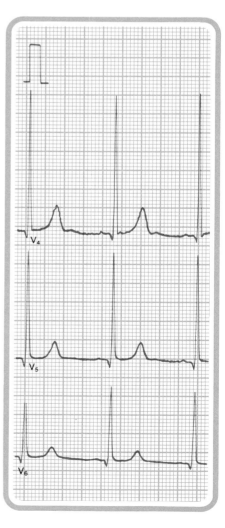

Right Ventricular Hypertrophy (RVH)

In all normal and in most abnormal electrocardiograms, the voltages generated by left ventricular depolarisation dominate the electrocardiographic appearances in every lead. Minor degrees of right ventricular enlargement have no appreciable effect on the appearances. However, the increased bulk of the right ventricle in more pronounced right ventricular hypertrophy results in a major increase in the voltage contribution of Phase 2 of ventricular depolarisation and this may become the dominant influence in many ECG leads.

The most obvious consequence of RVH is an increase in the voltage of the R wave in the right precordial leads (Figure 106). The most diagnostic feature is a dominant R wave in V_1[†] (the term "dominant R wave" implies that whatever the configuration of the QRS complex in V_1 the largest wave in that QRS complex is an R wave). The most readily understood configuration of the QRS complex in V_1 is an Rs complex (Figures 106 and 107). However, not uncommonly a small q wave may be present in V_1 in right ventricular hypertrophy (giving rise to a qR or a qRs complex – i.e. the QRS morphology may be different but the R wave is still dominant). An example is shown in Figure 108. The explanation for the presence of a q wave in V_1 is not fully understood. It may be that right ventricular hypertrophy involves the upper part of the interventricular septum and as a result of this the depolarisation of the interventricular septum initially passes upwards and backwards instead of forwards and downwards (Figure 109). This gives rise to an initial movement of the QRS vector away from V_1 and results in an initial negative wave (i.e. a q wave).

[†]A dominant R′ wave may be seen in V_1 in the presence of RBBB. It is important to exclude RBBB (by the fact that the total QRS duration is less than 0.12 sec) before RVH is diagnosed.

Figure 106

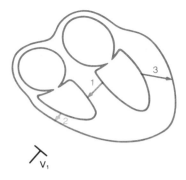

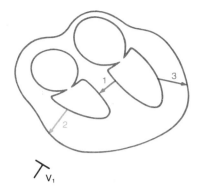

Normal

Right Ventricular Hypertrophy

(a) The timing, sequence and relative voltages of the three phases of ventricular depolarisation are as shown:-

(a) The timing and sequence of the three phases of ventricular depolarisation are normal. The voltage resulting from Phase 2 is substantially increased. That resulting from Phase 1 may also be slightly increased.

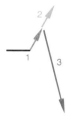

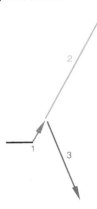

(b) The normal QRS complex in V$_1$ is of the rS pattern:-

(b) The normal rS configuration in V$_1$ is radically altered to produce a dominant R wave.

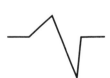

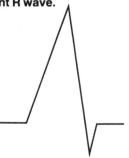

(c) The normal rS complex is followed by an iso-electric S-T segment. The T waves may be upright, flat or inverted.

(c) The abnormal Rs complex in V$_1$ is followed by a depressed S-T segment and an inverted T wave.

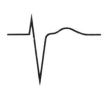

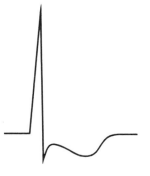

The ECG in Figure 107 would be reported as follows:–

"Sinus rhythm. The mean frontal plane QRS axis is +135°. There is a dominant R wave in V_1. There is clockwise cardiac rotation. The appearances are indicative of right ventricular hypertrophy. The form of the P waves in II suggests the possibility of right atrial hypertrophy".

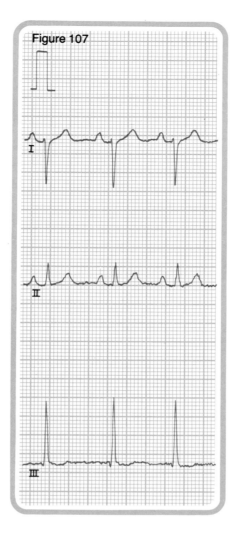

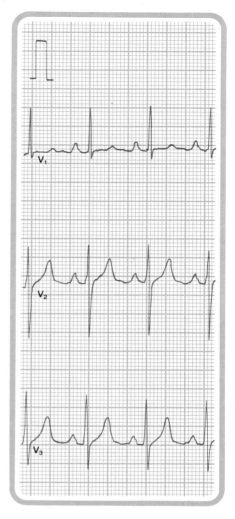

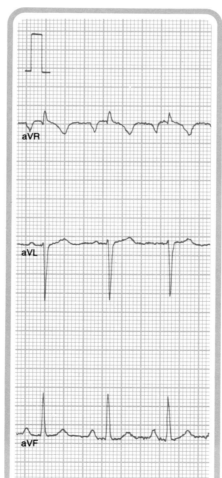

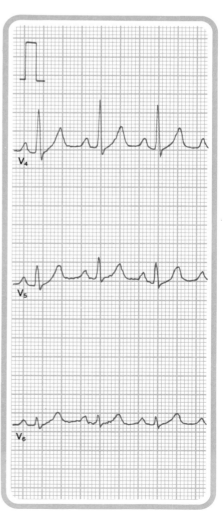

Figure 107

The rhythm is sinus. There is abnormal right axis deviation (+135°). There is a dominant R wave (an Rs complex) in V_1. There is therefore right ventricular hypertrophy. There is clockwise cardiac rotation. There are no S–T,T changes of right ventricular hypertrophy (see below). The P waves are tall and pointed in Lead II suggesting right atrial hypertrophy (see next section).

153

The ECG of Figure 108 would be reported as follows:–
"Sinus rhythm. The mean frontal plane QRS axis is $+135°$. There is a dominant R wave in V_1. There is pronounced clockwise cardiac rotation. There are non-specific S-T, T changes from V_1 to V_5. The appearances are those of right ventricular hypertrophy. There is evidence also of right atrial hypertrophy.

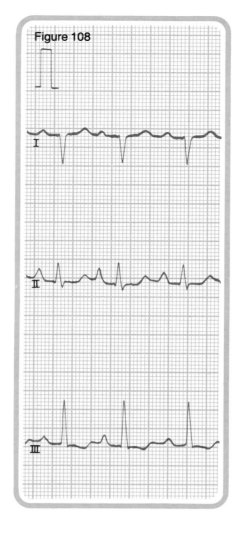

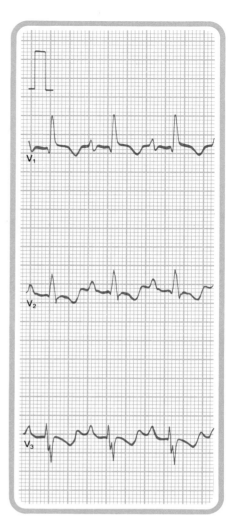

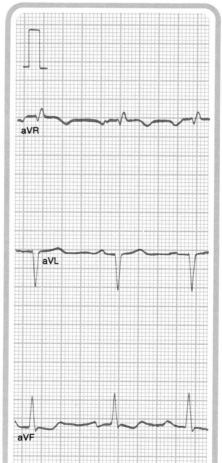

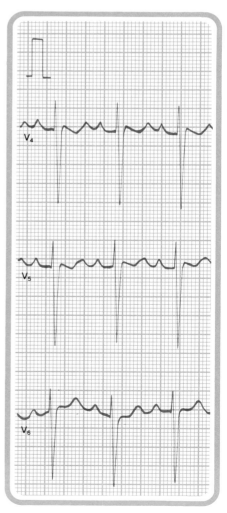

Figure 108

The rhythm is sinus. There is abnormal right axis deviation $(+135°)$. There is a dominant R wave (qR complex) in V_1. There is therefore right ventricular hypertrophy. There is clockwise cardiac rotation and a deep S wave in V_6. There is S-T segment depression from V_1 to V_4. The P waves are tall and pointed in Lead II, indicating right atrial hypertrophy (see pages 159 to 161). The P-R interval is prolonged 0.22 sec.

154

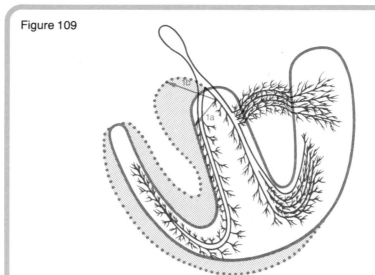

Figure 109

T_{V_1}

In the normal heart septal depolarisation passes forwards, downwards and to the right (arrow 1a). In the presence of right ventricular hypertrophy it can pass backwards, upwards and to the right (arrow 1b) to produce an initial part of the QRS complex moving away from V_1, i.e. an initial q wave.

The primary depolarisation (QRS) abnormality gives rise to secondary repolarisation changes in the form of S–T segment depression and T wave inversion in leads facing the right ventricle. These changes involve the right and mid-precordial leads.

Unlike left ventricular hypertrophy, right ventricular hypertrophy is accompanied by deviation of the axis beyond the normal range. Right ventricular hypertrophy is associated with right axis deviation. In addition, since the right ventricle is larger than normal, more of the right ventricular myocardium than usual underlies the precordial leads. The transition zone therefore moves further towards the left in the precordial series, i.e. there is usually pronounced clockwise cardiac rotation (pages 34 to 37). As a result of this the R wave size in the left precordial leads is reduced and as a result of the increased voltage of Phase 2 depolarisation the S wave in the left precordial leads is increased.

Diagnostic criteria for right ventricular hypertrophy

1. A frontal plane QRS axis more positive than +90°.
2. Dominant R wave in V_1 (Rs, R, RR′, qR or qRS).
3. Absence of evidence of anterolateral infarction* (see page 197).
4. QRS duration must be less than 0.12 sec †.

Note

*Anterolateral infarction is one cause of right axis deviation (page 197 and Table 2, page 156). In the presence of both anterolateral infarction and true posterior infarction the combination of abnormal right axis deviation and a dominant R wave in V_1 may occur and this may wrongly suggest right ventricular hypertrophy. However, the true diagnosis is indicated by the evidence of anterolateral infarction.

†If the QRS duration is 0.12 sec or longer there is bundle branch block which, in the presence of a dominant R wave in V_1, would be right bundle branch block. The diagnosis of right ventricular hypertrophy in the presence of right bundle branch block is difficult and unreliable.

Additional features frequently present in right ventricular hypertrophy

1. S–T segment depression and T wave inversion in some of the Leads V_1 to V_4.
2. Deep S waves in V_5, V_6 and also in I and aVL.
3. Evidence of right atrial hypertrophy (see page 159).

Problems in the differential diagnosis of right ventricular hypertrophy

As indicated earlier, right ventricular hypertrophy may be well advanced before any ECG changes become apparent.

The earliest change is usually a shift of the axis to the right. However, a mean frontal plane QRS axis more positive than $+90°$ occurs in a large number of conditions (see Table 2).

Table 2

Causes of mean frontal plane QRS axis more positive than $+90°$

Normal finding in infants and children
Occasional normal finding in tall, slim adults
Occasional finding in chronic lung disease
   (even in the absence of pulmonary hypertension)
Anterolateral myocardial infarction
Left posterior hemiblock
Right ventricular hypertrophy
Pulmonary embolism
Atrial septal defect

The second of the diagnostic criteria for right ventricular hypertrophy (the presence of a dominant R wave in V_1) also has several possible causes (see Table 3).

Table 3

Causes of increased R wave amplitude in V_1

Normal finding in children
True posterior myocardial infarction
Ventricular pre-excitation
Duchenne type muscular dystrophy
Right bundle branch block (occasionally)
Right ventricular hypertrophy

The **combination** of abnormal right axis deviation and a dominant R wave in V_1 makes it very highly likely that there is right ventricular hypertrophy. The likelihood is further increased by the presence of S-T segment depression and T wave inversion in the right precordial leads and by the presence of right atrial hypertrophy (see page 159).

Clinical Significance

The majority of conditions giving rise to right ventricular hypertrophy are conditions which produce systolic overload of the right ventricle – pulmonary stenosis, pulmonary hypertension (primary, or secondary to left ventricular insufficiency or to mitral valve disease) and Fallot's tetralogy. Only relatively rarely does chronic cor pulmonale give rise to right ventricular hypertrophy.

Diastolic overload of the right ventricle occurs in atrial septal defect, anomalous pulmonary venous return and tricuspid incompetence. The electrocardiographic appearances in diastolic overload of the right ventricle are indistinguishable from those in complete or incomplete right bundle branch block.

Bi-ventricular Hypertrophy

Bi-ventricular hypertrophy may be difficult or impossible to recognise from the electrocardiogram. The increased electrical forces of both Phases 2 and 3 ventricular depolarisation may cancel themselves out so that the precordial QRS complexes may appear completely normal. If both ventricles are enlarged, one more markedly so than the other, the pattern will be that of hypertrophy of the dominant ventricle. When both ventricles are hypertrophied to a similar degree many of the changes will cancel each other out. However, because of the increased ventricular wall thickness the time taken for depolarisation to spread from endocardium to epicardium within the ventricles will be increased and the total duration may be prolonged to 0.10 or 0.11 sec but not beyond this. In addition, T wave inversion may be apparent in any of the chest leads. Sometimes **the combination of signs of left ventricular hypertrophy with right axis deviation** (i.e. more positive than +90°) **will present and this combination, if chronically present, suggests bi-ventricular hypertrophy. Less frequently, combined ventricular hypertrophy may give rise to signs of right ventricular hypertrophy and an axis more negative than −30°.**

The essential points to note about bi-ventricular hypertrophy are as follows:-

1. . It may exist without diagnostic ECG changes.

2. The total QRS duration may be prolonged to 0.10 or 0.11 sec.

3. T wave inversion may be present in the precordial leads.

4. The combination of signs of left ventricular hypertrophy and an axis more positive than +90° is suggestive of bi-ventricular hypertrophy.

5. Occasionally the combination of signs of right ventricular hypertrophy with an axis more negative than −30° is found.

Clinical Significance

Bi-ventricular hypertrophy is found in severe rheumatic valve disease (aortic valve disease with pulmonary hypertension or mitral incompetence with pulmonary hypertension) cardiomyopathy and occasionally in congenital heart disease.

Atrial Hypertrophy

Just as ventricular hypertrophy produces recognisable changes in ventricular depolarisation (i.e. in the QRS complexes) and repolarisation (i.e. in the T waves), so atrial hypertrophy produces changes in the atrial depolarisation (P) wave. Since the atrial repolarisation (Ta) wave is not usually visible in the electrocardiogram, it is not surprising that recognisable changes in its form are not usually visible in atrial hypertrophy. Enlargement of the left or right atrium gives rise to an increase in the voltage and duration of the respective component of the P wave.

The Normal P Wave

It will be recalled (pages 43, 44 and 59) that right atrial depolarisation starts before left atrial depolarisation starts and finishes before left atrial depolarisation finishes. In normal circumstances atrial depolarisation begins as soon as depolarisation of the sino-atrial node spreads to activate the adjacent right atrial myocardium. Depolarisation then spreads simultaneously in all available directions through right atrial myocardium. The direction in which the greatest amount of atrial myocardium is available determines the direction in which the right atrial component of the P wave is best seen (Figure 110). This is usually towards Lead II in the limb leads and towards V_1 in the precordial leads. The first part of the left atrial myocardium to be depolarised is that point which is on the **shortest** route of depolarisation from the sino-atrial node (Figure 110). From this point, depolarisation spreads in all available directions through the left atrial myocardium. The direction in which the greatest amount of atrial myocardium is available determines the direction in which the left atrial component of the P wave is best seen. This is usually also towards Lead II in the limb leads but is away from V_1 in the precordial leads.

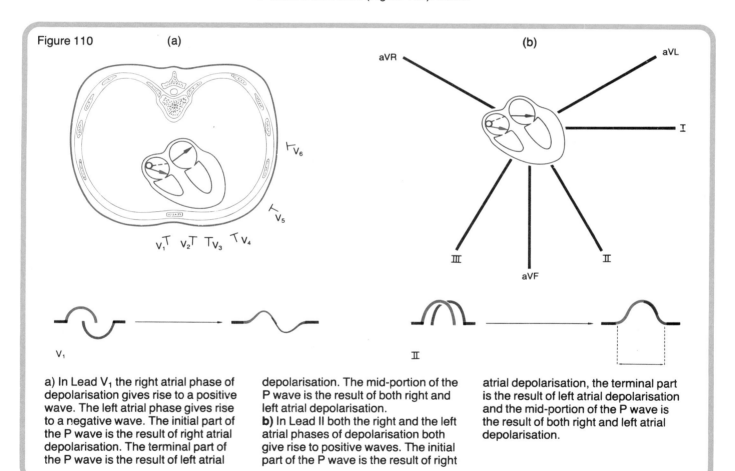

Figure 110   (a)   (b)

a) In Lead V_1 the right atrial phase of depolarisation gives rise to a positive wave. The left atrial phase gives rise to a negative wave. The initial part of the P wave is the result of right atrial depolarisation. The terminal part of the P wave is the result of left atrial depolarisation. The mid-portion of the P wave is the result of both right and left atrial depolarisation.
b) In Lead II both the right and the left atrial phases of depolarisation both give rise to positive waves. The initial part of the P wave is the result of right atrial depolarisation, the terminal part is the result of left atrial depolarisation and the mid-portion of the P wave is the result of both right and left atrial depolarisation.

Lead II therefore normally shows a uniphasic upright P wave which consists of overlapping right and left atrial components (Figure 110b), whereas V_1 normally shows a biphasic P wave with an initial positive and a subsequent negative component (Figure 110a).

In Lead II the normal P wave does not exceed 2.5mm in height or 0.12 sec in duration. In the normal P wave in V_1 the area of the negative component does not exceed the area of the positive component which precedes it.

Atrial Abnormality

The P wave is a much less well-defined wave-form than the QRS complex. Abnormalities of the P wave therefore tend to be less specific than those of the QRS complexes. Thus, while it is customary to speak of abnormal P waves as showing "hypertrophy" of the right or left atrium, there is, in fact, no means of distinguishing hypertrophy of a given atrium from ischaemia, infarction or inflammation of that atrium or from a conduction defect within the atrium. It may be therefore that the term "atrial abnormality" might be preferable to "atrial hypertrophy", but the latter term is widely used and will not easily be displaced. The important point to realise is that when there is evidence of (for example) left atrial hypertrophy, the only legitimate conclusion from the electrocardiogram is that the left atrium is in some way abnormal ("primary" interpretation). In the light of clinical data indicating the presence of mitral stenosis or of left ventricular hypertrophy, the presence of true left atrial hypertrophy might be inferred ("secondary" interpretation). In the absence of such data no assessment of the cause of the atrial abnormality can be made.

Right Atrial Hypertrophy

In right atrial hypertrophy the right atrial component of the P wave is increased in voltage and in duration. Since the right atrial component of the P wave is normally seen as a positive deflection both in Lead II and in V_1, the P wave height is increased in both of these leads. Since right atrial depolarisation is normally complete well before left atrial depolarisation is completed, the delay in the completion of right atrial depolarisation is not sufficient to prolong right atrial depolarisation beyond the end of left atrial depolarisation. Because of this the P wave duration is not increased (Figure 111a).

Figure 111

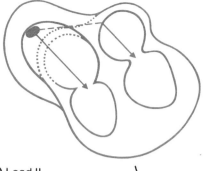

a) Lead II

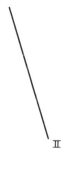

In right atrial hypertrophy the (initial) right atrial component of the P wave is increased in magnitude and in duration. The resultant effect on the P wave is an increase in the P wave height but not in its duration.
a) The resultant P wave in Lead II is abnormally tall and is pointed.
b) The resultant P wave in Lead V₁ has an abnormally tall (initial) positive component.

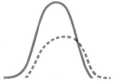

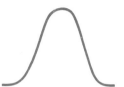

Normal P wave in II – right and left atrial components.

The P wave in II in right atrial hypertrophy – right and left atrial components. The right atrial component is increased.

The P wave in II in right atrial hypertrophy is abnormally tall.

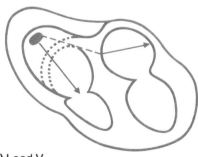

b) Lead V₁

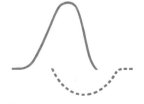

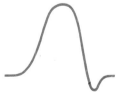

Normal P wave in V₁ – right and left atrial components.

The P wave in V₁ in right atrial hypertrophy – right and left atrial components. The right atrial component is increased.

The P wave in V₁ in right atrial hypertrophy has a tall initial positive component.

The primary electrocardiographic change in right atrial hypertrophy is therefore an increase in the voltage of the P wave in Lead II and an increase in the voltage of the initial positive part of the P wave in V_1. There is a good deal of variation in the dominant direction of right atrial depolarisation in the horizontal plane and as a result of this changes in the P wave height in V_1 do not reliably occur in right atrial hypertrophy. The diagnosis of right atrial hypertrophy can therefore only safely be made from the P waves in the frontal plane leads. Lead II usually shows the changes best. An example is shown in Figure 112. The ECG in Figure 112 would be reported as follows:-

"Sinus rhythm. The mean frontal plane QRS axis is +165°. There is right ventricular hypertrophy, right atrial hypertrophy and clockwise cardiac rotation".

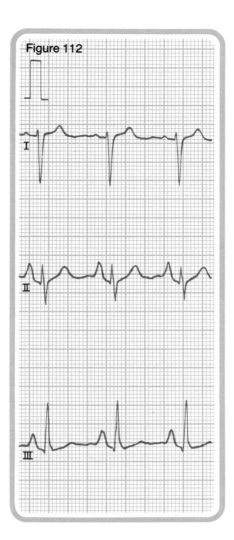

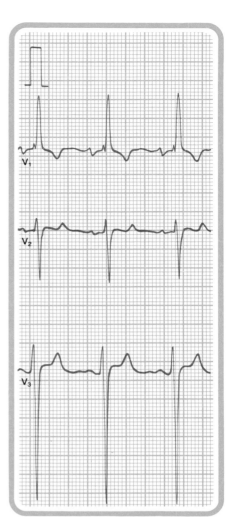

Figure 112

There is an abnormal degree of right axis deviation (+165°) and a dominant R wave in V_1. There is thus right ventricular hypertrophy. The P waves are tall and pointed in Lead II and are in excess of 3mm. There is thus right atrial hypertrophy. Right atrial hypertrophy very frequently accompanies right ventricular hypertrophy. The pronounced clockwise cardiac rotation is part of the right ventricular hypertrophy.

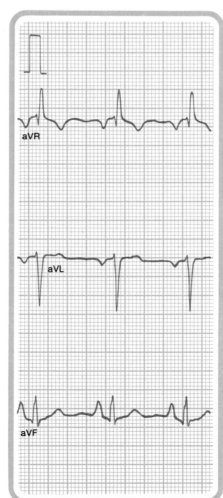

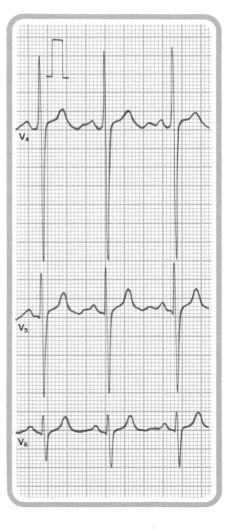

161

Criterion for right atrial hypertrophy

The P wave height is 3mm or more in Leads II, III or aVF (Leads III and aVF are included because the P wave vector is sometimes directed more closely towards either of these leads than along Lead II, i.e. the P wave axis is often $+75°$ or more positive than this).

Associated findings

In association with right atrial hypertrophy, the positive part of the P wave in V_1 is often greater than 1.5mm tall. There is usually evidence of right ventricular hypertrophy. There is often also a prominent atrial repolarisation wave (see pages 166 and 167).

Clinical Significance

As indicated earlier, the electrocardiographic finding of "right atrial hypertrophy" strictly speaking only defines the presence of right atrial abnormality. Changes similar to those in hypertrophy also occur in ischaemia or infarction of the right atrium although the latter two are rare clinical events. The presence of associated right ventricular hypertrophy makes it much more likely that the right atrial hypertrophy pattern on the electrocardiogram does indicate true hypertrophy of the right atrium. Right atrial hypertrophy occurs in all conditions which give rise to right ventricular hypertrophy and in addition it occurs in tricuspid stenosis.

Left Atrial Hypertrophy

The electrocardiographic changes produced by left atrial hypertrophy are those changes produced by an increase in the voltage and duration of the left atrial depolarisation wave. Since the terminal part of the normal P wave is produced by left atrial depolarisation, it follows that the total P wave duration is prolonged in left atrial hypertrophy.

In addition, the P wave tends to be bifid in Lead II and biphasic in V_1 (Figure 113). In V_1 the area of the (terminal) negative component exceeds the area of the (initial) positive component. An example of left atrial hypertrophy is shown in Figure 114.

Figure 113

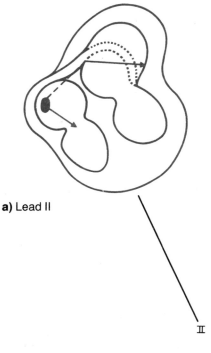

a) Lead II

In left atrial hypertrophy the left atrial (terminal) component of the P wave is increased in magnitude and in duration. The resultant effect on the P wave is to increase the size of the terminal portion and also to increase the total P wave duration.

a) The resultant P wave in Lead II is broadened (more than 0.12 sec) and bifid with a tall second component.

b) The resultant P wave in Lead V₁ is broadened and biphasic. The area of the (terminal) negative component is larger than the area of the (initial) positive component.

II

Normal P wave in II – right and left atrial components.

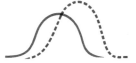

The P wave in II in left atrial hypertrophy – right and left atrial components. The left atrial component is increased.

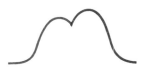

The P wave in II in left atrial hypertrophy is notched and broad. The second component may be tall.

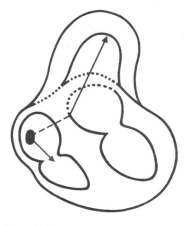

b) Lead V₁

T_{V_1}

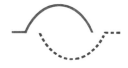

Normal P wave in V₁ – right and left atrial components.

The P wave in V₁ in left atrial hypertrophy – right and left atrial components. The left atrial component is increased.

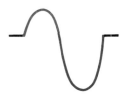

The P wave in Lead V₁ in left atrial hypertrophy has a dominant negative (terminal) component.

The ECG in Figure 114 would be reported as follows:- "Sinus rhythm. The mean frontal plane QRS axis is +75°. The P waves are broad and bifid in Lead II and there is a dominant negative component to the P wave in V_1. The changes are indicative of left atrial hypertrophy (strictly "left atrial abnormality"). In other respects the record is within normal limits".

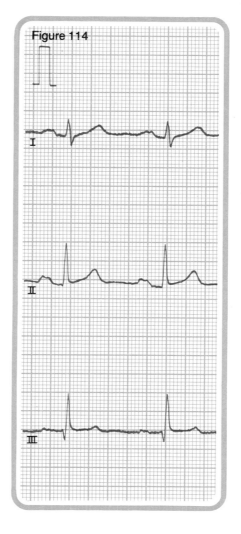

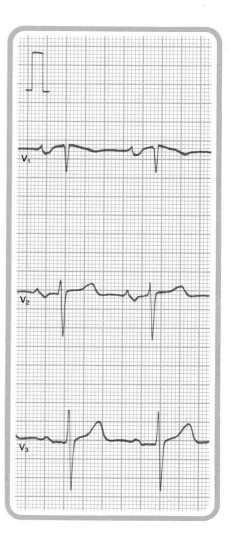

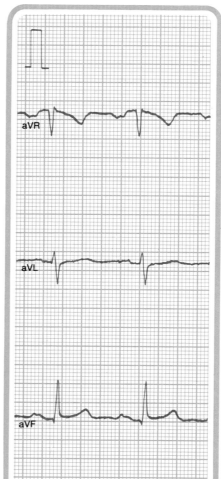

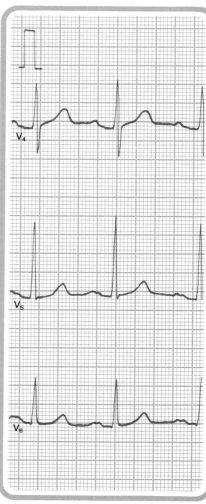

Figure 114

The rhythm is sinus. P waves are bifid in Lead II. The P wave duration in Lead II is prolonged at 0.15 sec (best seen in the second T wave in Lead II). The P waves in V_1 are clearly biphasic. In this lead there is a small, brief (and rather sharp looking) initial positive component followed by a deeper and very much broader negative component. The area of the negative component clearly exceeds that of the positive component.

164

Criteria for left atrial hypertrophy

1. The P wave is notched and exceeds 0.12 sec in duration in Leads I, II, aVF or aVL.
2. The P wave in V_1 has a dominant negative component (i.e. either it is entirely negative or alternatively the area of the (terminal) negative component exceeds that of the (initial) positive component).

(Either criterion suggests the diagnosis. If both are satisfied the diagnosis is more likely still).

Features commonly associated with left atrial hypertrophy

Just as right atrial hypertrophy is frequently found in association with right ventricular hypertrophy, so left atrial hypertrophy is frequently found in association with left ventricular hypertrophy. In patients with pure mitral stenosis, left atrial hypertrophy may occur in association with **right** ventricular hypertrophy.

Clinical Significance

Left atrial hypertrophy occurs in any condition associated with left ventricular hypertrophy and it also occurs in mitral stenosis. It is frequently found in association with systemic hypertension even when there is no electrocardiographic evidence of left ventricular hypertrophy in that condition. It may also be found in association with aortic stenosis, aortic incompetence, mitral incompetence, hypertrophic cardiomyopathy and chronic ischaemic heart disease.

As discussed earlier (under the heading of right atrial hypertrophy) the term "atrial hypertrophy" is less justifiable than "atrial abnormality". The primary electrocardiographic interpretation of the presence of broad bifid P waves in Lead II or a dominant negative component to the P wave in V_1 is that there is some *abnormality* of the left atrium. If it is known that there is mitral stenosis or left ventricular hypertrophy then true left atrial hypertrophy might well be inferred ("secondary" interpretation). The electrocardiogram itself merely provides evidence of abnormality of the left atrium and cannot distinguish between atrial hypertrophy, atrial ischaemia and atrial infarction. When electrocardiographic evidence of left atrial hypertrophy is found in a person with ischaemic heart disease it is likely that the common explanation is ischaemia or infarction of the atrium.

Bi-atrial Hypertrophy

The diagnosis of bi-atrial hypertrophy is not as difficult as the diagnosis of bi-ventricular hypertrophy since the hypertrophy of each individual atrium affects predominantly a different part of the P wave whereas hypertrophy of each individual ventricle affects the same part of the QRS complex. Bi-atrial hypertrophy may therefore be diagnosed whenever the criteria for both left and right atrial hypertrophy are fulfilled.

Diagnostic criteria for bi-atrial hypertrophy

1. P waves in the limb leads which are **both** 3mm or greater in height, and **also** in excess of 0.12 sec in duration.
2. The presence of a large biphasic P wave in V_1 with an (initial) upright portion of 2mm or more in height, and a (terminal) negative portion at least 1mm deep and 0.04 sec in duration.
3. The presence of a tall peaked P wave 2mm or more in height in V_1 in combination with wide (i.e. more than 0.12 sec in duration) notched P waves in the limb leads or in the left precordial leads.

(Any one criterion suggests the diagnosis. The more criteria are fulfilled the more likely the diagnosis becomes).

Clinical Significance

Bi-atrial enlargement is found in conditions giving rise to bi-ventricular enlargement. This includes congenital heart disease, hypertrophic cardiomyopathy and pulmonary hypertension occurring either with aortic valve disease or with mitral incompetence. The reservations expressed about the use of the term "atrial hypertrophy" with reference to hypertrophy of individual atria apply equally well with reference to hypertrophy of both atria.

Atrial Repolarisation Wave

It was pointed out (page 5) that electrical recovery of myocardium must occur following depolarisation of that myocardium before any subsequent repeat depolarisation is possible. In the case of the ventricular myocardium, depolarisation and repolarisation are both recognisable from the surface electrocardiogram. The **QRS complex is, in fact, the surface electrocardiographic manifestation of ventricular myocardial depolarisation** and **the T wave is the surface electrocardiographic manifestation of ventricular myocardial repolarisation** (though it should be noted that ventricular myocardial repolarisation is actually taking place during the S-T segment and, in some parts of the heart, even before the QRS complex is completed). **The P wave is the surface electrocardiographic manifestation of atrial myocardial depolarisation.** The process of repolarisation of the atrial myocardium does not give rise to a recognisable wave on the surface electrocardiogram (i.e. it has no surface electrocardiographic manifestation) even though repolarisation must necessarily occur before any subsequent, repeat depolarisation of the atrial myocardium is possible. The atrial repolarisation wave is called the "atrial T wave" or "Ta" wave. It is normally a shallow, smooth negative wave which, since it occurs at the same time as the much larger QRS complex, is normally totally obscured by the latter. It becomes apparent on the surface electrocardiogram only when it is increased in size. When the Ta wave becomes prominent it increases both in depth and in duration (Figure 115). It may then be apparent as a dip in the trace, seen both **before** and **after** the QRS complex. It is easily confused with a depressed S-T segment but recognition that the depression starts **before** the QRS complex should prevent this misunderstanding. Its appearance may be likened to a QRS complex standing slightly left of centre in a shallow saucer.

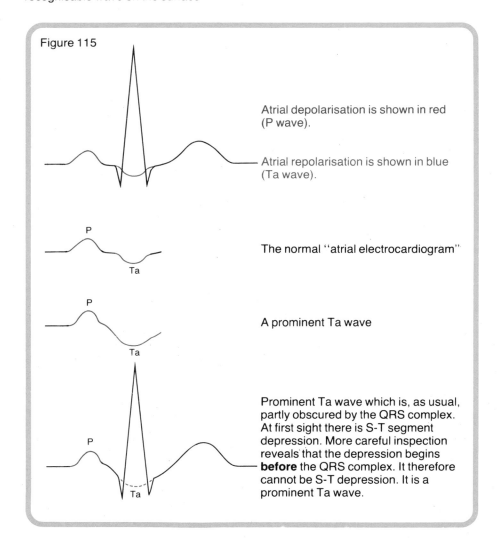

Figure 115

Atrial depolarisation is shown in red (P wave).

Atrial repolarisation is shown in blue (Ta wave).

The normal "atrial electrocardiogram"

A prominent Ta wave

Prominent Ta wave which is, as usual, partly obscured by the QRS complex. At first sight there is S-T segment depression. More careful inspection reveals that the depression begins **before** the QRS complex. It therefore cannot be S-T depression. It is a prominent Ta wave.

Causes of Prominent Atrial Repolarisation Waves

By far the commonest cause of an exaggerated Ta wave is **sinus tachycardia.** An example is shown in Figure 116. The ECG of Figure 116 would be reported as follows:-
"Sinus tachycardia. Rate 165/min. Prominent atrial repolarisation wave simulating S-T depression in some leads. Allowing for the heart rate, the record is within normal limits".

Prominent Ta waves may also occur in **right atrial hypertrophy.** Close inspection of Figure 112 shows a prominent Ta wave well seen in Leads II and aVF. Prominent Ta waves also occur in atrial infarction (see page 199).

Rarely a normal Ta wave can be seen in cases of complete heart block when the QRS complex does not obscure the wave.

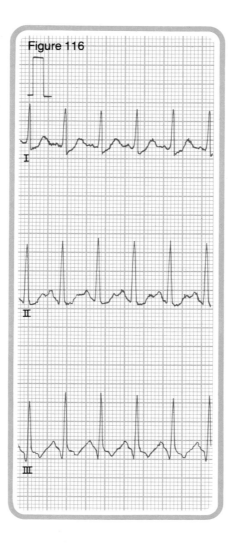

Figure 116

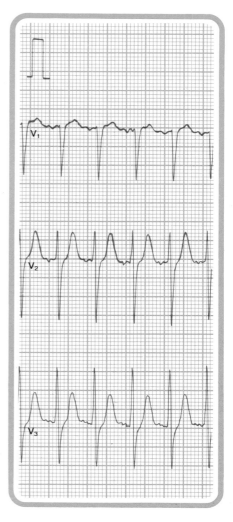

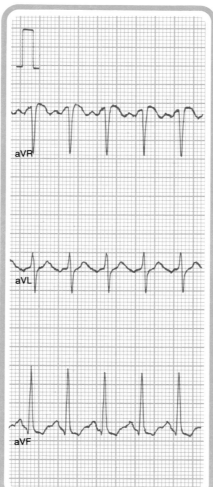

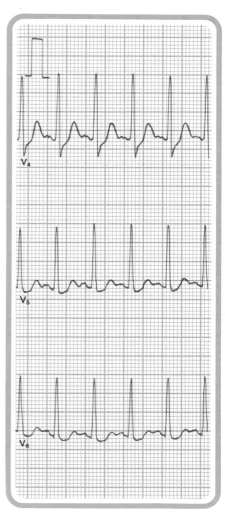

Figure 116

A 12-lead electrocardiogram taken just after the completion of an exercise test. The rhythm is sinus tachycardia and the heart rate is 165/min. There is apparent S-T depression in I, II, aVF and V_4-V_6, but closer inspection (especially in II where the T and Ta vectors are usually best seen) reveals that the negativity begins **before** the QRS complexes. It is a prominent Ta wave. There is no significant S-T abnormality and the exercise test is negative.

Ischaemic Heart Disease

The electrocardiogram is used more often in the investigation of suspected ischaemic heart disease than in that of any other condition. Since the viability of every part of the myocardium and of the conducting tissue is dependent upon the adequacy of perfusion of the tissue, it follows that coronary atheroma can induce ischaemic damage in any part of the myocardium or conducting tissue. **Ischaemia of the myocardium** may give rise to changes in the P waves, QRS complexes, S-T segments or T waves in any lead of the electrocardiogram and **ischaemia of the conducting tissue** can cause any conceivable arrhythmia. The range of cardiographic abnormalities which can occur in ischaemic heart disease is therefore vast. However, **it is perfectly possible to have severe, extensive, stenosing atheroma of the coronary arteries without there being any recognisable abnormality in the 12-lead electrocardiogram.** It must be remembered that the electrocardiogram provides information only about the **myocardium** (via the configuration and dimensions of P waves, QRS complexes, S-T segments and T waves) and about the **specialised conducting tissue** (via the electrocardiographic evidence of the cardiac rhythm). Electrocardiographic evidence of ischaemic heart disease is always **inferential.** If no ischaemic damage to the myocardium or conducting tissue has occurred (either permanently or transiently) the electrocardiogram can play no part in confirming or refuting a clinical impression of ischaemic heart disease. **For example, 50-75% of patients with unequivocal angina pectoris have normal resting 12-lead electrocardiograms when first seen.**

These two facts – namely that **almost any** ECG abnormality may occur in ischaemic heart disease and that even in the presence of severe ischaemic heart disease there may be **no abnormality** – bedevil attempts to acquire a balanced understanding of the electrocardiogram as a diagnostic tool in ischaemic heart disease. Nevertheless, it is possible to recognise the more important and the common electrocardiographic manifestation of ischaemic heart disease and these manifestations will be dealt with in this chapter.

The Electrocardiogram in Acute Myocardial Infarction

Changes in QRS complexes, in S-T segments or in T waves may occur in acute myocardial infarction and many of these changes may persist.

However, the only definitive, diagnostic changes of myocardial infarction (whether recent or old) are changes in the QRS complexes.

The QRS Complexes in Infarction

Two QRS abnormalities may be indicative of myocardial infarction. These are:-

1. Inappropriately low R wave voltage in a local area.

2. Abnormal Q waves.

Whilst these two changes may seem very dissimilar, they are actually part of the same process. The **development of a negative wave** (Q wave) and **the reduction in size of the positive wave** each result from loss of positivity which, in turn, is the result of necrosis of myocardium. This is so, simply because QRS changes of infarction are related to the reduction in the amount of, or to the total absence of, living myocardium underneath the exploring electrode. The size of the positive wave in each precordial lead is, both in normal and in abnormal circumstances, related to the thickness of viable myocardium underneath the electrode. In normal circumstances this thickness increases progressively from right to left in the precordial series (Figure 117).

Note

Figures in this chapter depicting the horizontal cross-section of the heart in the approximate level of the precordial leads omit the atria for the sake of simplicity. They show cross-sections through the ventricles below the level of the atrio-ventricular valves. (In this plane the right ventricular cavity is seen to be crescent-shaped and to be "wrapped round" the left ventricle). This simplification of the diagram is necessary to demonstrate the importance of depolarisation of the posterior wall of the heart on the appearances in the precordial leads when there is anterior infarction.

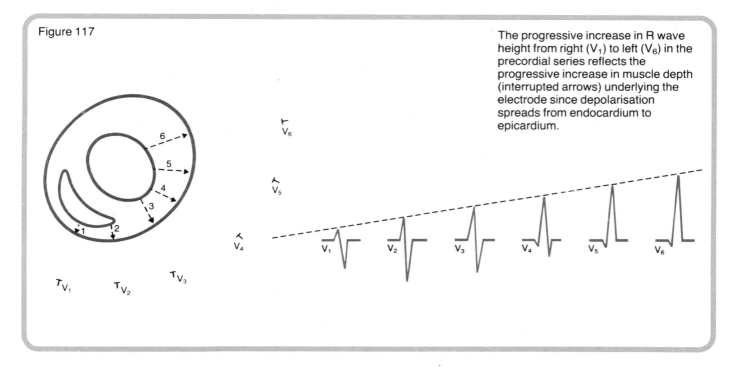

Figure 117

The progressive increase in R wave height from right (V_1) to left (V_6) in the precordial series reflects the progressive increase in muscle depth (interrupted arrows) underlying the electrode since depolarisation spreads from endocardium to epicardium.

Loss of R wave voltage

If infarction (i.e. total loss of viability) of part of the thickness of the left ventricular myocardium occurs in that part of the left ventricle underlying electrodes V_3 to V_5, the result will be a reduction in the R wave voltage under these electrodes (Figure 118).

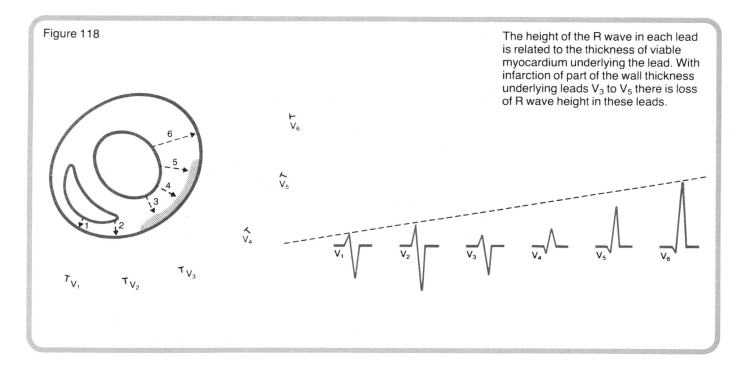

Figure 118

The height of the R wave in each lead is related to the thickness of viable myocardium underlying the lead. With infarction of part of the wall thickness underlying leads V_3 to V_5 there is loss of R wave height in these leads.

Loss of R wave height can only be judged to be present if **either** a previous record is available showing a significantly greater R wave height in the appropriate leads before the infarction occurred **or** the leads involved are two or more of the leads V_2-V_5. The criteria cannot be applied to V_1 or to V_6 since it is necessary to interpolate between these leads in order to estimate what the true R wave height should be (dotted line, Figure 117). At least two leads within the group V_2-V_5 must show evidence of R wave reduction for this criterion to be used to indicate myocardial infarction since (as noted on page 45) occasionally in a normal precordial series one R wave may be smaller in V_2, V_3 or V_4 than in the lead to its immediate right in the precordial series (i.e. V_1, V_2 or V_3 respectively). Theoretically it is possible to have reduction in R wave height in V_5 alone in myocardial infarction, but in most cases infarction involves myocardium underlying at least two leads.

Note

Infarction must **not** be diagnosed on the basis of an R wave height in V_5 or V_6 less than that in V_4 for this is a common normal variation related to the greater depth of lung lying between V_5 and V_6, on the one hand, and the heart, on the other hand, compared with that lying between V_4 and the heart (Figure 42, page 33). However, infarction may be diagnosed from reduced R wave voltage in V_5 and V_6 if a record prior to infarction is available to indicate the true initial R wave height.

Abnormal Q waves and QS complexes

When infarction involves the full thickness of the myocardium ("transmural" infarction – i.e. from endocardium to epicardium) there will be **total** loss of R waves in leads overlying the infarcted zone (Figure 119).

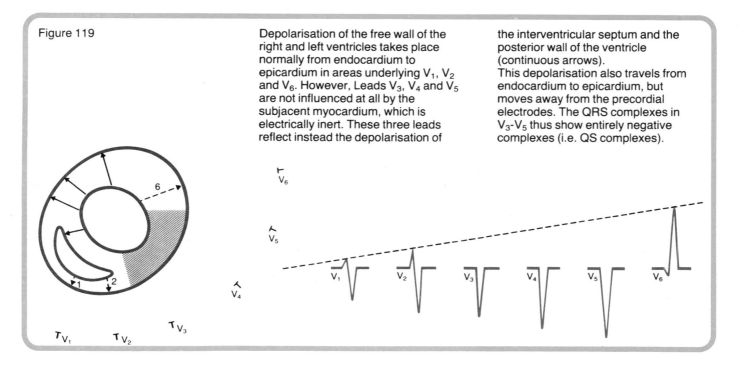

Figure 119

Depolarisation of the free wall of the right and left ventricles takes place normally from endocardium to epicardium in areas underlying V₁, V₂ and V₆. However, Leads V₃, V₄ and V₅ are not influenced at all by the subjacent myocardium, which is electrically inert. These three leads reflect instead the depolarisation of the interventricular septum and the posterior wall of the ventricle (continuous arrows).

This depolarisation also travels from endocardium to epicardium, but moves away from the precordial electrodes. The QRS complexes in V₃-V₅ thus show entirely negative complexes (i.e. QS complexes).

Total loss of R waves in the precordial leads gives rise to entirely negative waves, i.e. by definition (page 5) to QS complexes. These negative waves are the result of depolarisation of the posterior wall of the ventricle travelling from endocardium to epicardium (and therefore away from the anterior leads). These depolarisation waves from the posterior wall of the heart are, in normal circumstances, obscured by the dominant depolarisation of the anterior wall of the ventricles which lie much closer to the precordial leads.

When infarction involves less than the full thickness of the myocardium but still involves a major part of the wall thickness, less severe changes occur in which the R waves, whilst appreciably reduced in size, are still present and there are abnomal Q waves (see later, page 174) but, since there are residual R waves, no actual QS complexes (Figure 120). The finding of abnormal Q waves and reduced R wave voltage is the commonest electrocardiographic appearance in established infarction.

Figure 120

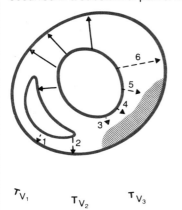

Depolarisation of the free wall of the left ventricle takes place normally from endocardium to epicardium in areas underlying electrodes V₁, V₂ and V₆. However, infarction has occurred in a substantial part of the left ventricular wall thickness in areas underlying electrodes V₃, V₄ and V₅. As a result of this the R wave voltage is **substantially** diminished in these leads. The size of the residual R waves in Leads V₃-V₅ is related to the thickness of remaining viable myocardium (interrupted arrows 3, 4 and 5). The situation differs from that shown in Figure 118 only in degree, i.e. in the extent of the wall thickness involved in infarction. In this case most of the wall thickness is involved and the thickness of the remaining viable myocardium is insufficient to overcome the effects of the posterior left ventricular wall depolarisation passing away from the precordial leads giving rise to deep, broad Q waves.

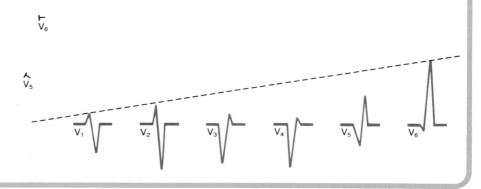

The reduction in R wave voltage is the result of reduction in the thickness of viable myocardium underlying the recording electrode. This reduction in viable myocardial thickness in the anterior wall of the ventricle permits the influence of the posterior wall depolarisation to dominate and abnormal Q waves develop in the relevant precordial leads (produced by depolarisation of the posterior wall travelling from endocardium to epicardium away from the anterior leads).

The reduction in R wave voltage can only be recognised if **either** a previous record is available showing a significantly greater R wave height in the appropriate leads before the infarction occurred, **or**

the leads involved are two or more of the leads V_2 to V_5 (see page 170).

We therefore have four possible QRS changes indicative of infarction:-
1. Reduced R wave voltage (where this can confidently be ascertained)
2. Abnormal Q waves without any conclusive evidence of R wave reduction
3. Reduced R wave voltage in association with abnormal Q waves and,
4. QS complexes

These four changes are part of a common process and represent increasing thickness of infarction. With a non-uniform thickness of infarction, combinations of these findings may occur (Figure 121).

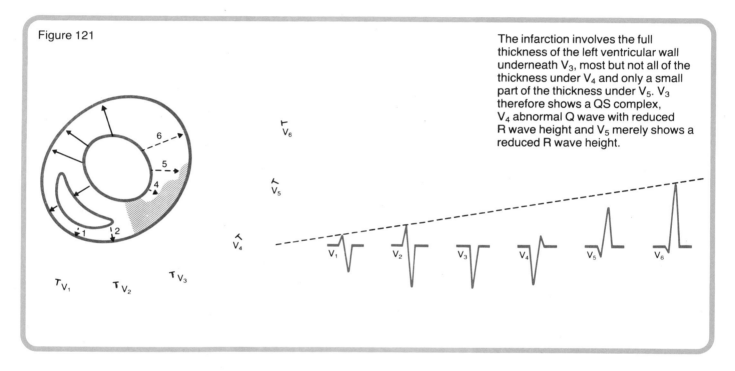

Figure 121

The infarction involves the full thickness of the left ventricular wall underneath V_3, most but not all of the thickness under V_4 and only a small part of the thickness under V_5. V_3 therefore shows a QS complex, V_4 abnormal Q wave with reduced R wave height and V_5 merely shows a reduced R wave height.

At this stage it is important to redefine the situations in which Q waves and QRS complexes are normal or abnormal.

Normal Q waves

In the precordial leads the normal q wave is found only to the left of the interventricular septum (since it is produced by septal depolarisation) passing from left to right (page 32)). When the heart position is indeterminate (pages 34–37) these normal q waves will be seen in V_4, V_5 and V_6 (Figure 46). With pronounced clockwise cardiac rotation they may appear in V_6 only or possibly only in leads even further to the left (Lead I and aVL) (Figures 46 and 47). In the presence of counter-clockwise cardiac rotation they may be seen from V_2 to V_6 (Figure 46), or with extreme counter-clockwise cardiac rotation from V_1 to V_6 (Figure 47).

In the limb leads the normal septal q waves will be seen in those leads which show a left ventricular configuration. The leads involved will depend upon the axis of the heart. When the heart is horizontal, i.e. the axis is in the region of zero to $-30°$ (page 53), the normal qR complex of the left precordial leads will be transmitted to Leads I and aVL and these leads will show normal q waves. When the heart is vertical (i.e. the axis is in the region of $+60°$ to $+90°$ (page 53)), the normal qR complex of the left precordial leads will be transmitted to Leads II and aVF and these leads will show normal q waves. With an axis in the region of $0°$ to $+60°$ Leads I and II will show normal q waves.

Normal QS complexes

QS complexes indicate that the whole process of depolarisation of viable ventricular myocardium takes places away from the lead in question. Since in all parts of the ventricles depolarisation is from endocardium to epicardium, it follows that **any lead which "looks into" the cavity of the heart will see QS complexes.** This is the usual, normal situation in the case of aVR and, depending on the axis of the heart, can also be normal for III or for aVL (Figure 122).

Figure 122

The arrow indicates the direction of the mean frontal plane QRS axis in each case.

Note in this figure that the heart is shown to be **physically** vertical or horizontal, this is intended to facilitate understanding of what is an **electrical** rather than a physical concept. For example the horizontal heart is one in which the main (left ventricular) electrical forces are directed horizontally and to the left.

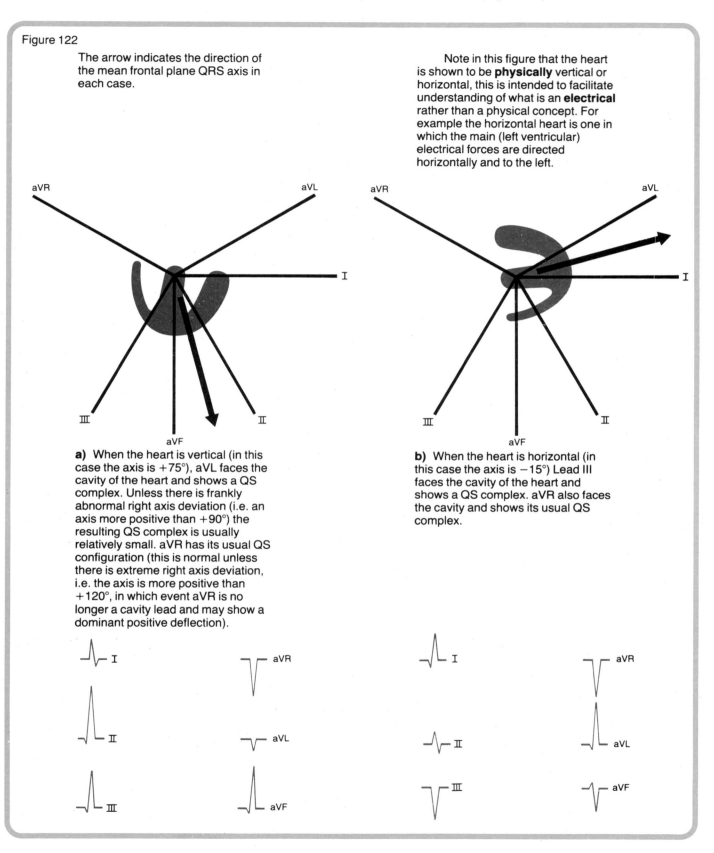

a) When the heart is vertical (in this case the axis is +75°), aVL faces the cavity of the heart and shows a QS complex. Unless there is frankly abnormal right axis deviation (i.e. an axis more positive than +90°) the resulting QS complex is usually relatively small. aVR has its usual QS configuration (this is normal unless there is extreme right axis deviation, i.e. the axis is more positive than +120°, in which event aVR is no longer a cavity lead and may show a dominant positive deflection).

b) When the heart is horizontal (in this case the axis is −15°) Lead III faces the cavity of the heart and shows a QS complex. aVR also faces the cavity and shows its usual QS complex.

Thus when the heart is vertical (Figure 122 (a)) Leads II, III and aVF show **normal septal q** waves (qR complexes), and aVL shows a **normal QS complex.** (aVR shows a QS complex as usual).

When the heart is horizontal (Figure 122 (b)) Leads I and aVL show normal **septal q waves,** and III shows a **normal QS complex** (aVR shows a QS complex as usual).

In pronounced clockwise cardiac rotation V_1 (and very occasionally V_2) may also show QS complexes (Figure 47).

Abnormal QS complexes

QS complexes in leads other than those looking into the cavity of the heart are abnormal.

Abnormal q waves

Q waves may be recognised to be abnormal because of:-

1. Abnormal width (duration) **or**

2. Abnormal depth (relative to the following R wave).

Q waves of 0.04 sec or longer duration **are abnormal** (provided they are not normal QS complexes – *vide supra*).

Q waves with a depth which is more than 25% of the height of the ensuing R wave are abnormal (Figure 123).

Figure 123

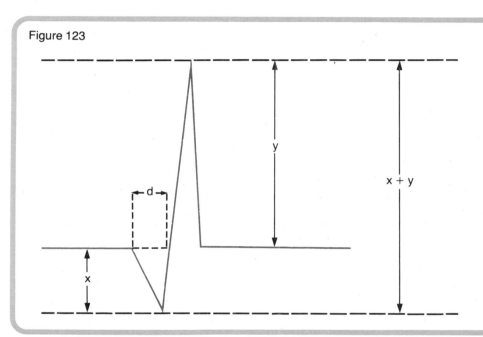

A qR type of QRS complex is shown diagrammatically. The q wave duration (d) is measured from the onset of the q wave to the point where the upstroke of the R wave crosses the horizontal line. The q wave depth is x. The criterion for abnormality is that $x > y/4$ (i.e. for normality $x \leqslant y/4$). Note that the height of the r waves (y) is not the same as the total QRS height (x+y). The criterion for abnormality could also be stated as $x > \frac{x+y}{5}$, and this is exactly the same criterion.

The essential electro-cardiographic criteria for the diagnosis of myocardial infarction from the QRS complexes are therefore as follows:-

1. Reduction in r wave height (from a normal level assessed either by a previous record antidating infarction or by interpolation in the precordial leads)*
or

2. The occurrence of QS complexes in V_1*, V_2, V_3, V_4, V_5, V_6, I, II, aVF, aVL[+]
or

3. Abnormally deep or abnormally wide q waves in V_1*, V_2, V_3, V_4, V_5, V_6, I, II, aVF, aVL[+]. q waves are abnormal if **either** they equal or exceed 0.04 sec in duration **or** if their depth exceeds one quarter of the height of the ensuing R wave.

Notes

1. * Reduction in r wave height cannot be used as a criterion in the limb leads for r wave height in the limb leads is dependent upon the mean frontal plane QRS axis and the range of possible positions for the normal axis is appreciable.

2. * In the presence of pronounced clockwise rotation QS complexes may appear normally in V_1 and occasionally in V_2.

3. [+] In the presence of a vertical heart QS complexes may be present normally in aVL.

4. Lead III is omitted from these considerations. This is because Lead III can have a deep Q wave even when the ECG is completely normal (when the heart is horizontal (above) or whenever the positive wave in aVL exceeds that in aVF (page 54)).

5. In the presence of left bundle branch block or ventricular pre-excitation none of the above criteria may be used.

Examples of electrocardiograms showing abnormal q waves are shown in Figures 124 and 125.

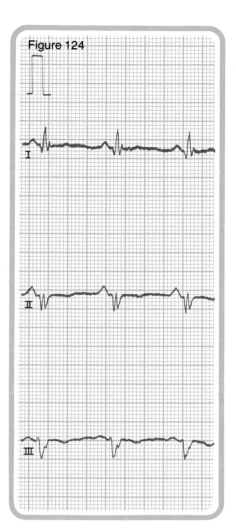

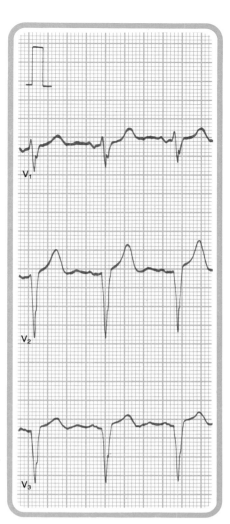

Figure 124

The rhythm is sinus. The r wave in V_1 is normal. The r wave in V_2 is smaller than that in V_1. This may in itself be an abnormality, indicative of infarction, but occasionally in a normal electrocardiogram the r wave in one of the leads V_2, V_3 or V_4 may be smaller than that in the leads immediately to its right in the precordial series in the transition zone area (page 45). V_3, V_4 and V_5 show QS complexes indicative of transmural infarction in the area of myocardium underlying these electrodes. V_6 shows a Qr complex. The r wave is clearly smaller than it should be (even though we cannot "bracket" this r wave with those from leads on either side of it), and the Q wave is abnormally deep (it has a depth exceeding one quarter the height of the ensuing r wave) and is also abnormally wide (in this case it is clearly more than 0.04 sec in duration). On the basis of **either** of these criteria the Q waves are abnormal. Superficial examination suggests that there are abnormal Q waves in Leads II, III and aVF but close examination reveals a small initial r wave in each of these leads (difficult to see in Lead II except in the third QRS complex in that lead). It may well be that these r waves have been reduced in height as a result of infarction, but one cannot be sure of this. In the case of the limb leads such dramatic variations in r wave appearances can simply represent variations in the frontal plane axis. The axis in this case is very abnormal at $-75°$. In the absence of definitive evidence of inferior (see page 180) infarction, this axis most probably indicates left anterior hemiblock (page 197).

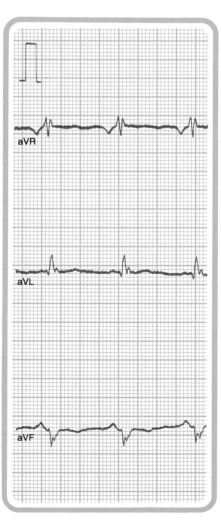

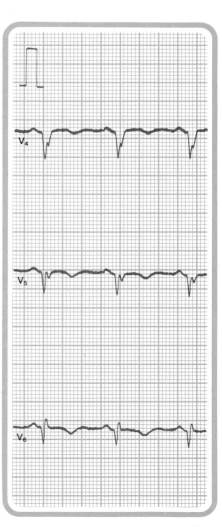

175

Figure 125

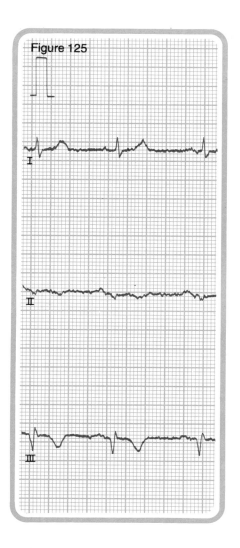

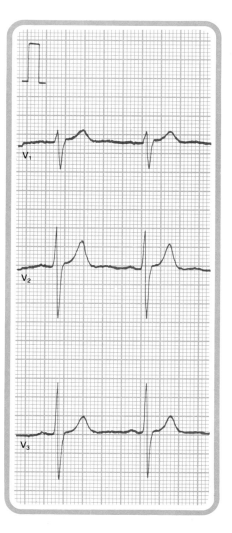

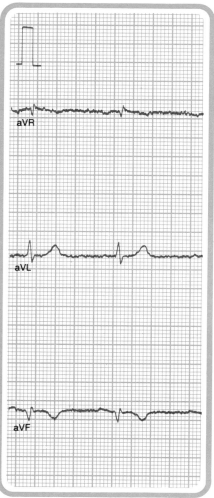

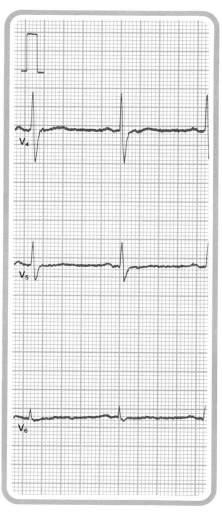

Figure 125

The rhythm is sinus. The R wave in the left precordial leads looks abnormally small but one cannot be **totally** confident of the signficance of this without a previous record for comparison. In the normal ECG the R wave in V_6 is often smaller than that in V_5, and that in V_5 is often smaller than that in V_4 (page 33 and Figure 42). However, it is unusual for the R wave in V_4 to be smaller than that in V_3. In addition the R wave in V_6 is very much smaller than one normally sees. The **probability** therefore is that the R waves in the left precordial leads are abnormally small. This **could** indicate infarction but **one cannot be sure of this.** However, there are definitively abnormal Q waves in Leads II, III and aVF (in each case the Q waves are abnormally deep (more than one quarter of the height of the ensuing R wave) and abnormally wide (clearly exceeding 0.04 sec)). These Q waves therefore indicate infarction.

The S-T Segment Changes of Infarction

It has already been stressed that it is only the QRS changes which provide **definitive** evidence of infarction. However, in the early stages of infarction S-T segment elevation usually occurs and may occasionally be dramatic in degree. Such changes are indicative of **injury** rather than **infarction.** The injury state is an unstable one. Acute S-T segment elevation **always** resolves to some extent (and **usually** resolves completely). The resolution of the acute S-T segment elevation is **usually** accompanied by development of the QRS changes of frank infarction, but **occasionally** the S-T segment elevation may resolve without the development of these diagnostic changes of infarction.

The essential change of myocardial injury is S-T segment elevation above the iso-electric line. The iso-electric line is the horizontal line indicating the position of the recording pen when there is no cardiac activity, i.e. between heart beats (that is between the end of the T wave and beginning of the next P wave). The normal S-T segment does not deviate by more than one millimetre above or below the iso-electric line (page 42). In the early stages of acute myocardial infarction, S-T segment elevation occurs (Figure 126).

The S-T segment shift is produced by injury to the myocardial cell membrane. As a result of that injury the current flow across the membrane is disturbed. The disturbance only occurs in injured myocardium, the pattern in healthy myocardium being unchanged. The normal iso-electric S-T segment in any lead depends upon the balance between normal myocardium in parts of the heart facing (close to) and opposite (remote from) a given lead. When the injury current flows in the cell membrane of part of the myocardium, the balance is disturbed and S-T segment shift occurs.

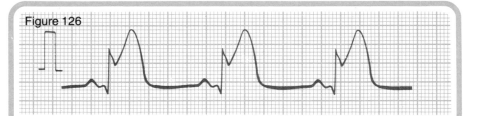

Figure 126

The rhythm is sinus. The rate is relatively slow. Because of the slow rate a clear iso-electric line is visible between the end of each T wave and the beginning of each P wave. The S-T segment is clearly elevated some 5mm above the iso-electric line.
Note 1
As explained earlier (page 42) in the presence of tachycardia, there may be no interval between the end of the T wave and the beginning of the next P wave and no iso-electric line would be visible. In that event, S-T segment elevation may only be regarded as significant if it is striking (Figure 52).

Note 2
Minor degrees of apparent S-T segment elevation may be present in leads in which the S-T segment merges imperceptibly into the T wave. This is often the case in normal records in the right precordial leads. One should be very cautious about regarding minor degrees of S-T segment shift in V_1 and V_2 as being significant (e.g. V_2 Record 11, page 82; V_2 Record 14, page 85; V_2 Record 24, page 95).

Abnormal S-T segment elevation of the type described occurs in leads facing the infarction, both in transmural myocardial infarction and in sub-epicardial infarction. As will be seen later (page 182) **"reciprocal" S-T segment depression** may be seen (at the same time as the above primary changes) in leads precording from positions opposite to the infarct. **Primary S-T segment depression** may be seen in leads facing in the infarct when the infarct is sub-endocardial (page 183).

The T Wave Changes of Infarction

A whole variety of T wave changes may occur in association with myocardial infarction. These include flattening of the T waves, di-phasic T waves, inverted T waves and abnormally tall T waves. None of these changes is specific. There is a tendency to regard non-specific T wave changes as unimportant, i.e. to equate "non-specific" with "not significant". This is quite unjustifiable. "Non-specific" simply means that a specific cause cannot be assigned to a change which is **definitely abnormal.** For example, minor T wave flattening may be the only ECG abnormality in a patient with severe coronary artery disease. Non-specific T wave changes occur in myocardial ischaemia, ventricular hypertrophy, intraventricular conduction defects, myocarditis, cardiomyopathy, pericarditis, electrolyte disturbances (particularly potassium changes) in response to certain drugs (especially digitalis) in hypothyroidism, subarachnoid haemorrhage, occasionally in pregnancy and even in response to drinking cold water. Since changes in body position can affect the physical position of the heart within the thorax, such changes in position can affect the QRS axis and therefore also the T wave axis. Such slight changes in axis (which are usually of the order of 15-30°) can produce changes in the T waves in the limb leads. By convention, of course, the standard 12-lead electrocardiogram is recorded with the patient in the recumbent position. It can be seen from the list of possible causes of T wave changes given above that though these changes are abnormal (i.e. they are not found in the vast majority of normal persons) they may occasionally (though unusually) have a non-pathological explanation. The most obvious two examples of this are pregnancy and drinking cold water. In these cases the explanation is usually apparent! It would certainly be unwise, for example, to diagnose pregnancy on the basis of such changes! Equally one cannot be **certain** that pregnancy is the cause unless one has a record taken for the pregnancy and one subsequent to the pregnancy, neither of which shows the T wave change in question. This is another example of the importance of primary and secondary interpretation of the electrocardiogram (page 109).

The most typical T wave change of acute myocardial infarction is deep, symmetrical T wave inversion (Figure 127).

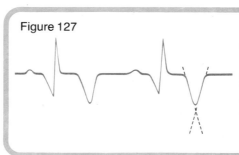

Figure 127

There is an abnormal Q wave. The S-T segment is normal but there is deep, symmetrical T wave inversion. The "symmetry" refers to the equality of the angles downstroke and upstroke of the T wave.

Deep-symmetrical T wave inversion may occur in association with the sequential changes of acute transmural or sub-epicardial myocardial infarction, but may also occur in the absence of QRS changes (i.e. as a primary change in sub-endocardial infarction). In such a case the T wave changes are usually apparent in many leads.

Abnormal T waves in inferior* infarction

The criterion for normality of the T waves in the limb leads was quoted on page 56 as being a T wave axis not differing from the QRS axis by more than ±45°. At that stage (and again on page 58) it was indicated that, **in the special situation of inferior myocardial infarction,** negative (inverted) T waves in II and aVF are regarded as abnormal even if the angle between the mean frontal plane QRS and T axes does not exceed 45°.

Examples are seen in Record 26, page 97 and in Figure 125. Both examples show abnormal q waves in II, III and aVF indicative of inferior infarction and the T waves are inverted in these leads. This is abnormal even though the frontal plane QRS axis and the frontal plane T axis do not differ by more than 45°. (In Record 26 the QRS axis is −30° and the T wave axis −75°. In Figure 125 the QRS axis is −45° and the T wave axis is −45°.)

Note

* The location of changes in myocardial infarction is described later (page 180).

The Sequence of Changes in Acute Myocardial Infarction

Although any part or all of the spectrum of changes described above may occur in myocardial infarction, a common, typical sequence of changes is recognised. The more completely the described changes are present and the more closely the usual sequential patterns are followed, the more confident one can be of the diagnosis and of the timing of the infarction. The sequential changes of acute myocardial infarction in a single lead are shown in Figure 128.

Figure 128

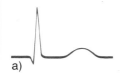 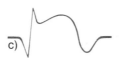 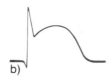 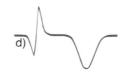 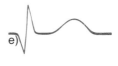

a) Shows the control, normal appearances in a lead, which by the QRS morphology, clearly lies over the left ventricle.

b) Within **hours** of the clinical onset of infarction there is S-T segment elevation. At this stage no QRS changes or T wave changes have occurred. Although such a pattern is frequently spoken of, loosely, as showing "acute infarction", no definitive evidence of infarction is shown. There is evidence of myocardial damage. There is an unstable situation. In the vast majority of cases evolutionary changes of infarction follow. Occasionally the record returns to normal.

c) Within **days** the R wave voltage has fallen and abnormal Q waves (in this case both in duration and in depth relative to the R wave height) have appeared. These changes are sufficient to prove the occurrence of infarction. In addition T wave inversion has appeared. The S-T elevation is less pronounced than in (b).

d) Within **one or more weeks** the S-T segment changes revert completely to normal. The R wave voltage remains reduced and the abnormal Q waves persist. Deep symmetrical T wave inversion may develop at this stage. In some patients this pattern remains permanently, in others it progresses to the appearances shown in (e).

e) **Months** after the clinical infarction the T waves may gradually return to normal. The abnormal Q waves and reduced R wave voltage persist.

Note the following:
1. S-T elevation is an unstable situation and indicates a recent event. It nearly always precedes evolutionary changes of infarction.
2. Reduced R wave voltage and the development of abnormal Q waves indicate infarction. These changes are usually permanent. Occasionally even these changes may regress. When this occurs it does not indicate regeneration of myocardium, but rather shrinkage of the extent of scar tissue underlying the electrode with the pulling closer together of adjacent areas of healthy myocardium. As a result of this shrinkage of scar tissue, leads which after an infarction show either abnormal q wave (or reduced R waves) may subsequently show r waves (or increase in R wave size). This is termed "regeneration of the R waves". As noted above it does not indicate regeneration of myocardium.
3. QRS evidence of infarction with elevated S-T segments indicates recent infarction (i.e. within days). QRS evidence of infarction with normal S-T segments and deep, symmetrical T wave inversion indicates infarction of intermediate age (weeks or a month or two). QRS evidence of infarction with normal S-T segments and T waves indicates old (months to years) infarction.
4. Occasionally, all evidence of infarction may be lost with the passing of time – due to shrinkage of scar tissue.

The Location of Changes in Myocardial Infarction

Primary electrocardiographic changes of the type described will occur in leads overlying the infarct. The leads in which such primary changes occur will, conversely, indicate the location of the infarct. This is shown in Table 4 and illustrated in Figures 129 and 130.

Table 4

Location of Infarction	Leads showing Primary Changes
	Typical Changes
Anterior Infarction Anteroseptal	V_1, V_2, V_3
Anterior	Some of the group V_1-V_3 plus some of the group V_4-V_6
Anterolateral	V_4, V_5, V_6, I, aVL, and possibly II
Extensive anterior	V_1, V_2, V_3, V_4, V_5, V_6, I, aVL
High lateral	aVL (plus high precordial leads)
Inferior Infarction Inferior	II, III, aVF
Inferolateral = (apical)	II, III, aVF, V_5, V_6 and sometimes also I and aVL
Inferoseptal	II, III, aVF, V_1, V_2, V_3
	Other Changes (see text)
Posterior Infarction	V_1, V_2 (Inverse of the usual changes elsewhere)
Subendocardial Infarction	Any lead (usually multiple leads)

High lateral infarcts show in aVL only, but if high precordial leads are used they may show similar changes. These leads are placed in the same horizontal distribution as the standard precordial leads but are placed one (labelled V'1, V'2, V'3 etc) or two (labelled V"1, V"2, V"3 etc) interspaces higher.

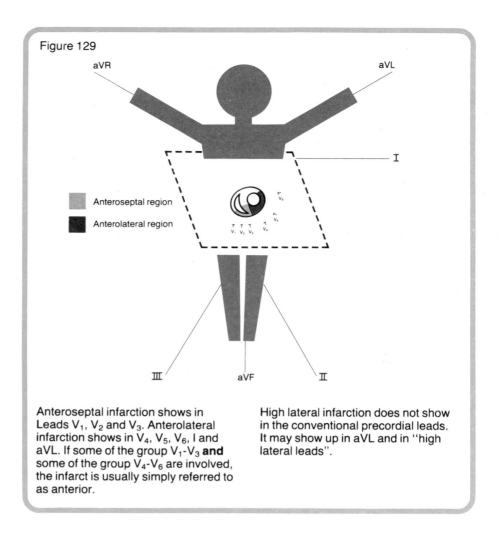

Figure 129

Anteroseptal region

Anterolateral region

Anteroseptal infarction shows in Leads V₁, V₂ and V₃. Anterolateral infarction shows in V₄, V₅, V₆, I and aVL. If some of the group V₁-V₃ **and** some of the group V₄-V₆ are involved, the infarct is usually simply referred to as anterior.

High lateral infarction does not show in the conventional precordial leads. It may show up in aVL and in "high lateral leads".

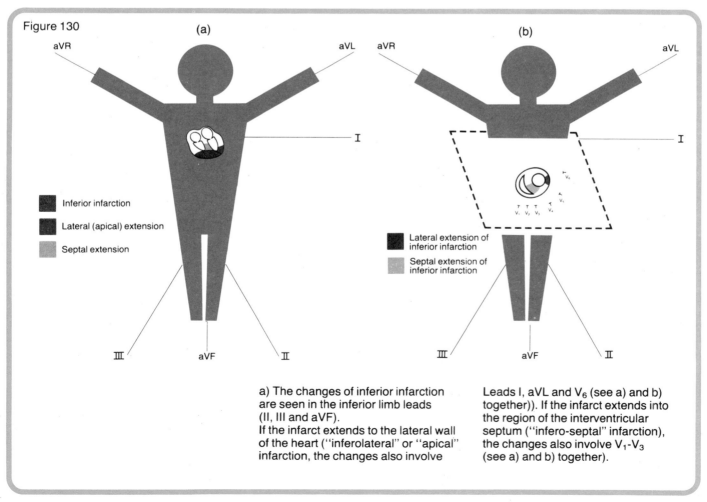

Figure 130

(a)

(b)

Inferior infarction

Lateral (apical) extension

Septal extension

Lateral extension of inferior infarction

Septal extension of inferior infarction

a) The changes of inferior infarction are seen in the inferior limb leads (II, III and aVF).
If the infarct extends to the lateral wall of the heart ("inferolateral" or "apical" infarction, the changes also involve

Leads I, aVL and V₆ (see a) and b) together)). If the infarct extends into the region of the interventricular septum ("infero-septal" infarction), the changes also involve V₁-V₃ (see a) and b) together).

Reciprocal Changes

In addition to the primary changes which occur in leads facing the infarcted area, "reciprocal" changes occur in leads opposite to the infarction. Reciprocal changes are the inverse of primary changes, i.e. S-T segment depression instead of S-T segment elevation and tall-pointed T waves instead of symmetrical T wave inversion. The reciprocal changes can easily be visualised by turning the primary changes upside down (Figure 131).

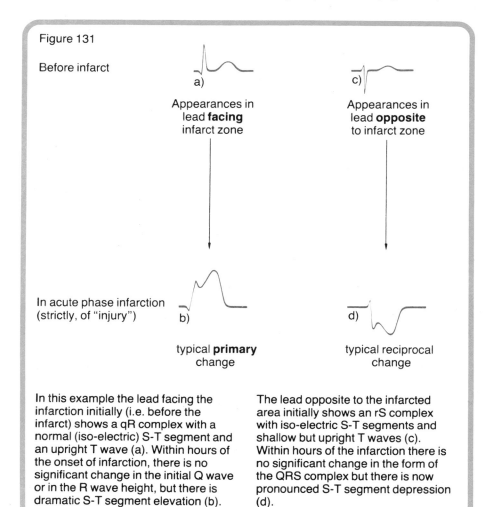

Figure 131

Before infarct

a)

Appearances in lead **facing** infarct zone

c)

Appearances in lead **opposite** to infarct zone

In acute phase infarction (strictly, of "injury")

b)

typical **primary** change

d)

typical reciprocal change

In this example the lead facing the infarction initially (i.e. before the infarct) shows a qR complex with a normal (iso-electric) S-T segment and an upright T wave (a). Within hours of the onset of infarction, there is no significant change in the initial Q wave or in the R wave height, but there is dramatic S-T segment elevation (b).

The lead opposite to the infarcted area initially shows an rS complex with iso-electric S-T segments and shallow but upright T waves (c). Within hours of the infarction there is no significant change in the form of the QRS complex but there is now pronounced S-T segment depression (d).

The inferior limb leads on the one hand and the precordial leads, together with Leads I and Lead aVL, on the other hand are mutually "opposite" in that primary changes in one of these groups will frequently be accompanied by reciprocal changes in the other group. Although, as we shall see later, S-T segment depression may, when present alone, be a primary change, it is safe to assume that **when S-T segment elevation is present in one group of leads and S-T segment depression in another, in the same cardiogram, the elevation is the primary and the depression the secondary change.**

True Posterior Infarction

Infarction showing primary changes in II, III and aVF is properly termed inferior infarction, for these are the "inferior" limb leads. Previous terminology referred to this as "posterior" infarction, but this was anatomically incorrect. **True** "posterior" infarction is relatively rare and is not easily recognised since no leads in the conventional 12-lead recording are posteriorly situated. It can only be recognised by looking in the **anterior** leads for **reciprocal** changes. There are no primary changes since there are no true posterior leads. The evidence of true posterior infarction is therefore the presence of abnormally tall and broad R waves in V$_1$ (reciprocal to abnormally deep and broad Q in a posterior lead, if one existed). If the infarct is very recent S-T depression may be present in V$_1$, if it is of intermediate age, tall T waves may be present in V$_1$, V$_2$ and V$_3$ may be similarly affected (Figure 132).

Figure 132

True posterior infarction showing in V$_1$

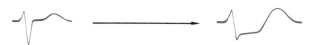

| Normal appearance prior to infarction | Appearance in acute stage of true posterior infarction. The r wave has become taller and broader (the reciprocal of abnormally deep and broad q waves in leads showing primary changes). The S-T segment is depressed (the reciprocal of S-T elevation in leads showing primary changes). The T waves are taller than normal (the reciprocal of T wave inversion). |
| True posterior infarction. This is most easily recognised in V$_1$. The R wave becomes broader and taller than normal (its breadth exceeds 0.04 sec) | and in the initial stages there is also S-T segment depression and increase in height of the T waves. |

True posterior infarction is often accompanied by inferior or by anterolateral infarction. An example is shown in Figure 141.

Subendocardial Infarction

Most infarcts are regional, intramural infarcts (sub-epicardial or transmural). When the term "myocardial infarction" is used without a qualifying adjective, **regional** infarction is implied. **Sub-endocardial** infarcts are relatively rare. When they do occur they not infrequently encircle the interior of the left ventricle and are therefore **zonal** rather than regional infarcts. The electrocardiographic evidence consists of **primary** S-T segment depression (i.e. S-T segment depression in some leads without simultaneous S-T segment elevation in other leads, with the possible exception of cavity leads) or of deep-symmetrical T wave inversion without any change in the QRS complexes. Each of these changes can be produced by myocardial ischaemia without infarction and for this reason the diagnosis of sub-endocardial infarction cannot be made on a single electrocardiogram alone. Either a single such record accompanied by clinical or enzyme evidence of infarction (i.e. necessarily accompanied by secondary interpretation) or serial records which **persistently** show primary S-T segment depression or deep symmetrical T wave inversion is required for the diagnosis to be made. When the primary change is S-T depression it will be visible in all or most leads with the exception of the cavity leads (aVR is always a cavity lead, aVL is a cavity lead when the heart is vertical, and aVF is a cavity lead when the heart is horizontal). The cavity leads alone may show reciprocal S-T segment elevation. This is the only exception to the rule that "when S-T segment elevation and S-T depression are both present in the same recording, it is the elevation which is the primary change". By definition, cavity leads inevitably show QS complexes.

The Changes in Myocardial Ischaemia

Relative hypoxia of the myocardium, from local ischaemia, may occur in the absence of necrosis (infarction). Such changes may occur in relation to **exertion** (physical stress), in response to **emotion** (psychological stress) or **spontaneously** (i.e. in the absence of overt stress). Significant myocardial ischaemia can exist without any recognisable ECG abnormalities. When electrocardiographic changes do occur in relation to myocardial ischaemia they are confined to the S-T segments and T waves. **Myocardial ischaemia, in the absence of infarction, does not give rise to any changes in the QRS complexes.**

The following electrocardiographic changes may occur in myocardial ischaemia:-

1. Flattening of the T waves.
2. Inversion of the T waves.
3. Abnormally tall T waves (i.e. inferred increase in T wave height).
4. "Normalisation" of primarily abnormal T waves.
5. Sloping S-T segment depression.
6. Horizontal S-T segment depression.
7. S-T segment elevation.
8. Combinations of the above.

Flattening of the T Wave

One of the commonest findings in ischaemic heart disease is flattening (i.e. reduction in the voltage of) the T waves. Since there are no **definitive** criteria for the normal T wave height (page 40 and pages 56-58) it can only be stated that the T waves appear to be of low voltage. This is a non-specific change and may be associated with almost any condition affecting the myocardium or pericardium – ischaemia, ventricular hypertrophy, intraventricular conduction problems, electrolyte disturbances, drug effects, myocarditis, cardiomyopathy, hormone disturbances, pericarditis and even obesity. An example of such non-specific T wave flattening is seen in Record 12, page 83 (in Leads V_4, V_5 and V_6 and in all of the limb leads), in Record 22, page 93 (the T waves are of low voltage in all 12 leads of this record, but this is to be expected since the QRS voltages are low. Prominent U waves are seen in V_2 and V_3 – see page 149) and in Record 27, page 98 (in Leads V_4-V_6 and the limb leads). Though such T wave flattening is one of the commonest T wave changes in ischaemic heart disease its presence does not **prove** the existence of ischaemic heart disease, even if the changes occur in relation to stress.

Inversion of the T Wave

The term "T wave inversion" refers to negative T waves in leads in which the T wave is usually upright. The term is most properly applied in the precordial leads where negative T waves are always abnormal if present in any of the Leads V_3-V_6. Negative T waves in either V_1 or V_2 are abnormal if they were formerly upright in those leads (page 40) and negative T waves in V_2 are abnormal if the T waves are upright in V_1.

The term "T wave inversion" is also frequently applied when negative T waves are found in Leads I, II or aVF where the T waves are usually upright. However, it should be remembered that in the limb leads normality or otherwise of the T waves applies to **all** the leads collectively and not to each lead individually (page 58). In this respect the limb leads differ fundamentally from the precordial leads and one should strictly speaking refer not to T wave inversion in any given limb lead but to an abnormal angle between the mean frontal plane and T wave axes (pages 56-58).

T wave inversion is a non-specific change which can occur in myocardial ischaemia, ventricular hypertrophy, intraventricular conduction problems, electrolyte disturbances, drug effects, myocarditis, cardiomyopathy, intracranial haemorrhage, mitral valve prolapse, pulmonary embolism, pericarditis, after episodes of tachycardia and after Stokes-Adams seizures. T waves which are **deeply and symmetrically** inverted are likely to be of ischaemic origin. Abnormal T waves are shown in Record 3 (page 73). The T wave inversion in V_5 and V_6 is abnormal in this record. One may refer loosely to T wave inversion in I and aVL in this record, but more strictly the angle between the mean frontal plane QRS and T wave axes is abnormal (more than 45°) and thus in fact the limb lead T waves are abnormal (i.e. they are all abnormal). There is no QRS abnormality in this record and the T wave changes are therefore, by definition, **primary.** They could still have any of the causes listed above including myocardial ischaemia. They are not **diagnostic** of ischaemia.

In Record 5 (page 75) the T waves in the limb leads are abnormal and there is T wave inversion in V_4-V_6. However, in this case the precordial QRS complexes are abnormal. It is likely that the T wave changes are **secondary** to the QRS abnormality (which in this case is left ventricular hypertrophy).

Abnormally Tall T Waves

Since there are no accepted absolute criteria for normality of T wave height in any lead there can be no definitive criterion for abnormally tall T waves. The term cannot sensibly be applied at all to the limb leads for the T waves in all the limb leads are either (collectively) normal or (collectively) abnormal depending on the relationship of the T wave axis to the QRS axis (pages 56-58).

In the precordial leads the tallest T wave is usually in V_3 or V_4, the smallest in V_1 and V_2 and in general from V_3 to V_6 the T wave is not less than 1/8 and not more than 2/3 of the height of the R wave. Abnormally tall T waves can only be gauged against these approximate criteria. An example of an ECG which shows T waves of definitely abnormal height is shown in Figure 133.

Strikingly tall T waves are not definitely abnormal. They may be found as a normal variation in healthy individuals. In the precordial leads they may be indicative of ischaemia of the posterior wall of the heart (they are the inverse of the T wave inversion which would be shown in posterior leads directly over the ischaemic area if such leads existed). They also occur in the precordial leads in cases of recent true posterior infarction (again as the inverse of the T wave inversion which would be shown in posterior leads over the infarcted area if such leads existed). Tall precordial T waves are also seen in hyperkalaemia, in cases of intracranial haemorrhage, in left ventricular hypertrophy and in left bundle branch block (in both of the latter cases the abnormality of the QRS complex usually clearly indicates the diagnosis).

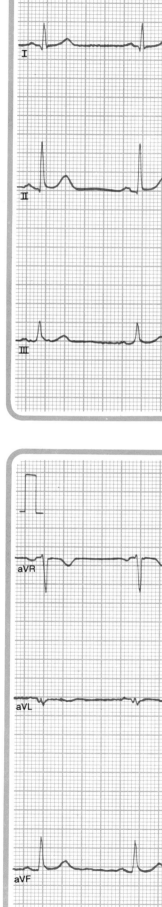

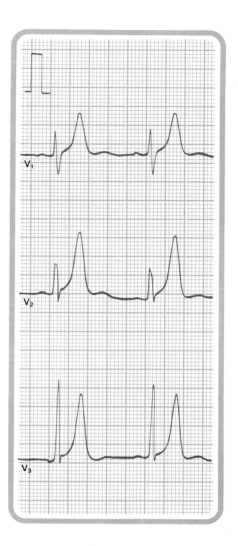

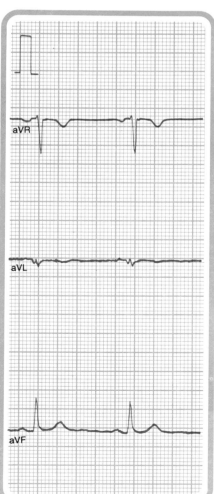

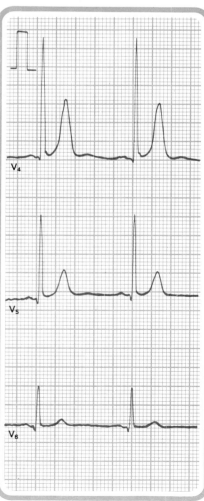

Figure 133

The rhythm is sinus. The T waves are upright in all the precordial leads. This feature is quite normal. The T waves are quite tall from V_1-V_4 and particularly so in V_2 and V_3. The T waves here are abnormally tall. This patient had ischaemia of the posterior wall of the ventricle proved by caesium scanning.

Normalisation of T Waves

If the T waves in certain leads are chronically inverted in a patient with ischaemic heart disease it occasionally happens that the T waves become upright during a further ischaemic episode, whether that ischaemic episode occurs spontaneously or in relation to emotional or physical stress. This process is referred to as "normalisation" of the T wave. It is definitely abnormal and is almost always indicative of myocardial ischaemia.

Primary Sloping S-T Segment Depression

The term "primary" indicates that the S-T segment depression is not secondary to S-T segment elevation in other leads, i.e. there is no simultaneous S-T segment elevation in other leads.

Downward sloping S-T segment depression is a non-specific abnormality which can be produced by ventricular hypertrophy, intraventricular conduction problems, cardiomyopathy, myocarditis, digitalis, hyperkalaemia and pericarditis as well as myocardial ischaemia. Sloping S-T segment depression occurring in association with the QRS changes of ventricular hypertrophy or intraventricular conduction defect should be regarded as part of the diagnosis relevant to the particular QRS abnormality. For example, the sloping S-T segment depression seen in Leads I, II, aVL and V_4–V_6 in Record 5 (page 75) should be seen as part of the appearance of left ventricular hypertrophy for the record shows definite QRS changes of that condition. Likewise the sloping S-T segment depression seen in Leads I, aVL, V_5 and V_6 in Record 7 (page 77) should be seen as part of the appearance of left bundle branch block for the record shows definite QRS changes of that condition. The sloping S-T segment depression seen in V_5 and V_6 in Record 12 (page 83) is seen in the absence of any QRS abnormality and is therefore primary. The cause of the S-T segment depression therefore cannot be determined from the electrocardiogram. Secondary interpretation (page 109) must be used, i.e. the **probable** cause should be assessed from the clinical picture. The **definitive** cause cannot be assessed. For example if the depression occurred in relation to stress and in association with chest pain, if there is no evidence of hyperkalaemia and the patient is not on digitalis, ischaemia is a probable cause.

Primary Horizontal S-T Segment Depression

The term "primary" indicates that the S-T segment depression is not secondary to S-T segment elevation in other leads, (i.e. there is no simultaneous S-T segment elevation in other leads) and is not occurring in association with the kind of QRS changes which often give rise to S-T depression (e.g. those of ventricular hypertrophy or of bundle branch block). (In cases where there are primary QRS abnormalities with appropriate secondary S-T changes, if new S-T segment changes develop without any changes in the QRS complexes these new changes are also deemed primary).

The finding of primary horizontal S-T segment depression is very strongly suggestive of subendocardial ischaemia or infarction. It is not nearly such a non-specific feature as most of the other S-T and T wave changes discussed above. Horizontal S-T segment depression may occur in spontaneous ischaemic episodes or in relation to angina induced by physical or emotional stress. It is not possible from a single record to say whether the S-T segment depression is induced by **ischaemia** of the myocardium or by **infarction** of the subendocardium. When subsequent records show return of the S-T segment to normal, it can be inferred that the horizontal S-T segment depression found in earlier records must have been indicative of ischaemia of the myocardium rather than of infarction of the subendocardium. When the changes are persistent it is likely that there has been infarction of the subendocardium. In addition, secondary interpretation may help. For example, if the levels of cardiac enzymes show an increase, the S-T segment depression is more likely to be indicative of infarction.

Subendocardial infarction is usually zonal rather than regional (page 183) and horizontal S-T segment depression is often seen in many leads – in fact frequently in all leads except those looking into the cavity of the heart.

S-T Segment Elevation

S-T segment elevation is usually part of the pattern of acute myocardial injury and often precedes the development of definitive changes of regional myocardial infarction. Occasionally primary S-T segment elevation may occur in relation to what is known as "Prinzmetal angina" or "variant angina". This is a form of angina which differs from the usual variety in several ways. The pain is not usually aggravated by exertion or by emotion, it tends to be more intense and more prolonged than exertional angina. It often occurs at the same time of day. If an ECG is obtained during an attack there may be transient S-T segment elevation which does not progress through the usual evolutionary changes of infarction (when S-T segment change occurs in relation to the usual form of angina – induced by exertion or emotion – it is usually S-T segment depression). The episodes are often associated with arrhythmias. Coronary angiography in such patients often shows a high grade obstruction in at least one major proximal coronary artery. Where the coronary arteries appear angiographically normal, coronary artery spasm in a similar site is thought to be responsible.

Primary S-T segment elevation in relation to anginal episodes is rare since "Prinzmetal angina" is rare.

Combinations of S-T Segment and T Wave Changes

Various combinations of the above-described S-T segment and T wave changes may occur. Usually such combinations are non-specific and frequently consist of flat or sloping S-T segment depression together with flattening of the T waves or possible inversion of the terminal part of the T wave ("Terminal T wave inversion").

Exercise Stress Testing

The object of stress test electrocardiography (which is almost synonymous with exercise electrocardiography – see below) is to create a haemodynamic situation in which part, at least, of the ventricular myocardium becomes hypoxic if the patient has stenosing atheroma of the coronary arteries. If the extent and severity of the myocardial hypoxia is sufficient to induce diagnostic changes in the electrocardiogram, the stress test will be positive. If not, the stress test will be negative. Depending upon the severity of the stress induced, the false negative rate of the procedure may be in the region of 10-30% (i.e. not infrequently a completely normal electrocardiogram may be obtained at the end of a rigorous stress test procedure despite the presence of significant coronary atheroma. It follows that a negative stress test does **not** exclude significant coronary artery disease).

Although the morbidity and mortality of the test are both extremely low, they are not zero and the physician must realise that there is at least a small risk in stressing a patient, whom he suspects of having ischaemic heart disease, to the point of myocardial ischaemia. If all appropriate precautions (including the provision of **adequate** cardio-pulmonary resuscitative procedures) are available, the mortality rate of the procedure is about 0.01% and the morbidity rate (i.e. the necessity for subsequent hospital admission for non-fatal complications) is about 0.02%. **Adequate** cardio-pulmonary resuscitative procedures include not only the immediate availability of the appropriate equipment and trained personnel, but also adequate in-patient back-up procedures with coronary and respiratory intensive care.

Although some centres do conduct exercise stress tests when the resting electrocardiogram is abnormal, interpretation of records from such tests is even more difficult than when the resting record is normal. Since the **primary** aim of exercise electrocardiography is to look for diagnostic evidence of ischaemic heart disease and since such evidence is often difficult or impossible to evaluate if the resting record is abnormal, in the author's opinion there is no point in exercise stress testing **for diagnostic purposes** if the resting record is abnormal. There is, however, a second reason for exercise stress testing – namely the assessment of a patient's exercise capability. If this is the reason for the test the electrocardiogram is used as a safety monitor rather than as a diagnostic aid. In this event the test can usefully be applied even when the resting record is abnormal (however, see later under "precautions"). These two aims, namely **the diagnosis of ischaemic heart disease** and the **assessment of exercise capability** are often blurred and are obscured by loose thinking. This reduces the precision of the observations and leads to uncertainties about the result.

Types of Stress Test

1. Master Two-step. This test requires only modest equipment. It involves walking up and down a two-step platform (similar to the type used in athletic medal presentation ceremonies). The patient climbs the two steps at one end, descends them at the other end and walks briskly round on the level in a circle to start again. This test is much less frequently used than formerly. The work load remains constant during the test and it is sometimes difficult to obtain a level of exercise sufficient to achieve an adequate heart rate response.

2. Atrial Pacing. In this test cardiac stress is applied by means of controlled tachycardia induced by atrial pacing using a temporary transvenous pacing electrode introduced into the right atrium. It has the advantage of producing rapid and accurate control of the heart rate (and unlike the situation with stress tests, the tachycardia can be stopped abruptly if necessary). However, it has major drawbacks – it is unphysiological (in exercise there is an appreciable peripheral vasodilatation, an increase in cardiac output and in stroke volume whereas in atrial pacing the cardiac output changes little and the stroke volume falls as the heart rate is increased) and it is an invasive procedure requiring full cardiac screening and catheterisation facilities. It is certainly not suitable for general usage.

3. Graded Exercise Test. This is the most commonly used procedure and involves the use of a treadmill or bicycle ergometer. The former is preferable (though more expensive) since all patients are accustomed to walking and few to cycling. The fundamental difference from the Master Two-step is that the work load is graded.

Protocol for a Graded (Treadmill) Exercise Test

There are numerous multistage exercise protocols available. There is no ideal protocol – the needs vary both as far as the patient and as far as the institution are concerned. The initial workload should be well within the patient's normal exercise capability. The final workload should be sufficient to achieve the target heart rate (see below). Intermediate workloads should be sufficient to provide a smooth progression of exercise levels.

The following protocol was devised by the author for use in the Manchester Royal Infirmary.

Manchester Royal Infirmary – Exercise Protocol

Precautions

1. Continuous supervision is necessary during and immediately after the procedure. **The test should only be carried out in the presence of a doctor and a technician or assistant.**

2. A defibrillator in good working order must be available.

3. Emergency drugs must be available, including glyceryl trinitrite, atropine and lignocaine.

4. Full emergency back-up facilities including the possibility of endotracheal intubation and coronary and respiratory intensive care should be available.

5. The patient should have the nature of the test explained to him and his informed consent obtained.

6. The patient should not currently be taking treatment with digitalis or beta-blockers. The former may produce ECG changes which increase during exercise, rendering interpretation of the test difficult. The latter usually precludes the achievement of an adequate heart rate response. Occasionally, diuretics, antidepressants and sedatives may cause false-positive responses.

7. It is important to ensure that the patient has not recently had a heavy meal.

8. It is important to exclude congestive heart failure, severe hypertension, history of myocardial infarction within the preceding 2–3 months and a history of recent (i.e. within weeks) onset of chest pain or recent change in the pattern of pain suggestive of crescendo angina or unstable angina.

9. The heart rate, the precordial ECG (usually a modified V_5 lead) and preferably also the blood pressure should be monitored during the procedure.

If the appropriate (rather more sophisticated) equipment is available the full 12-lead ECG should be monitored during the procedure.

Procedure

1. A standard 12-lead ECG is obtained and inspected by the supervising doctor. If this record shows evidence of S-T segment elevation or depression or serious arrhythmia (including ventricular tachycardia, multiple ventricular ectopics, R-on-T ectopics, atrial tachycardia, atrial flutter and possibly atrial fibrillation) the test must not proceed. As indicated earlier, if the resting record is abnormal the value of proceeding with the test for diagnostic purposes is very limited.

2. After thorough preparation of the skin, the precordial electrode is applied. A modified V_5 electrode is probably best if the equipment only permits a single lead to be monitored during the test. The modified V_5 lead is produced by connecting the positive end of the bipolar system to the usual V_5 location (page 27) and the negative end at some suitable site such as the manubrium sterni. If possible the full 12-lead system should be connected throughout the test. In female patients with large breasts, the breasts may need to be supported by some suitable garment to minimise motion artefact. In male patients with hairy chests local shaving may be necessary. (It is unusual for both of these preparatory steps to be necessary!).

3. A resting record is taken from the monitoring precordial lead. If the standard 12-lead electrocardiogram was satisfactory, the modified V_5 appearances should also be satisfactory. A further rhythm strip is obtained from this modified V_5 lead with the patient standing. (Where monitoring facilities with all 12 leads are available, the full 12-lead record should be taken with the patient standing, at rest, on the treadmill.)

4. If possible, arrangements should be made to monitor the blood pressure during the test. This is best done by the usual sphygmomanometric technique, but it is unreasonable to expect to be able to measure anything other than the **systolic** blood pressure.

5. Exercise then proceeds as indicated in Table 5 below:-

Table 5

Stage	Duration of stage (min)	Total elapsed time (min)	Speed km/h	mph	Gradient (%)	Work load (METS*)	Recreational activities of equivalent level
1	1	1	3	1.9	0	2	Casual walking
2	3	4	3	1.9	10	5	Casual cycling
3	3	7	4	2.5	12	6–7	Jogging
4	3	10	5.5	3.4	14	8–9	Running
5	3	13	7	4.4	16	16	Squash

EXERCISE IS STOPPED
IF AN ABNORMALITY DEVELOPS
or
IF THE TARGET HEART RATE IS ACHIEVED

Otherwise, exercise continues from one stage to another without interruption. The indications for stopping exercise are given on page 190.

6. Following the completion or cessation of exercise the patient is transferred quickly to a bed for the post-exercise observations. If a 3-lead ECG machine is used the 12-lead record is taken in the following order:
first, V_4, V_5, V_6,
then, I, II, III,
then, aVR, aVL, aVF,
finally V_1, V_2, V_3.

If full 12-lead ECG monitoring is available throughout the test a 12-lead record is taken with the patient standing at rest on the treadmill immediately after cessation of exercise and before transfer to the bed.

Note

* The unit "MET" refers to a metabolic equivalent, i.e. they are multiples of the basal metabolic rate. Healthy, sedentary individuals can usually exercise to 10-11 METS and beyond and healthy, physically active individuals to 16 METS and beyond. Most patients with true angina develop indications for stopping the test at or before the 8 MET level.

Where a single channel machine is used the same order is followed i.e. V_4, V_5, V_6, I, ... V_2, V_3.

The reason for this order is that the left precordial leads are the most likely leads to show a positive response, followed by the standard limb leads, then aVL and aVF and finally the right precordial leads. In the immediate post-exercise situation the haemodynamic state is changing rapidly and it is important to use those leads most likely to show changes as soon as possible in case any changes which occur are short-lived.

The full 12-lead recording is repeated 2 minutes, 4 minutes and 6 minutes after the end of exercise. The order of recording the 12 leads is not critical at this juncture.

Indications for stopping the exercise test
1. Development of an abnormality

Clinical Indications
The patient requests it. (He feels he has "had enough").
Excessive fatigue
Excessive dyspnoea
Dizziness
Pallor, clammy skin, exhaustion
Reduction in blood pressure and/or heart rate despite increasing work loads.
Worrying Arrhythmias
Frequent ventricular ectopic beats
Multifocal ventricular ectopic beats
Ventricular tachycardia
Atrial tachycardia
Atrial flutter
Atrial fibrillation

Evidence of Ischaemia
Increasing anginal pain
Significant (more than 1mm) S-T segment shift (depression or elevation)
Equipment Failure
Monitoring system faults
Defibrillator faults
Treadmill faults
2. Achievement of heart rate

The "target" heart rate is related to the age of the patient. The most rigorous tests set a target of 85–90% of the predicted maximal exertional heart rate in normal subjects of the appropriate age. In general, the author prefers to use slightly lower heart rates as given below in Table 6:-
(The 85-90% maximal target rates are also quoted for comparison)

Table 6

Patient age	Target heart rate	("85-90% Maximal" target heart rates)
<40	170	175
40-50	160	170
50-60	155	165
60-70	150	160

Interpretation of the exercise test
1. Features diagnostic of the positive test

The only **definitive** criteria for positive exercise electrocardiograms are:
a) horizontal S-T segment depression of 1mm or more.
b) horizontal S-T segment elevation of 1mm or more.
c) downsloping or upsloping S-T segment elevation or depression of 1mm or more.

In each case the S-T segment shift must persist for 0.08 sec or more in each complex.

When these changes occur they are usually apparent in the early post-exercise record and usually revert to normal within a few minutes.

In 10% of positive cases the changes are seen only **during** exercise and will be missed if, as is often the case, records can only be taken after the end of exercise. (Sophisticated and expensive recording equipment is needed to obtain artefact-free interpretable ECG recordings during exercise). In most positive cases, however, S-T segment shift begins during exertion and continues for the first few minutes at the end of exercise. In a small proportion of positive cases (perhaps 5%) S-T segment shift only appears **after** the completion of the exercise. S-T segment elevation is much less common that S-T segment depression (perhaps 1 or 2% of positive cases). This response is usually indicative of the presence of severe stenoses in major proximal branches of the coronary systems.

S-T segment shift should ideally be measured against the true iso-electric line (the T-P interval (page 42)) but this is not always practicable in the context of exercise electrocardiography for, if the target heart rate is achieved, no T-P interval remains. (The target heart rate is more likely to be achieved when the coronary arteries are normal or when there is only mild coronary atheroma). If the heart rate is very rapid and no T-P interval is visible, the S-T segment can, of necessity, only be assessed against the P-R segment.
In the presence of significant coronary atheroma, left ventricular performance on exercise will often be compromised and the patient will frequently not be able to achieve the target heart rate. In this event it is usually possible to compare the S-T segment with the true iso-electric line – i.e. the T-P interval.

Figure 134 shows a negative exercise test and Figure 135 shows a positive exercise test.

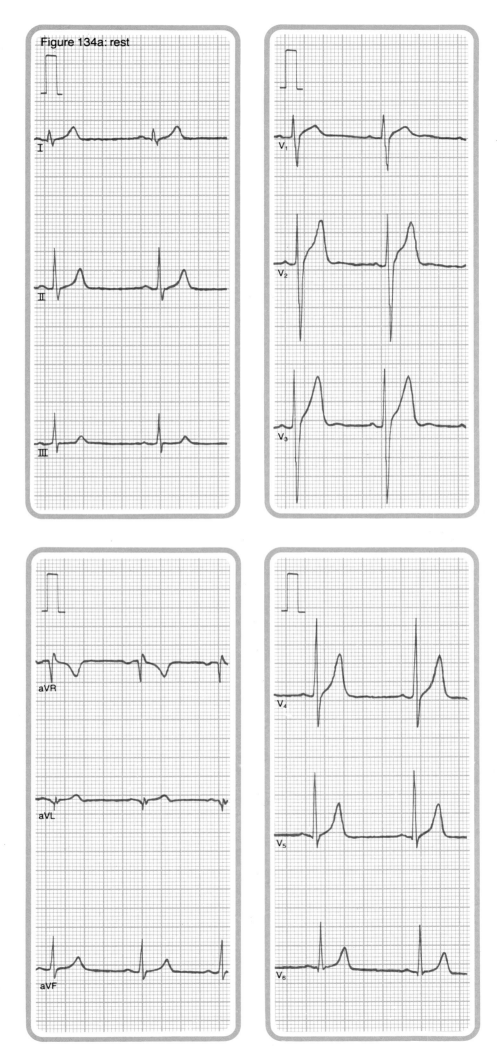

Figure 134a

The resting record is within normal limits. The q wave in aVL is normal since the heart is vertical (axis +75°) and aVL is therefore a cavity lead (Figure 62, page 55). The resting heart rate is 59/min.

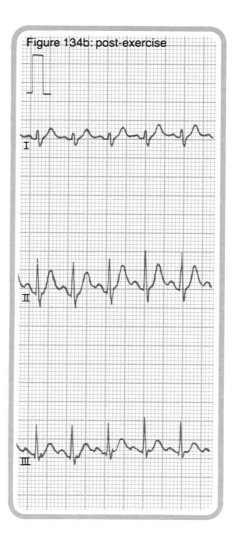

Figure 134b: post-exercise

I

II

III

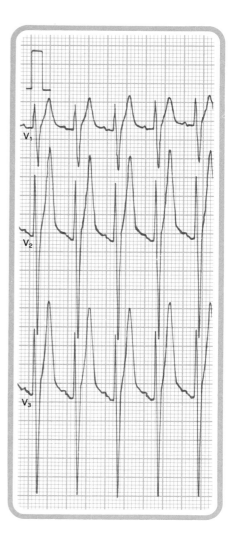

V₁

V₂

V₃

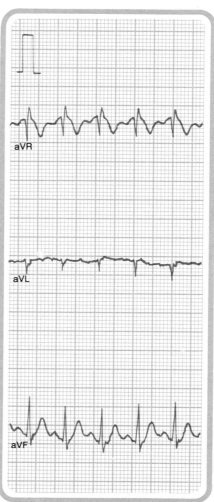

aVR

aVL

aVF

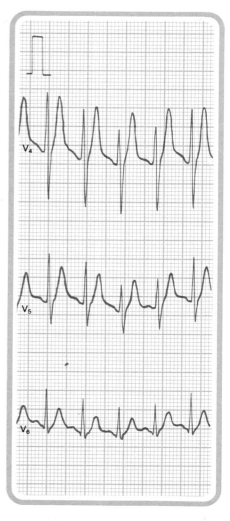

V₄

V₅

V₆

Figure 134b

The immediate post-exercise record is also within normal limits. The patient was a 42-year-old man. The heart rate achieved was 168/min and the patient thus achieved the target heart rate. There were no indications for stopping the exercise prematurely. There is no significant S-T segment shift (see criteria above) and the exercise test is therefore negative. Some changes do occur but these do **not** signify abnormality. Prominent atrial repolarisation (Ta) waves are seen (easily recognised in Leads II, III, aVF and V₆). The T waves in V₁–V₃ are taller following exercise than at rest, but this is not abnormal. (Had the T waves been abnormal, i.e. inverted, before exercise and had become upright following exercise, this would have been abnormal).

Subsequent records taken over the next 10 min after exercise likewise showed no abnormality. The Ta wave gradually diminished and the T waves in the right precordial leads gradually returned to their former size.

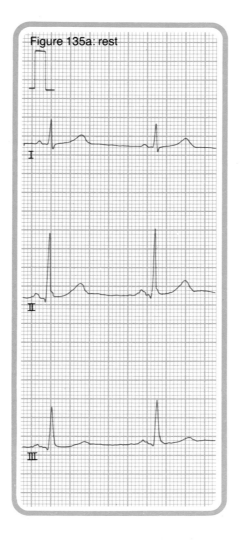

Figure 135a: rest

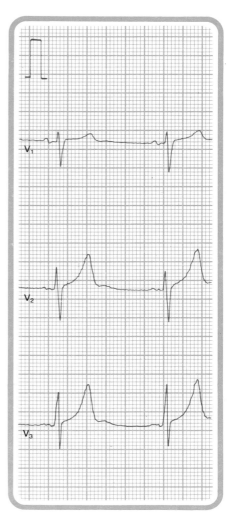

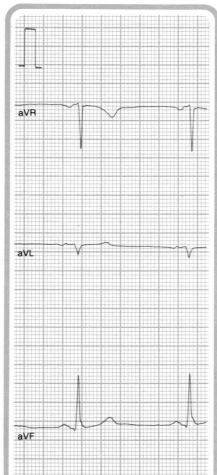

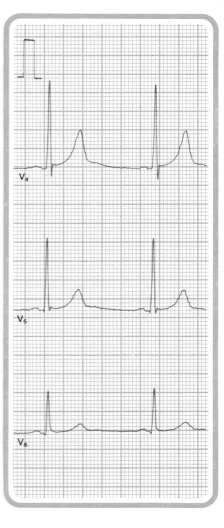

Figure 135a

The resting record is within normal limits (the deep negative wave in the QRS in aVL (it is an S wave since there is a small initial r wave – but it would still be normal even if it were a Q wave) is due to the fact that the heart is vertical – the axis is +75°). The T waves in V_2 and V_3 are rather tall but this is not definitely abnormal. The resting heart rate is 52/min.

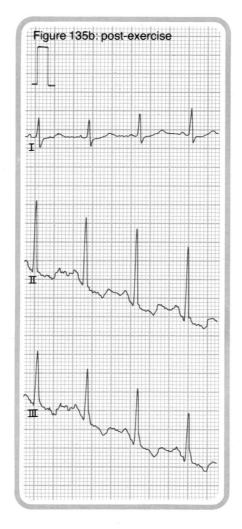

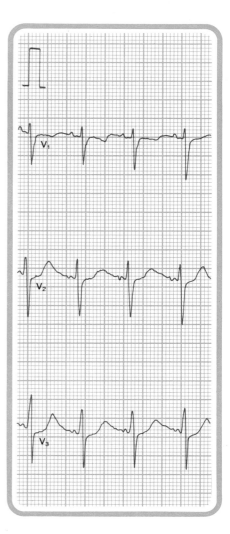

Figure 135b: post-exercise

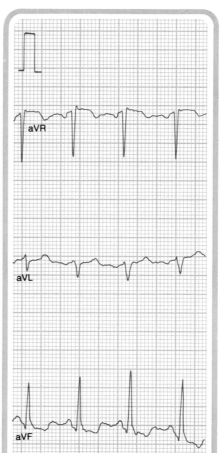

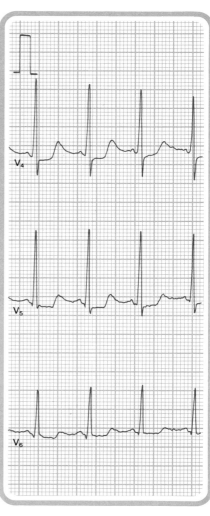

Figure 135b

The immediate post-exercise heart rate is only 115/min. The patient was unable to complete the exercise programme because of the development of anginal pain. There is 2mm S-T depression clearly seen in V_4 and V_5. There is lesser S-T depression in V_6 and aVF. Assessment of S-T changes in II and III is not possible because of the sloping S-T segment.

At coronary angiography the patient had a localised 90% occlusion of the proximal part of the anterior descending branch of the left coronary artery.

2. Factors strongly suggestive of a positive test

a) "Normalisation" of previously inverted T waves.

b) Development of terminal T wave inversion or of U wave inversion (see below).

c) Development of ventricular tachycardia or of multiple ventricular ectopic beats.

d) Development of increased R wave amplitude in the precordial leads.

e) Development of hypotension (a clinical not an electrocardiographic response, of course).

3. Features with no definitive diagnostic value

(i.e. important negative points)

a) Development of atrial or nodal arrhythmia.

b) Development of first degree heart block or Wenckebach phenonomen.

c) Development of intraventricular block – right or left bundle branch block, anterior or posterior hemiblock, bifascicular block etc.

d) T wave flattening or inversion.

e) Increase in U wave height (see below).

f) Sloping S-T segment shift if not both a) more than 1 mm in height, and b) 0.08 sec or longer in duration.

g) Changes in P wave morphology.

The U Wave

The U wave is a small, rounded positive deflection occurring immediately after the T wave. It is often seen in normal records but in normal circumstances is almost always inconspicuous. It is part of the repolarisation process (as are the S-T segments and T waves), but its precise mode of genesis is uncertain. The amplitude of the normal U wave is related to that of the preceding T wave. The U wave is normally 5-25% of the height of the preceding T wave. Because of this relationship, it follows that the U wave is usually tallest in V_2, V_3 and V_4. In these leads it may occasionally reach 2 mm in height though the average height of the normal U wave in these leads is less than 0.5 mm. The normal U wave is usually upright in the limb leads except for 'cavity' leads (i.e. in almost all hearts, aVR, in the case of vertical hearts, aVL, and in the case of horizontal hearts, Lead III).

Small (normal) U waves are seen in V_2, V_3, V_4, V_5 and Lead II of Record 2 (page 72). When the U wave is inverted it is abnormal. When the U wave exceeds the height of the preceding T wave it is abnormal – as in Leads V_2 and V_3 of Record 15 (page 86).

Conditions giving rise to increased height of the U wave or to U wave inversion are listed on page 263.

False-positive and false-negative exercise electrocardiograms

There are several factors which may give rise to false-positive or false-negative exercise tests, i.e. which may give rise to tests which wrongly suggest the presence or the absence respectively of ischaemic heart disease. Most of these factors should not present a real problem – for they are usually obvious in advance and when they are so recognised there is little point in going ahead with the investigation for the results are bound to be equivocal. The factors are as follows:-

1. Factors giving rise to false-positive tests

a) Intraventricular conduction defects.

b) Ventricular pre-excitation (see pages 212 to 220).

c) Overt ventricular hypertrophy.

d) Valve disease (which may be giving rise to "occult" ventricular hypertrophy, i.e. hypertrophy not apparent in the resting record).

e) Hypertension (for reasons given in d) above).

f) Pulmonary hypertension (for reasons given in d) above).

g) Cardiomyopathy (congestive or hypertrophic) and myocarditis.

h) Electrolyte disturbances – especially hypokalaemia.

i) Hypothyroidism.

j) Concurrent drug administration – especially digitalis but also including quinidine, procainamide, diuretics, antidepressants and sedatives.

k) Pericarditis.

l) Mitral valve prolapse.

m) Post-prandial changes.

n) Hyperventilation.

o) Pre-existing and non-specific S-T, T changes.

p) Pectus excavatum.

2. Factors giving rise to false-negative tests

a) Concurrent administration of beta-blocking drugs. The use of these drugs prevents the achievement of the target heart rate which is the commonest cause of false-negative responses.

b) Other anti-anginal drugs may occasionally give rise to false-negative responses.

c) An inadequate exercise level with inappropriately low maximal heart rate.

d) Previous physical training – this may result in a **relative** inadequacy of the maximal heart rate achieved, i.e. a higher heart rate target should be set.

In the absence of the above factors, false-negative exercise electro-cardiograms can still be found despite the presence of significant coronary disease.

Correlation of exercise electrocardiography with the presence of coronary artery disease

Pathological studies reveal that when the test is positive (i.e. there is significant S-T segment shift related to exertion) the patients **usually** have severe and extensive coronary atheroma.

A rigorously conducted negative exercise test does not, however, exclude significant coronary atheroma.

Coronary angiographic studies confirm that the exercise test can be negative despite the presence of significant atheroma in the coronary vessels and it also demonstrates that positive stress tests are more likely to be achieved in multi-vessel rather than in single-vessel disease.

The test does have prognostic value when asymptomatic subjects are screened. Those with positive stress tests have mortality rates 4 or 5 times higher than those with negative tests and the excess of mortality is roughly proportional to the depth of the S-T segment depression produced.

Diagnosis of Myocardial Infarction

At this stage it is appropriate to repeat the diagnostic criteria for myocardial infarction. It will be recalled that myocardial infarction can only be diagnosed on the basis of the appropriate QRS abnormalities (pages 168 *et. seq.*).

Diagnostic criteria[†] for myocardial infarction

A **definitive** diagnosis of myocardial infarction from the electrocardiogram can only be made on the basis of abnormalities of the QRS complex. These diagnostic abnormalities are as follows:-

a) q waves which **either** are 0.04 sec or longer in duration (excluding aVR and III) **or** have a depth which is more than one quarter of the height of the ensuing R wave (excluding aVR and III).

b) qs or QS complexes[*] (excluding aVR and III).

c) local area of inappropriately low R wave voltage (where this can confidently be ascertained).

Additional features frequently associated with myocardial infarction

These changes include S-T segment and T wave changes and also the development of specific changes related to the local effects of infarction (e.g. intraventricular conduction disturbances and cardiac arrhythmias).

a) S-T segment elevation (usually with slight curvature, convex upwards) occurs in leads facing the infarcted zone. This is a transient change often occurring within hours of the onset of symptoms, usually being the first electrocardiographic **manifestation** of acute infarction (though not actually being **diagnostic** of it) and usually lasting for days only. Prolonged (weeks or months) S-T segment elevation of minor degree may occur in extensive infarction and in the presence of a ventricular aneurysm.

b) S-T segment depression (usually with a slight curvature) occurs as a "reciprocal" change in leads "opposite to", i.e. remote from, the infarcted area during the time that primary S-T segment elevation persists.

c) Horizontal S-T segment depression may occur as a primary change (i.e. without concurrent S-T elevation in other leads) in subendocardial infarction.

Note

† These criteria are, strictly speaking, the criteria for loss of viable, electrically active myocardium. The commonest cause is myocardial infarction but any disease directly causing myocardial necrosis or replacement of electrically active by inactive myocardium can give rise to similar appearances. Thus fibrosis induced by cardiomyopathy or replacement of myocardium by amyloid tissue can give rise to similar appearances in the QRS complexes (see pseudo-infarction pattern, page 198). It follows that secondary as well as primary interpretation is important for a definitive diagnosis. The primary interpretation really just defines loss of viable myocardium. However, when the full, evolving, time-sequential pattern of myocardial infarction (page 179) is shown, definitive diagnosis by primary interpretation is possible.

* qs or QS complexes are normal for any lead "looking into" the cavity of the heart ("cavity leads"). aVR is almost always a cavity lead and usually shows a QS complex. Lead aVL is often a cavity lead when the heart is vertical and Lead III is often a cavity lead when the heart is horizontal, and in these respective circumstances aVL or III will usually show a qs complex. V_1 is often and V_2 is occasionally, a cavity lead if there is pronounced clockwise cardiac rotation. In such circumstances V_1 and possibly also V_2 may show QS complexes.

It is by far the most **typical** change of subendocardial infarction but it is not **specific** to it for it occurs also in subendocardial ischaemia and in exertional angina.

d) Downsloping or upsloping S-T segment depression may occur in leads overlying or adjacent to areas of infarction. The change is quite non-specific but in this context probably reflects local myocardial ischaemia.

e) Deep symmetrical T wave inversion frequently occurs overlying and adjacent to areas of acute myocardial infarction. The change does not usually occur in the first 24 hours (being later than the S-T segment change). It may persist for weeks. It is also seen in relation to ischaemia without infarction and may also be the sole manifestation of subendocardial infarction.

f) Shallow or asymmetrical T wave inversion is a non-specific change. It frequently occurs in areas adjacent to infarction but can occur in many other conditions (page 184).

g) Abnormally tall T waves may occur in leads "opposite to" the infarcted area (this change is most frequently seen in the precordial leads in true posterior infarction). This change can occur in true posterior ischaemia without infarction and can also occur in hyperkalaemia and in intraventricular conduction disturbances.

h) Terminal T wave inversion may occur with acute myocardial infarction – usually at about the time when there is recognisable S-T segment elevation. This change may be the same process as U wave inversion.

i) Low voltage T waves or **T wave flattening** is a non-specific change. It frequently occurs in areas adjacent to infarction but can occur in many other conditions.

j) Cardiac arrhythmias frequently occur in relation to infarction. Since any part of the myocardium or conducting tissue may be involved in the infarction, any arrhythmia is possible. There may be **disturbances of function at the sino-atrial node** (sinus tachycardia, sinus bradycardia, sinus arrhythmia, sino-atrial block, sinus arrest, nodal-escape beats, nodal-escape rhythm), **disturbances of conduction** (first, second or third degree atrio-ventricular block, right bundle branch block, left bundle branch block, left anterior hemiblock, left posterior hemiblock), **ectopic arrhythmias** (atrial ectopic beats, atrial tachycardia, atrial flutter, atrial fibrillation, nodal ectopic beats, nodal tachycardia, ventricular ectopic beats, ventricular tachycardia, ventricular fibrillation) and finally there may be any **combination of the above.** (Obviously, in the case of ventricular fibrillation, any concomitant rhythm disturbance would be both occult and irrelevant). The arrhythmias are described in Section 3.

k) Axis shift. Left ventricular depolarisation is the dominant influence in determining the form of the QRS complexes in all normal and in most abnormal electrocardiograms (page 22) and plays by far the most important role in determining the mean frontal plane QRS axis (pages 22-24). Myocardial infarction involves loss of viable myocardium, usually from the left ventricle. In the frontal plane, the mean forces of left ventricular depolarisation are directed downwards and to the left so that a typical normal frontal plane QRS axis is $+60°$ (pages 22-24). The normal range for the frontal plane axis in adults is $-30°$ to $+90°$ (page 53). When there is necrosis of these parts of the left ventricular myocardium which normally give rise to components of the depolarisation wave at extremes of this normal range, the loss of components at **one extreme** tends to give rise to a **mean** QRS axis at or beyond the other **extreme.** Thus since the myocardium of the inferior wall of the left ventricle normally contributes a component of ventricular depolarisation directly inferiorly in the frontal plane (i.e. towards aVF) the loss of this myocardium as in inferior infarction, tends to give rise to a mean frontal plane QRS axis directly more superiorly, but still to the left. Therefore, **the development of inferior infarction is often accompanied by the simultaneous development of abnormal left axis deviation.** This is a direct consequence of loss of the inferiorly directed component of left ventricular depolarisation and does not imply the development of left anterior hemiblock (pages 133 and 175). In like manner, **the development of antero-lateral myocardial infarction is often accompanied by the development of abnormal right axis deviation.** This is a direct consequence of the loss of the superiorly and leftward directed component of left ventricular depolarisation and does not imply the development of left posterior hemiblock (page 137).

(Figure 141 shows an example of inferior infarction giving rise to abnormal left axis deviation and Figure 96 an example of left anterior hemiblock giving rise to abnormal left axis deviation). The essential difference between the two on the frontal plane leads is the presence of an abnormal Q wave (actually QS complex in Figure 141) in aVF in inferior infarction, compared with an rS in aVF in LAH. Figure 137 shows an example of antero-lateral infarction giving rise to an abnormal degree of right axis deviation. (This does not imply the development of left posterior hemiblock).

Pseudo-infarction Patterns

As explained earlier, abnormal q waves or abnormal QS patterns, particularly if associated with S-T segment shift and T wave changes, are the most reliable electrocardiographic indications of myocardial infarction. However, similar changes are occasionally seen in patients without coronary artery disease. It is important to be aware of these "pseudo-infarction patterns".

Conditions associated with absence of, or reduction in the size of, the r waves in the right precordial leads, thus simulating infarction

a) **Chronic lung disease.** As a result of the pronounced clockwise cardiac rotation which occurs in this condition the r waves in the right and mid-precordial leads may be small or absent.

b) **Spontaneous pneumothorax.** This may produce changes similar to those in chronic lung disease.

c) **Left ventricular hypertrophy.** May give rise to reduction in r wave size (and occasionally to absence of r waves) in the right precordial leads. Record 5 (page 75) shows an example of left ventricular hypertrophy in which there are small r waves in V_1-V_3 and a sudden increase in R wave height in V_4. (This type of R wave progression can occasionally be indicative of anteroseptal infarction but in this case is due to left ventricular hypertrophy).

(Left bundle branch block may also give rise to abnormally low r wave voltages in the right precordial leads in just the same way as LVH (e.g. see Record 7, page 77 and compare with Record 5, page 75) but this is not rightfully considered a "pseudo-infarction pattern" since the presence of criteria for the diagnosis of left bundle branch block precludes the diagnosis of myocardial infarction (page 125 and page 250) except in special circumstances (pages 251 and 252)).

It is worthwhile to compare the r wave progression in the precordial leads in Record 4, page 74 (normal), Record 5, page 75 (LVH), Record 7, page 77 (LBBB) and Record 8, page 79 (Anteroseptal infarction).

Conditions in which abnormal q waves may occur, thus simulating infarction

a) **Cardiomyopathy.** In **hypertrophic cardiomyopathy** the interventricular septum may be markedly thickened (substantially increasing the "Phase 1" voltage of ventricular depolarisation). As a result, the septal q waves are increased in size and abnormal q waves may appear – particularly in Leads V_4, V_5, V_6, I and aVL.

In **congestive cardiomyopathy** abnormal q waves may occur in any lead. These q waves are usually the result of patches of fibrosis in localised areas of the myocardium.

Other **myocardial diseases** may give rise to abnormal q waves. These diseases include:-
Amyloidosis
Scleroderma
Primary or secondary tumours
Myocarditis
Friedreich's ataxia
Progressive muscular dystrophy.

b) **Left bundle branch block.** This often gives rise to QS complexes in the inferior limb leads (as in Record 28, page 99) and often in the right precordial leads (Record 28 shows abnormally small r waves in the right precordial leads).

These changes occur because of reversal of the direction of septal depolarisation. For this reason it is unwise to diagnose infarction in the presence of left bundle branch block unless previous records are available showing left bundle branch block **before** the infarction.

c) **Ventricular pre-excitation.** In this condition the direction of septal depolarisation is reversed and abnormal q waves may appear in the limb leads or in the precordial leads (e.g. Figure 150, page 217).

d) **Pulmonary embolism.** In this condition abnormal q waves may develop in III and aVF. This change has been attributed to dilatation of the right ventricle with consequent changes in the orientation of the interventricular septum so that the right side of the septum is directed superiorly. When this happens Phase 1 of ventricular depolarisation is directed away from III and aVF and initial q waves appear in these leads. In contrast to the situation in inferior infarction, such q waves do not usually appear also in II and they tend to be small in aVF. Occasionally, in massive pulmonary embolism, abnormal q waves may appear across the precordial leads.

Conditions in which S-T segment and T wave changes occur, thus simulating infarction

a) **Hyperkalaemia.** This may give rise to very tall T waves in the precordial leads. Sometimes there may be associated S-T elevation and reduction in R wave height. Such changes only occur in severe (pre-terminal) hyperkalaemia.

b) **Intracranial haemorrhage.** The commonest changes associated with intracranial haemorrhage are S-T segment and T wave changes, but abnormal q waves can be seen.

c) **Pericarditis.** The widespread distribution of the S-T, T changes in pericarditis and the absence of QRS changes usually means that confusion with infarction is unlikely (see pages 231 and 232).

d) **Myocardial Contusion.** Non-penetrating injuries of the myocardium may give rise to local injury or necrosis. Accordingly S-T or T wave changes or q wave development may occur. If the conducting tissue is involved A-V conduction problems may develop. The overall picture may closely mimic infarction but the clinical story usually prevents confusion (illustrating again the importance of secondary interpretation).

Most of these conditions will be considered in detail in the section on miscellaneous abnormalities.

Ventricular Aneurysm

It is widely taught that **persistent** S-T segment elevation (i.e. S-T elevation which occurs in relation to acute infarction but which does not settle after the first few days or weeks as is usually the case) is indicative of the presence of a ventricular aneurysm. Since "ventricular aneurysm" is a haemodynamic concept rather than an anatomical one it is not surprising, in the author's view, that electrocardiography provides no reliable basis whatsoever for the diagnosis. All patients who sustain myocardial infarction and survive, develop a fibrous non-contractile scar in the infarcted area. In a normal heart the whole perimeter of the left ventricular wall moves inwards during systole. After myocardial infarction the infarcted zone either moves inwards less than it did formerly (hypokinesia) or not at all (akinesia). An aneurysm exists when the infarcted zone moves **outwards** during systole (dyskinesia). It would, (again in the author's judgement) be a remarkable thing if this difference in mechanical movement of dead tissue (i.e. between akinesia or hypokinesia on the one hand, and dyskinesia on the other hand) were to be conveniently signified by a particular ECG change! There is no denying the fact that persistent S-T segment elevation does show a significant **correlation** with proven ventricular aneurysm (**proof** of the existence of an aneurysm is only possible by ventricular angiography) but the correlation is relatively weak – only two-thirds of patients with definite ventricular aneurysms have persistent S-T segment elevation and probably less than two-thirds of patients with persistent S-T segment elevation have ventricular aneurysms at angiography. The probable reason for the correlation is that the formation of a left ventricular aneurysm is more likely the more extensive the infarct. In the presence of extensive anterior infarction there will be little residual viable myocardium in the anterior cardiac wall. This wall therefore presents an electrical "window" through to the back of the heart. If there is ischaemia of the posterior wall of the heart (which might give S-T segment depression in a posterior lead) it will show S-T elevation in the anterior leads. Persistent S-T elevation in the anterior leads, together with evidence of extensive anterior infarction is thus simply a manifestation of extensive loss of viable myocardium from the anterior wall of the heart and of ischaemia of the posterior wall. Ventricular aneurysm formation is much more likely the more extensive is the loss of myocardium hence there is inevitably some degree of correlation. (This interpretation is by no means widely accepted. It is speculation by the author. The idea was acquired from Dr H B Burchell while the author was spending a year at the Mayo Clinic).

Atrial Infarction

There are no **diagnostic** changes of atrial infarction. Infarction of atrial myocardium is rare without simultaneous evidence of ventricular infarction. The most specific electrocardiographic sign of atrial infarction is elevation or depression of the P-R segment. This is because the atrial repolarisation wave (Ta wave or atrial T wave) which is the atrial equivalent of the ventricular T wave (page 166), tends to occur at the same time as the QRS complex. The P-R interval therefore corresponds in timing to the atrial equivalent of the S-T segment. Elevation of the P-R interval can therefore indicate acute atrial injury and depression of the P-R interval can indicate ischaemia of the atrium. A less specific but more sensitive indicator of atrial infarction is a bifid P in II or a biphasic P in V_1 with a dominant negative component (i.e. appearances of the type seen in left atrial hypertrophy). The electrocardiogram cannot reliably distinguish among left atrial hypertrophy, left atrial infarction and left atrial ischaemia. The occurrence of atrial arrhythmias also suggests the possibility of atrial infarction.

Examples of the 12-lead ECG in Ischaemic Heart Disease

It is a useful exercise at this stage to work through a range of different electrocardiographic appearances in patients with unequivocal ischaemic heart disease.

Figure 136

Report
"Sinus rhythm, the mean frontal plane QRS axis is +30°. Old anteroseptal myocardial infarction. Left atrial abnormality".

Explanation
The rhythm is sinus, the frontal plane QRS and T axes are normal (i.e. the QRS axis is within the normal range and the T axis (+15°) is within ±45° of the QRS axis). There is a small initial r wave in V_1. The r wave in V_2 should be significantly larger than that in V_1 but it is not. Occasionally this can occur normally in one lead – especially in the transition zone (page 45). However, in this case it is clearly abnormal since the r wave in V_3 is, if anything, smaller still – it is certainly not larger (as it should be). The r wave progression from V_1-V_3 is definitely abnormal. This abnormality cannot be explained by clockwise cardiac rotation since it is apparent in V_1-V_3 and yet there is a tall R wave in V_4 and the transition zone is between V_4 and V_5. It cannot be explained by left bundle branch block (page 124) since the latter is not present (the total QRS duration is normal and there are normal septal q waves in V_6). The only other feature which could account for it is ventricular pre-excitation (page 215). This is not present, for the P-R interval is normal. The appearances are therefore diagnostic of anteroseptal infarction. The age of the infarct cannot be determined with any accuracy. It is certainly "old" but this could indicate that it happened between a few months and many years ago. The area of the negative component of the P wave in V_1 exceeds the area of the positive component. This indicates left atrial abnormality. It could be atrial ischaemia or atrial hypertrophy. Since there is evidence of ventricular infarction and therefore of ischaemic heart disease, it may well be indicative of atrial ischaemia or infarction. The ECG does not distinguish between ischaemia, infarction and hypertrophy of the atria.

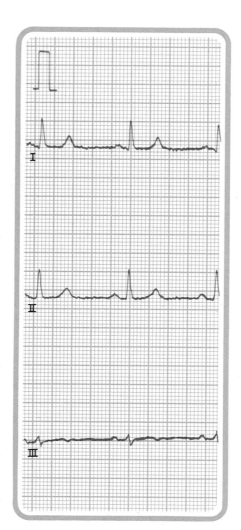

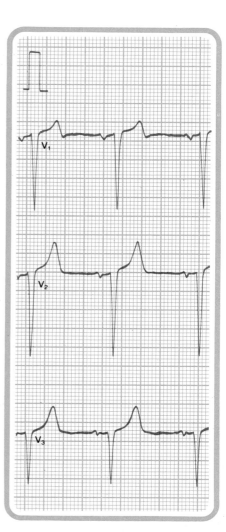

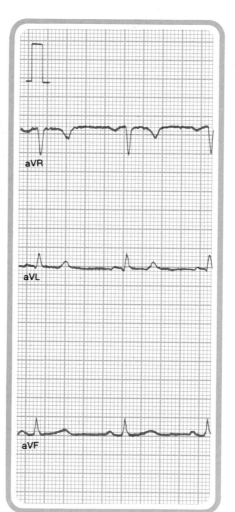

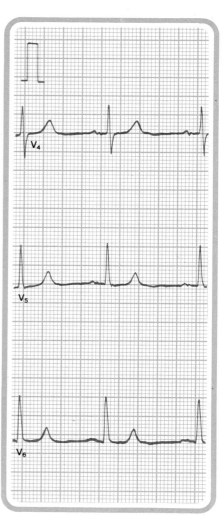

Figure 137

Report

"Sinus rhythm. The mean frontal plane QRS axis is indeterminate. There is evidence of recent extensive anterior myocardial infarction. The appearances are also consistent with true posterior ischaemic damage".

Explanation

There are definitely abnormal Q waves from V_2-V_6 and in I and aVL. (In each clearly indicates necrosis of the myocardium underlying V_2-V_6 and in the antero-lateral area. The pronounced S-T segment elevation in these same leads, with reciprocal S-T segment depression in III and aVF indicates that the necrosis is the result of infarction and that the infarct is recent – probably days old. The S-T segment depression in V_1 cannot be explained on the basis of a reciprocal change since it is very close to a lead showing primary changes (V_2). It could therefore be a primary change in itself and could indicate damage in the posterior wall of the left ventricle. At most the appearances in V_1 indicate ischaemic **damage** to the posterior wall of the left ventricle. There is no definite evidence of true posterior **infarction** since the R wave in V_1 is neither greater in height than the ensuing S wave is in depth, nor is it 0.04 sec or longer in duration.

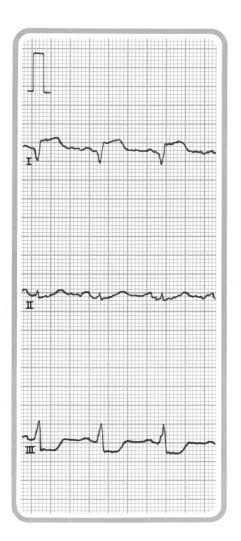

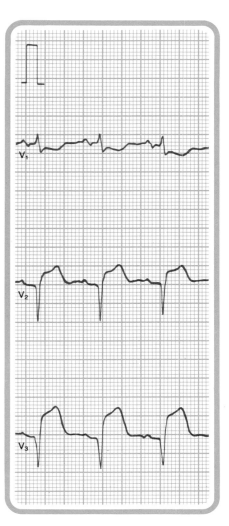

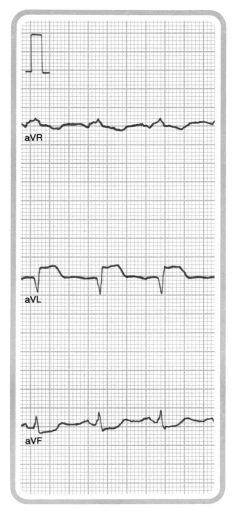

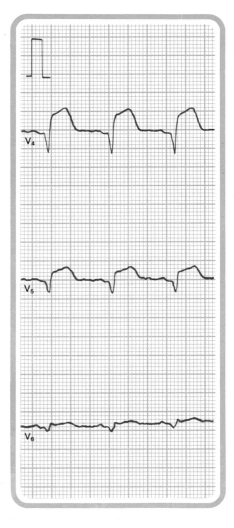

Figure 138

Report

"Sinus rhythm. The mean frontal plane QRS axis is −15°. There is evidence of relatively recent anterior myocardial infarction and of old inferior infarction".

Explanation

There are QS complexes from V_1-V_3 with abnormal q waves in V_4. There is no evidence of left bundle branch block or of ventricular pre-excitation and these appearances are therefore indicative of anterior infarction assuming that none of the causes of pseudo-infarction patterns is present (page 198). The QS complexes indicate transmural infarction underlying V_1-V_3. The abnormal q wave in V_4 indicates less than full thickness infarction underlying the electrodes. The R waves in V_5 and V_6 are probably smaller than they were prior to the infarction but without a record before the infarct, one cannot be confident of this. There is no definite S-T elevation and therefore the infarct is not very recent (i.e. it is more than days old). However, there is T wave inversion from V_1-V_5 and low voltage T waves in V_6, I and aVL. (Note that, as is often the case, the non-specific T wave changes are more widespread than the definitive QRS changes of infarction). The T wave changes indicate that the infarct is of intermediate age (i.e. more than days old but probably less than weeks old). There are QS complexes in aVF without S-T elevation or T inversion in this lead. This indicates the presence of old inferior infarction.

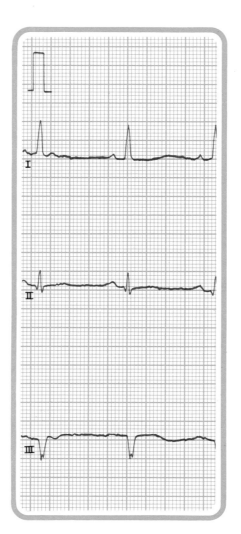

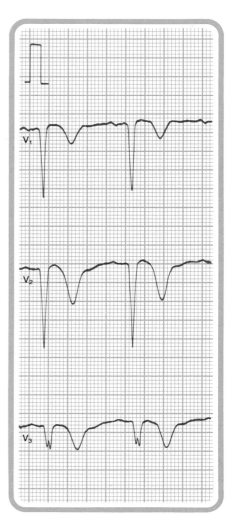

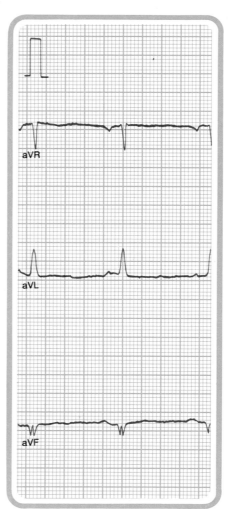

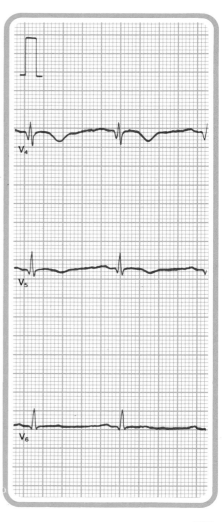

Figure 139

Report

"Sinus rhythm. The mean frontal plane QRS axis is +75°. There is evidence of recent infero-lateral myocardial ischaemic damage."

Explanation

The striking abnormality is the S-T segment elevation. This is most obvious in Leads II, III and aVF (the inferior leads). It is also apparent in V_4-V_6 (the lateral precordial leads). The changes are those of **damage** ("injury") to the myocardium on the inferior wall of the ventricle extending into the lateral wall. (This combination of localisation is sometimes referred to as "apical" (page 180)). There is S-T segment depression in I, aVL and V_1-V_3. This S-T segment depression is "reciprocal". There are no diagnostic QRS changes of infarction, though it is likely that such changes will appear within the next few days (page 179). The R wave voltages in the left precordial leads are smaller than one would expect and it is **possible** there has already been some true infarction in the lateral wall. However, one cannot be **certain** of this since the leads in question are not "bracketed" by undoubtedly normal appearances (for the simple reason that there are no precordial leads further to the left of V_6) and the appearance of the precordial QRS complexes could simply be a manifestation of clockwise cardiac rotation.

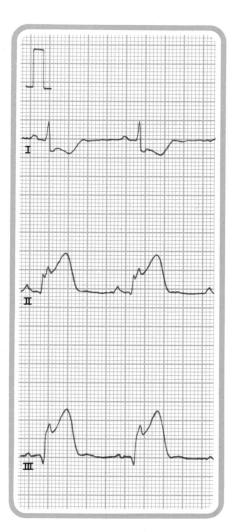

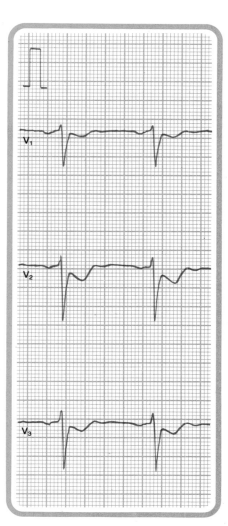

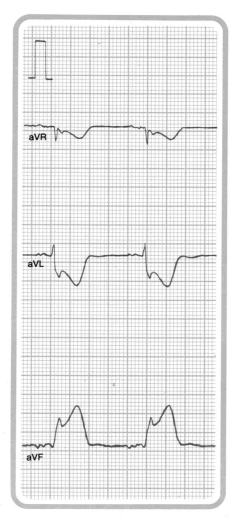

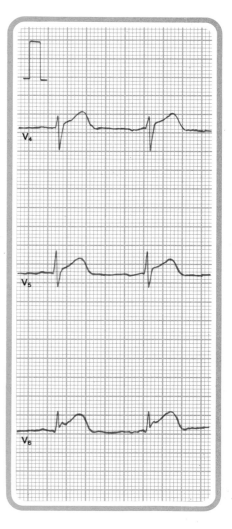

Figure 140

Report

"Sinus rhythm. The mean frontal plane QRS axis is −15°. There is evidence of inferior myocardial infarction of relatively recent origin. There is minimal S-T segment elevation in V_5 and V_6 with terminal T wave inversion in these leads, suggesting ischaemic damage to the antero-lateral wall of the ventricle. The tall T waves in V_2 and V_3 raise the possibility of true posterior ischaemia".

Explanation

The Q waves in aVF exceed 0.04 sec in duration and have a depth which substantially exceeds one quarter of the height of the ensuing R wave. In the absence of ventricular pre-excitation and left bundle branch block this is diagnostic of inferior infarction. As is frequently also the case in inferior infarction, prominent Q waves are also seen in III. However, the appearances in Lead III can never be used to diagnose infarction for the reasons given on pages 54 and 173 and 174. There is T wave inversion in the inferior limb Leads II, III and aVF. This is abnormal in this context (even though the frontal plane T wave axis, at −15°, is normal in its relationship to the frontal plane QRS axis). As explained on page 58, when there is definitive QRS evidence of inferior myocardial infarction, T wave inversion in the inferior limb leads is considered abnormal even if the angle between the mean QRS and T wave axes does not lie outside the normal limits of ±45°. These T wave changes are secondary to the QRS abnormality and indicate that the infarction is unlikely to be more than several weeks old. The slight S-T segment elevation in V_5 and V_6 is definitely abnormal as is the slight terminal T wave inversion in these leads. These changes indicate the presence of recent antero-lateral myocardial ischaemic damage. The T waves in V_2 and V_3 are tall. One cannot be sure that this is an abnormality (unless a prior record with lower T wave voltages is available for comparison). They **could** indicate true posterior ischaemia.

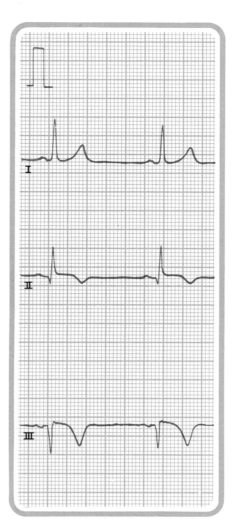

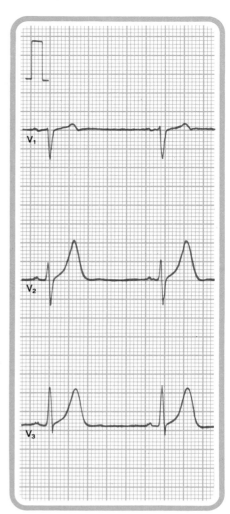

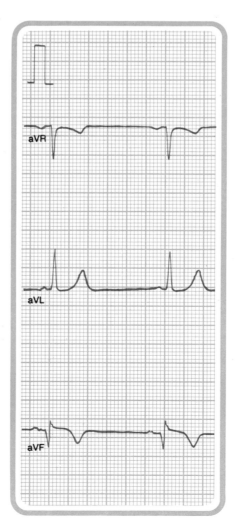

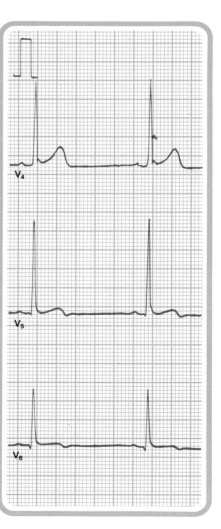

Figure 141

Report

"Sinus tachycardia. The mean frontal plane QRS axis is −45°. This is an abnormal degree of left axis deviation. There is evidence of old infero-lateral myocardial infarction. In addition there are signs of recent true posterior infarction. There is also evidence of left atrial abnormality".

Explanation

The rhythm is sinus but the rate exceeds 100/minute and there is therefore sinus tachycardia. There is an abnormal degree of left axis deviation (−45°). The two commonest causes of this are left anterior hemiblock and inferior myocardial infarction (page 135). There are clearly abnormal Q waves in II and aVF (and also, as is often the case, Lead III) indicating inferior myocardial infarction. This is therefore an adequate explanation for the left axis deviation and there is no need to invoke left anterior hemiblock. The T waves are upright indicating that at least several weeks have elapsed since the infarct occurred. The infarct could be anything from weeks to years in age. V_6 shows a clear infarct pattern, with abnormal Q waves, obvious reduction in R wave height (so striking that it is apparent even without "bracketing" with normal appearances in leads on each side of the one in question). The appearances indicate infarction of the lateral wall of the ventricle. There is still S-T elevation in this lead and the antero-lateral change is therefore recent (days). There is striking S-T depression from V_1-V_4. This cannot be a reciprocal change for it is far more pronounced and extensive than the concurrent S-T elevation (seen only in V_6). It is therefore likely to be a primary change. As such it could indicate subendocardial ischaemia (or infarction) or true posterior ischaemic damage. Since there is an abnormally tall and broad R wave in V_1 there is unequivocal evidence of true posterior infarction. The S-T segment depression is likely to be part of this and to indicate that the true posterior infarct is recent. (Theoretically the dominant R wave in V_1 could suggest right ventricular hypertrophy but there is no supporting evidence for this (right axis deviation, clockwise cardiac rotation, right atrial hypertrophy) and there is impressive evidence of extensive ischaemic heart disease). The form of the P waves in V_1 indicates left atrial abnormality.

Note

(The combination of abnormal left axis deviation and a dominant R wave in V_1 could suggest biventricular hypertrophy (page 157) but there is unequivocal evidence of infero-lateral infarction (abnormal q waves in II, aVF and V_6) and pronounced horizontal S-T changes in V_1-V_4, typical of myocardial ischaemia. There is therefore no need to invoke biventricular hypertrophy).

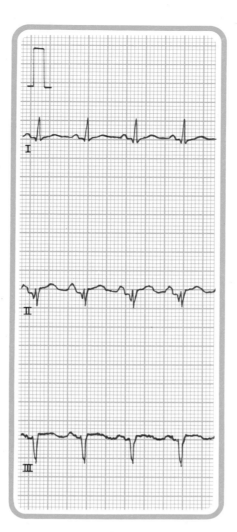
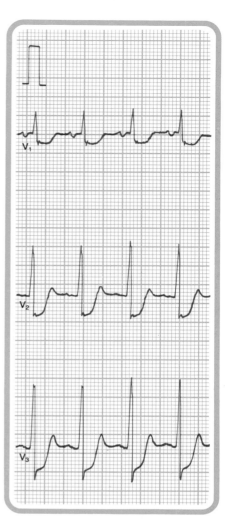
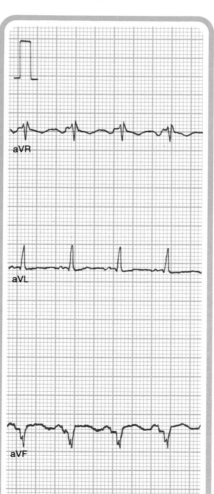
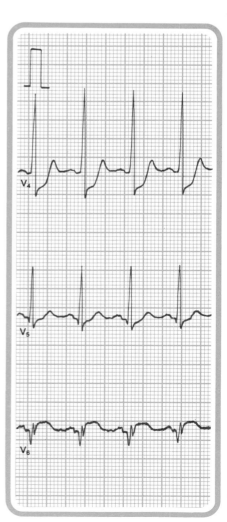

Figure 142

Report

"Sinus rhythm. The mean frontal plane QRS axis is +60°. The appearances in Leads II, III and aVF suggest recent inferior myocardial infarction. The deep symmetrical T wave inversion from V₂-V₆ and in I and aVL suggest subendocardial ischaemia or infarction".

Explanation

The electrocardiogram is clearly abnormal and certainly indicates ischaemic heart disease. There is a suggestion of S-T elevation in II and aVF, but the degree of S-T elevation is not beyond normal limits. There are pronounced q waves in II and aVF but they are not definitely abnormal. The terminal T wave inversion in II and aVF is definitely abnormal. Collectively these appearances suggest recent inferior infarction but the criteria for a definitive diagnosis have not been fulfilled. The deep symmmetrical T wave inversion from V_2-V_6 and in Lead I and aVL suggest subendocardial ischaemia or infarction. Only consecutive records or collateral clinical data (i.e. secondary interpretation) can distinguish between these two possibilities. Note that the upright T wave in aVR is also an abnormality – the T waves are usually negative in this lead. (However – the T waves should be considered **collectively** in the limb leads. The mean frontal plane T wave axis is 180°. The angle between the frontal plane T wave axis and the QRS axis is thus abnormal at +120°). The r wave progression from V_1-V_3 is very poor and it is therefore possible that there is partial thickness regional infarction in this area.

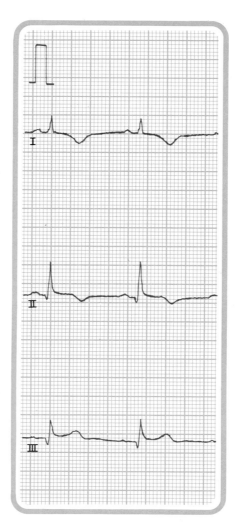

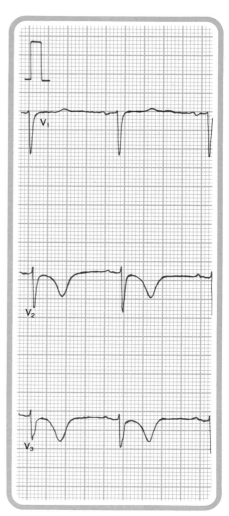

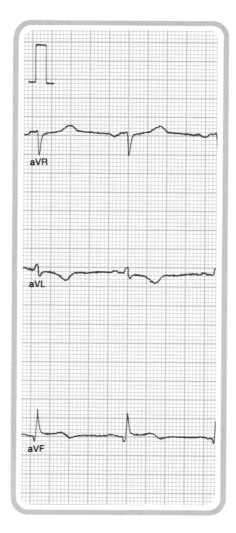

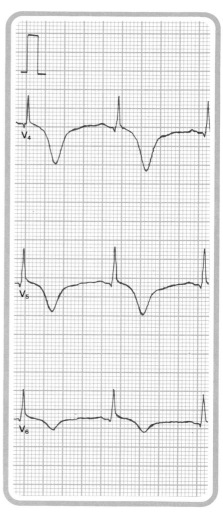

Figure 143

Report

"Sinus rhythm. The mean frontal plane QRS axis is +60°. The T waves in V_1-V_4 are abnormally tall. This is a non-specific change".

Explanation

The T waves are almost certainly abnormally tall in V_2 and V_3. No definitive criteria exist to establish this as a certainty. The possible causes include true posterior myocardial ischaemia, hyperkalaemia and normal variation. The use of relevant clinical data will permit secondary interpretation. This particular patient had been complaining of typical chest pain and it is therefore **likely** that there is true posterior ischaemia. The serum potassium level was normal. Note that the diagnosis cannot be made from the ECG alone. The clinical data do not **prove** that the tall waves indicate ischaemia – though they do suggest that there may well be ischaemia somewhere. The q waves in aVL are more than a quarter of the height of the ensuing r wave, but in this case aVL is almost a cavity lead – aVL is actually just at right angles to the frontal plane axis. The appearances in aVL should therefore be regarded as normal.

The fact that the R/S ratio in V_1 is unity (i.e. the R and S waves are of equal size) is also worthy of comment. Normally in V_1 the r wave is smaller than the S wave (page 32). The causes of an R wave in V_1 **larger** than the S wave include right ventricular hypertrophy and true posterior myocardial infarction (page 262 – of the other two causes, ventricular pre-excitation is ruled out by the ECG appearances (pages 212 to 220) and muscular dystrophy by the clinical picture (secondary interpretation)).

In the absence of an abnormal degree of right axis deviation, right ventricular hypertrophy cannot be diagnosed (page 155). The form of the QRS complexes in V_1 **could** be indicative of true posterior infarction.

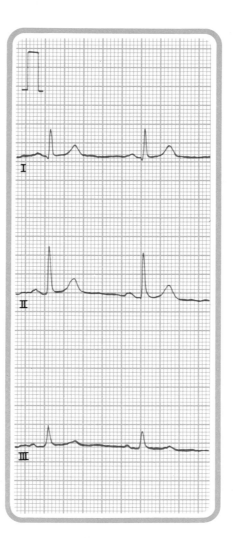

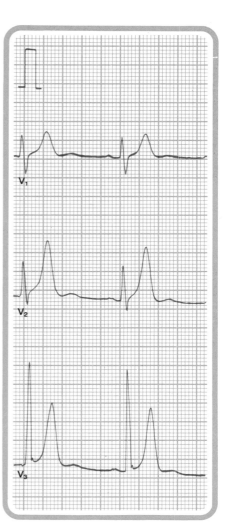

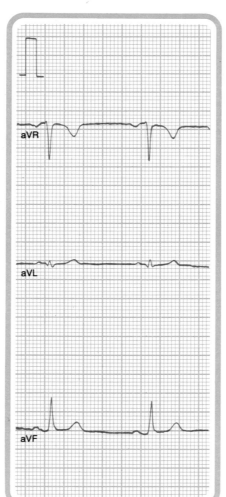

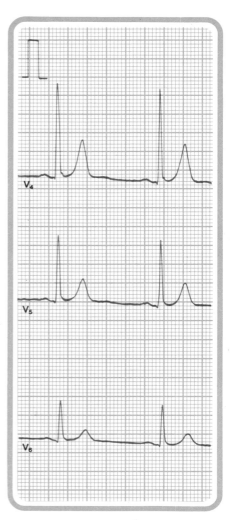

Figure 144

Report

"Sinus rhythm. The mean frontal plane QRS axis is +45°. There is T wave inversion in V_2, V_3 and aVL. The T waves are of low voltage in I, V_4 and V_5 and there is S-T segment depression in Lead I. The record is frankly abnormal but the changes are non-specific".

Explanation

The abnormalities are as listed in the report. The record is definitely abnormal, but a specific cause cannot be assigned. There are non-specific S-T, T changes in the precordial leads and in the limb leads (the mean frontal plane T axis is +105°, therefore the angle between the frontal plane QRS and T axes is abnormal). The patient was complaining of typical chest pain. Secondary interpretation therefore **suggests** but does not **prove** that the changes are ischaemic in origin.

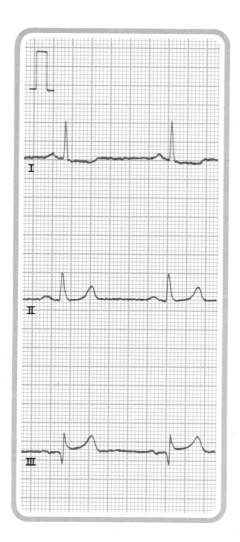

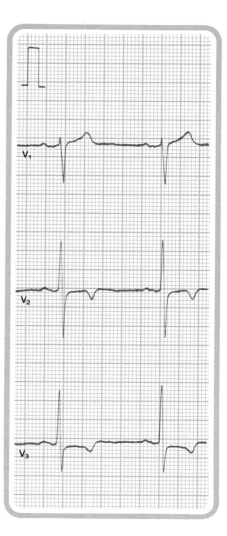

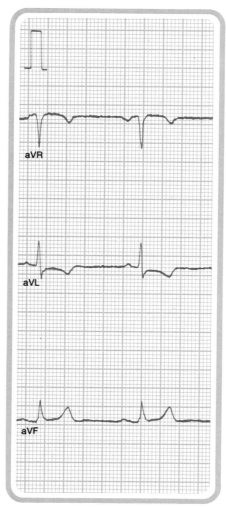

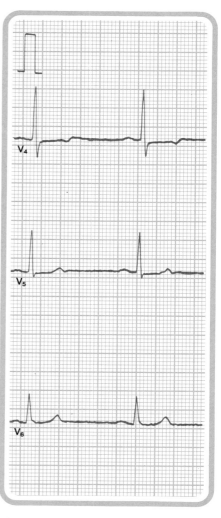

Figure 145

Report

"Sinus rhythm. There is left anterior hemiblock (the mean frontal plane QRS axis is −60°). There are non-specific S-T, T changes in Leads I, II and V_4-V_6. Abnormal U waves are seen in V_3-V_6."

Explanation

The two common causes of abnormal left axis deviation are left anterior hemiblock and inferior infarction. There is no evidence of inferior infarction (there are no q waves in II or aVF) and there is therefore left anterior hemiblock.

The S-T segment depression and T wave inversion in the leads facing the left ventricle are clearly abnormal, but are non-specific changes. The U waves in V_3-V_6 are abnormal since they are taller than the preceded T waves. The patient had a normal serum potassium level and a clinical history of recent ischaemic pain. The **probability** is, therefore, that the S-T, T and U wave changes are ischaemic in origin but one cannot be sure of this from the ECG appearances.

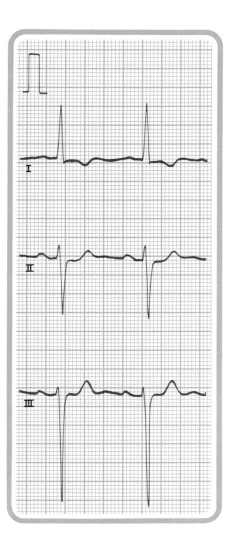

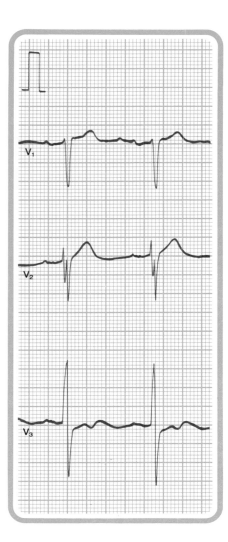

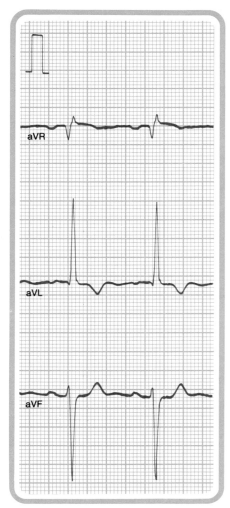

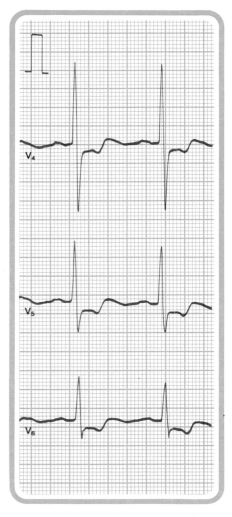

209

Figure 146

Report
*"Sinus rhythm. The mean frontal plane
QRS axis is +75°. There is evidence of
acute infero-lateral myocardial damage."*

Explanation
There is striking S-T segment elevation
in II, III and aVF and minimal S-T
elevation in V_5 and V_6. These changes
indicate infero-lateral (i.e. "apical")
myocardial damage. The S-T elevation in
the inferior leads is convex upwards. This
shape is typical of **ischaemic** damage.
The S-T segment depression in I, aVL
and V_1-V_3 is reciprocal to the primary S-T
elevation. There is no QRS evidence of
infarction.

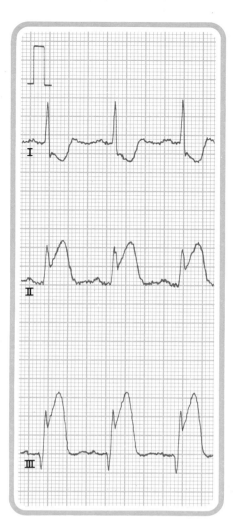

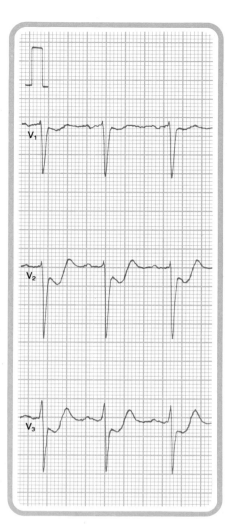

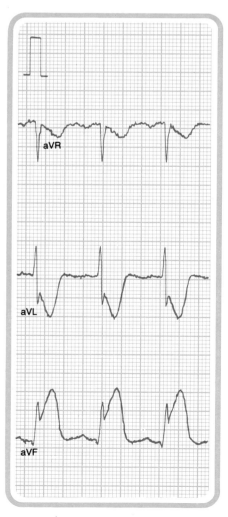

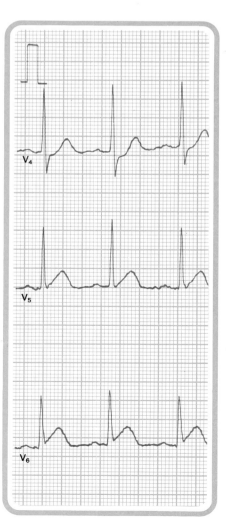

Figure 147

Report

"Sinus rhythm. The mean frontal plane QRS axis is −15°. There is evidence of relatively recent inferior myocardial infarction. There are non-specific S-T, T changes in V$_6$ and low voltage T waves in V$_4$ and V$_5$".

Explanation

There are abnormal Q waves in aVF indicating inferior infarction. There is S-T elevation in the inferior limb leads indicating that the infarct is recent. The T wave inversion in these leads is part of the pattern of recent infarction. There is slight S-T elevation in V$_6$ indicating involvement of the antero-lateral wall of the left ventricle in the infarction. There are non-specific T wave changes (flattening) in V$_4$ and V$_5$. The S-T segment depression in I and aVL is reciprocal.

Record 147 was taken from the same patient as Record 146, one day later. Note the **sequential** changes of inferior infarction. Note that the axis has shifted markedly to the left. Inferior myocardial infarction is one of the two common causes of shift of the axis to the left (in this case it has not actually become an abnormal degree of left axis deviation).

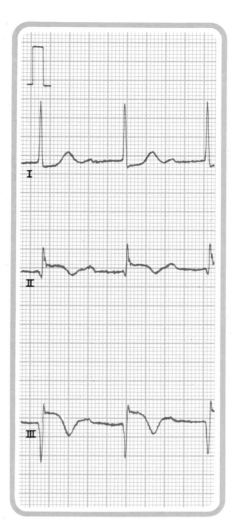

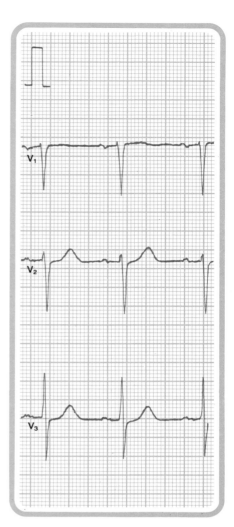

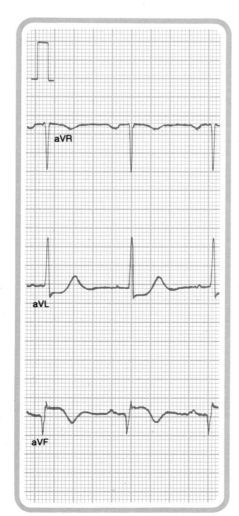

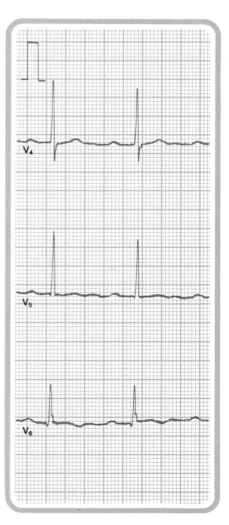

Miscellaneous Abnormalities

Ventricular Pre-excitation

This is a relatively rare condition and because of that fact it is usually dealt with towards the end of textbooks of electrocardiography. However, if the concept is not fully appreciated important diagnostic errors may occur.

The basic abnormality in ventricular pre-excitation is that the depolarisation wave, after passing through the atrial myocardium, activates the ventricles earlier than would be expected if the impulse travelled normally from atria to ventricles via the atrio-ventricular node and His bundle. For this reason ventricular pre-excitation is also known as **accelerated atrio-ventricular conduction.** In its most common form, the condition occurs as a result of the congenital presence of an "accessory" atrio-ventricular conduction pathway which conducts the impulse more rapidly than the A-V node and hence produces a rapid by-pass of the normal slow route. The P-R interval (the time interval between the first recognisable part of the P wave and the first recognisable part of the QRS complex) is shortened by the more rapid transmission of depolarisation, from atrial myocardium (P waves) to ventricular myocardium (QRS complexes).

As a consequence of the more rapid transmission of depolarisation from atrial myocardium to ventricular myocardium the P-R interval is shortened. As a result of the fact that the part of the ventricular myocardium to which the accessory atrio-ventricular pathway passes is the upper part of the right side of the interventricular septum and that this is the first part of the myocardium to be activated (whereas normally the left side of the upper part of the interventricular septum is the first part of the ventricular myocardium to be depolarised) **ventricular activation is interfered with and the QRS complex becomes distorted in shape and prolonged in duration. The combination of a short P-R interval and an abnormally shaped, abnormally long QRS complex comprises the electrocardiographic diagnosis of ventricular pre-excitation.**

The presence of two pathways for atrio-ventricular conduction (the **normal pathway** (through the A-V node, the His bundle and bundle branches) and the **accessory bundle**) leads to the possibility of the depolarisation wave passing from atria to ventricles down one pathway, back to the atria via the other pathway, then back to the ventricles via the first pathway etc. Such a cyclical, repetitive re-entry into the atrial and ventricular myocardium gives rise to paroxysmal tachycardia (e.g. atrial tachycardia or atrial flutter – see Section 3). **Patients with ventricular pre-excitation therefore have a tendency to episodes of paroxysmal tachycardia. This combination of (i) a short P-R interval, (ii) widening of the QRS complex with an abnormal configuration, and (iii) episodes of paroxysmal tachycardia, constitutes the Wolff-Parkinson-White (WPW) syndrome.** Note that the first two criteria are electrocardiographic and the third is clinical. All three are necessary for the diagnosis of the WPW syndrome. The presence of the two electrocardiographic criteria alone is often loosely regarded as diagnostic of the WPW syndrome, but strictly it is only diagnostic of ventricular pre-excitation, the physiological substrate which permits the paroxysmal tachycardia to occur. There are, in fact, several different types of ventricular pre-excitation. The different types have different electrocardiographic appearances and different anatomical substrates. The common type is WPW type pre-excitation.

The Mechanism of Accelerated Atrio-ventricular Conduction

Figure 148 (i) shows the normal pathway of atrio-ventricular conduction and Figure 148 (ii) the pathway in a typical case of ventricular pre-excitation.

(i) In normal conduction the depolarisation wave is initiated at the sino-atrial node and spreads in all directions through the atrial myocardium. That part of the atrial myocardium closest to the sino-atrial node (a) is the first part to be depolarised and this gives rise to the first part of the P wave. That part of the atrial myocardium most distant from the sino-atrial node (b) is the last part of the atrial myocardium to be depolarised and this gives rise to the last part of the P wave. The depolarisation wave reaches the atrio-ventricular node as soon as the myocardium adjacent to the A-V node (c) has been depolarised. This occurs at some time after the depolarisation of (a) and before that of (b), although the actual time at which the impulse reaches the A-V node cannot be recognised from the surface electrocardiogram. The route through the A-V node and His bundle provides the only pathway for depolarisation between atrial and ventricular myocardium. Since Purkinje arborisation begins earlier from the left bundle branch than from the right bundle branch (page 111) the interventricular septum is depolarised from left to right. This upper part of the interventricular septum is the first part of the ventricular myocardium to be depolarised (d) and this gives rise to the first part of the QRS complex (Figure 148 (i)).

(ii) In the presence of an accessory atrio-ventricular pathway (Figure 148 (ii)) there are two possible routes for transmission of depolarisation from atria to ventricles. The accessory pathway is depolarised at about the same time as the A-V node. However, the conduction through the accessory pathway is much faster than that through the A-V node.

Because of this, the first part of the ventricular myocardium to be depolarised is the **right** side of the interventricular septum and the septum is depolarised from right to left (e). The alteration in the initial direction of depolarisation of the ventricular myocardium changes the direction of the initial deflection in the QRS complex (from a negative to a positive wave – Figure 148 – compare e (ii) with d (i)). The initial part of the QRS complex (which begins before the completion of the P wave*) is slurred. This premature, slurred initial portion of the QRS complex (e) is called the "delta wave". The total QRS duration is prolonged since the normal pathways of intraventricular conduction are not followed (this is necessarily so since ventricular depolarisation does not start in the normal place). As a result of the simultaneous shortening of the P-R interval and lengthening of the total QRS duration, the total time from the onset of the P wave to the end of the QRS complex is approximately the same as normal (Figure 148 – compare (ii) with (i)). Since ventricular depolarisation is abnormal, ventricular repolarisation is also abnormal and there may be S-T segment depression and/or T wave inversion.

Note

* It should be clearly understood that the fact that the QRS complex normally starts well after the completion of the P wave is due to the very slow conduction in the A-V node. The depolarisation wave reaches the A-V node (c) well before the final part of the atrial myocardium is depolarised (b). The conduction velocity in the A-V node is very slow (page 111) and atrial myocardial depolarisation is normally complete before the depolarisation wave leaves the distal end of the A-V node. From this point, conduction through the His bundle and proximal part of the left bundle is very rapid (page 111).

It is illuminating to contrast the situation with that obtaining in complete left bundle branch block (Figure 148 (iii)). In this condition the pathway of atrio-ventricular conduction is normal (and therefore the P-R interval is normal). The septum is depolarised from right to left (and therefore the initial direction of the QRS deflection is opposite to normal). The pathway of

ventricular myocardial depolarisation is therefore necessarily abnormal, the time taken for this depolarisation is increased. The total QRS duration is therefore prolonged.

Figure 148 shows the similarities and differences between bundle branch block and ventricular pre-excitation and these features are emphasised in Table 7.

Figure 148

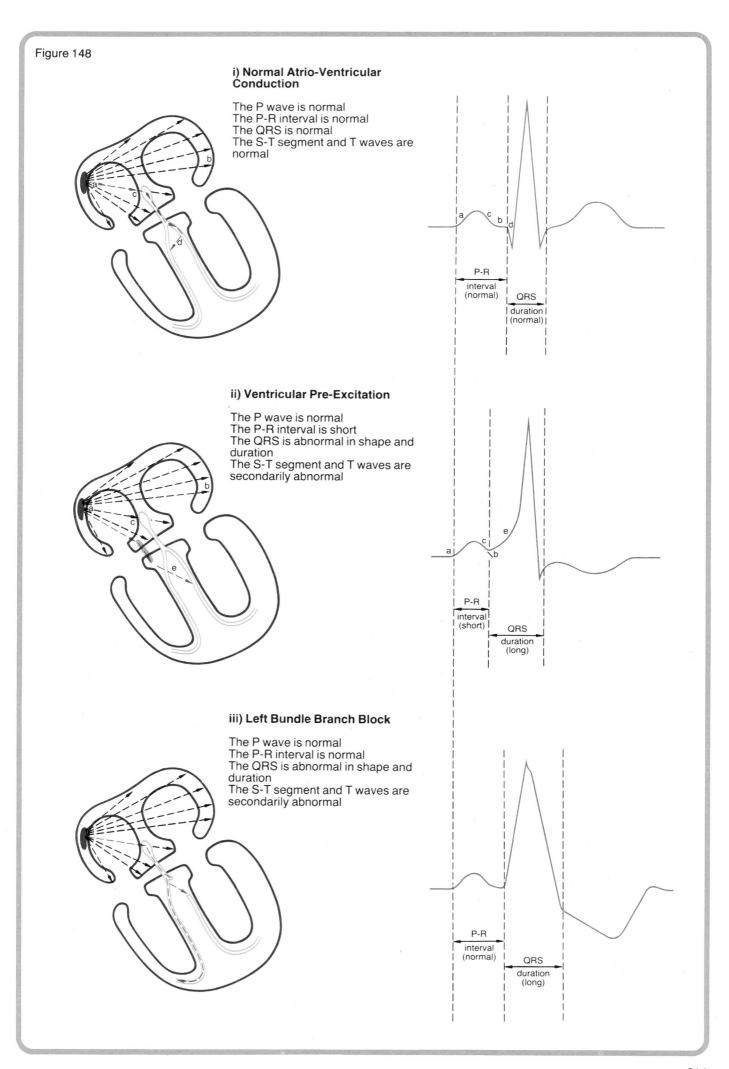

i) Normal Atrio-Ventricular Conduction

The P wave is normal
The P-R interval is normal
The QRS is normal
The S-T segment and T waves are normal

ii) Ventricular Pre-Excitation

The P wave is normal
The P-R interval is short
The QRS is abnormal in shape and duration
The S-T segment and T waves are secondarily abnormal

iii) Left Bundle Branch Block

The P wave is normal
The P-R interval is normal
The QRS is abnormal in shape and duration
The S-T segment and T waves are secondarily abnormal

Table 7

	Normal	Bundle Branch Block	Ventricular Pre-excitation
P wave	Normal	Normal	Normal
P-R interval	Normal	Normal	Abnormally short
Initial direction of QRS	Normal	Reversed	Reversed
Total QRS duration	Normal	Increased	Increased
Slurred delta wave	Absent	Absent	Present
Secondary S-T segment changes	Absent	Present	Present
Secondary T wave changes	Absent	Present	Present

Each of the electrocardiographic features of ventricular pre-excitation has its anatomical substrate as indicated in Table 8.

Table 8

ECG changes in pre-excitation	Anatomical substrate
Short P-R interval	Rapid A-V conduction through accessory pathway
Delta wave	Abnormal site of initiation of ventricular depolarisation
Prolongation of QRS duration	Abnormal site of initiation of ventricular depolarisation

Diagnostic criteria of WPW type pre-excitation

The criteria for the diagnosis of ventricular pre-excitation of the type found in the Wolff-Parkinson-White syndrome are as follows:-
1. A P-R interval of less than 0.12 sec (i.e. 0.11 sec or less*) in the presence of sinus rhythm†.
2. An abnormally wide QRS complex of more than 0.10 sec (i.e. 0.11 sec or more*).
3. The presence of initial (first 0.03 to 0.05 sec) slurring of the QRS complex.
These three criteria must **all** be fulfilled for a diagnosis of pre-excitation of the WPW type.

Additional features frequently present in WPW type pre-excitation
1. S-T segment depression and/or
2. Low-voltage T wave or T wave inversion.
3. Abnormal q waves or QS complexes may be seen in the absence of myocardial infarction (pages 216 to 220).
4. The r wave progression in the precordial leads may be abnormal (page 217).

Clinical Features Found in Association with the Full Clinical Picture of the Wolff-Parkinson-White Syndrome

1. Paroxysmal supraventricular tachycardia
or
2. Paroxysmal atrial fibrillation.

Note
* The limit of resolution of time measurements on the electrocardiogram recorded at normal speed is one quarter of one small square on the recording paper, i.e. 0.01 sec. (Thus "less than 0.12 sec" is equivalent to "0.11 sec or less" and "more than 0.10 sec" is equivalent to "0.11 sec or more").

† In the presence of atrial ectopic rhythms the P-R interval can be abnormally short simply because of the arrhythmia.

The electrocardiographic findings of WPW type pre-excitation are found in something of the order of 0.5% of routine electrocardiograms.

An example of WPW type ventricular pre-excitation is shown in Figure 149.

Note the superficial resemblance of Figure 149 to the appearances in left bundle branch block – compare Figure 149 with Figure 87 (page 123). The duration and configuration of the QRS complexes and the S-T segment and T wave appearances are virtually identical in the two cases. The fundamental difference lies in the **combination** of the short P-R interval and the delta wave. The delta wave is an early, slurred take-off of the QRS complex before the completion of the P wave (compare also Figure 148). The similarities between the QRS complexes in left bundle branch block and in this type of ventricular pre-excitation occur because in both cases the ventricular depolarisation is initiated abnormally from the upper and **right** side of the interventricular septum.

The delta wave is often directed superiorly (i.e. away from the inferior leads). In such a case the inferior leads will show a broad, slurred q wave (the delta wave in this case) which might lead to a wrongful diagnosis of inferior infarction. An example is shown in Figure 150.

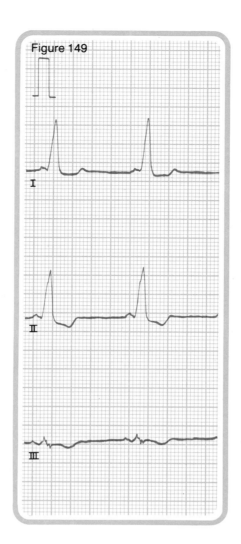

Figure 149

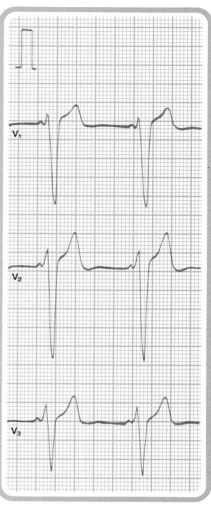

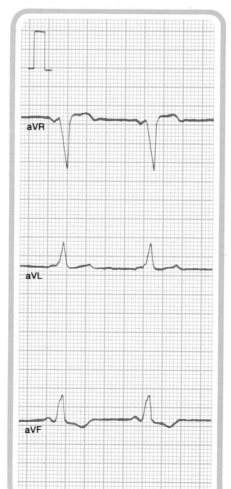

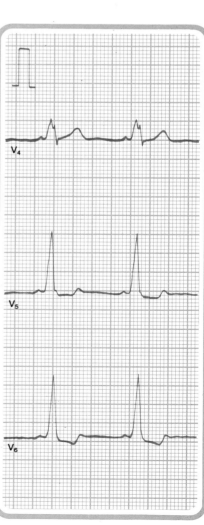

Figure 149

The rhythm is of sinus origin. The P-R interval is abnormally short at 0.06 sec (well seen in the second complex in V_1). The total QRS duration is abnormally long at 0.18 sec (well seen in both QRS complexes in V_2).

The initial slurring of the QRS complex (the delta wave) is well seen in I, V_2, V_3 and V_4. (One might expect that the delta wave would be visible in all leads, but it is always a small wave and is often inconspicuous in leads at right angles to the direction of the depolarisation giving rise to the delta wave). Non-specific S-T segment depression and T wave flattening are seen in I, II, III, aVF, V_5 and V_6.

Practical Note

The risks of serious mis-diagnosis of the electrocardiogram are substantially reduced if the following simple rules are followed:-

1. In the presence of left bundle branch block, do not diagnose myocardial infarction.

2. In the presence of pre-excitation, do not diagnose left bundle branch block or myocardial infarction.

In both cases the diagnosis of infarction **can** sometimes be made despite the prior presence of one of the two abnormalities (pre-excitation or bundle branch block), but special conditions may need to be fulfilled (such as the availability of previous records) and for the non-expert, the problem is best avoided. Under-diagnosis of the ECG is a much less serious sin than over-diagnosis.

It has been acknowledged earlier (page 212) that several different types of ventricular pre-excitation exist. Indeed the Wolff-Parkinson-White type pre-excitation has itself been divided into Types A, B and C.

In **Type A** the delta wave vector is directed anteriorly (thus the initial slurred part of the QRS complex will be positive in the anterior leads). In such a case the delta wave is positive in all the precordial leads. The remainder of the QRS is also positive in these leads. The QRS complex in V_1 has a morphology similar to that in right bundle branch block or right ventricular hypertrophy and there is often right axis deviation.

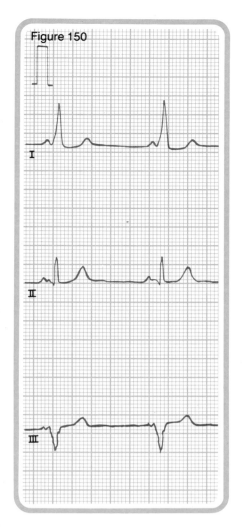

Figure 150

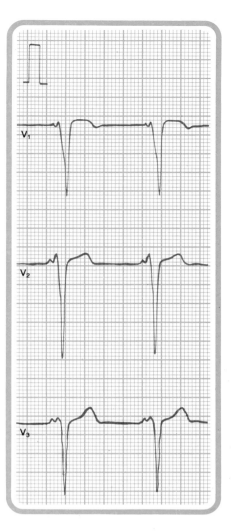

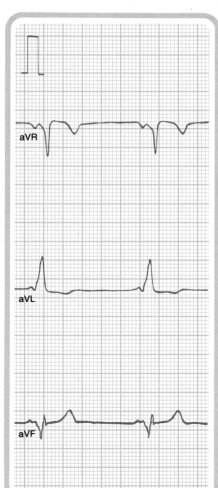

Figure 150

The rhythm is of sinus origin. The P-R interval is short at 0.05 sec (well seen in the second beat in V_2). The QRS duration is prolonged at 0.14 sec (well seen in I). There is a slurred initial part to the QRS complex (the delta wave) well seen in I, aVL and V_6. Abnormal Q waves are seen in aVF. In the absence of ventricular pre-excitation this would indicate inferior infarction. In the presence of pre-excitation it has no such significance. There is nothing in this record to indicate the presence of infarction.

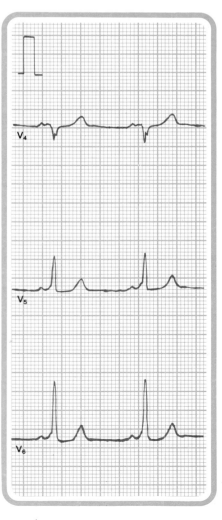

In **Type B** the delta wave vector may be negative or positive in the right precordial leads, but the dominant QRS deflection is negative in the right and positive in the left precordial leads, and the morphology of the QRS complex resembles that of left bundle branch block. Type B is much commoner than Type A and Figures 149 and 150 both show examples of Type B. In each case the delta wave is positive in V_1-V_3. When it is negative in these leads QS complexes will occur. Figure 151 shows an example of Type A. Both the delta wave and the main QRS deflections are upright from V_1-V_5. In both types the r wave progression in the precordial leads will often be abnormal. Unless the presence of ventricular pre-excitation is recognised this too may lead to a false diagnosis of myocardial infarction.

In **either Type A or Type B** the delta wave vector may be directed superiorly – in which case abnormal q waves will appear in any of the Leads II, III and aVF.

Type C is much rarer even than Type A. In this type the delta wave is negative in V_5 and V_6 but positive in V_1 to V_4.

It cannot be emphasised too strongly that abnormal q waves or QS complexes in ANY lead do not indicate myocardial infarction if there is evidence of ventricular pre-excitation.

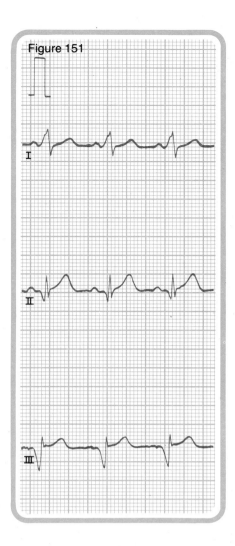

Figure 151

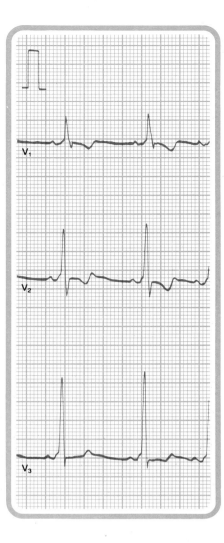

Figure 151

The rhythm is sinus. The P-R interval is abnormally short at 0.08 sec (well seen in V_1 and V_2). The total QRS duration is abnormal at 0.12 sec (well seen in V_2 and V_3) and there is a delta wave (well seen in I, aVL, V_1-V_5). The q waves in II, III and aVF are abnormal but do **not** indicate infarction. The S-T segment abnormalities in V_1-V_3 are a result of the pre-excitation. The dominant R wave in V_1 is not indicative either of right ventricular hypertrophy or of true posterior infarction – it is a result of the ventricular pre-excitation.

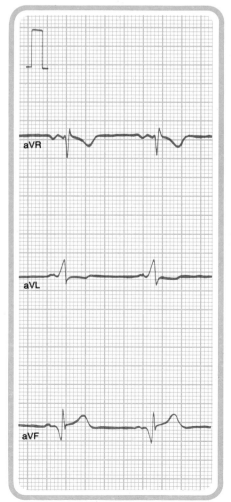

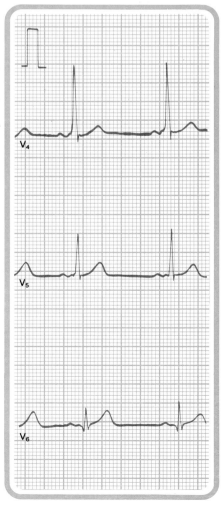

Doubt has recently been expressed about the validity of the classification of ECG patterns in ventricular pre-excitation. Numerous anatomical possibilities, each with its own resulting ECG pattern, are now known to exist.

Other Types of Ventricular Pre-excitation

In addition to the WPW type, other forms of pre-excitation exist. The next most common type is the **Lown-Ganong-Levine (LGL) syndrome.**

> The **electrocardiographic criteria** for the LGL type pre-excitation
> 1. A P-R interval (in the adult) of less than 0.12 sec (i.e. 0.11 sec or less[*]
> 2. A normal QRS duration with no delta wave.

Patients with pre-excitation of the LGL type have a tendency to episodes of paroxysmal supraventricular tachycardia (in the same way as those with WPW type pre-excitation). Patients who have the electrocardiographic features of LGL type pre-excitation, together with the **clinical criterion** of having had episodes of paroxysmal tachycardia have the LGL syndrome.

Note that since the QRS complexes are normal, the electrocardiographic findings are not confused with bundle branch block or myocardial infarction.

An example of the ECG appearances in LGL syndrome is seen in Figure 152.

In the LGL syndrome the accessory pathway is thought to run from the atrial myocardium to the distal part of the A-V node or to the beginning of the His bundle, thus short-circuiting the normal A-V nodal delay (with consequent reduction in the P-R interval) whilst permitting normal intraventricular conduction (with consequent normality of the QRS complex).

Note

[*] The limit of resolution of time measurements on the electrocardiogram recorded at normal speed is one quarter of one small square on the recording paper, i.e. 0.01 sec.

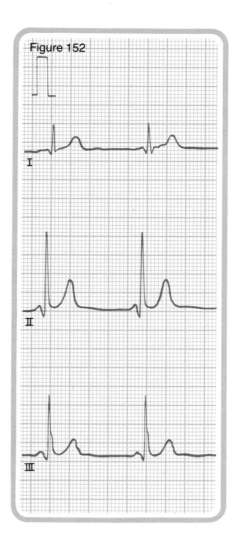

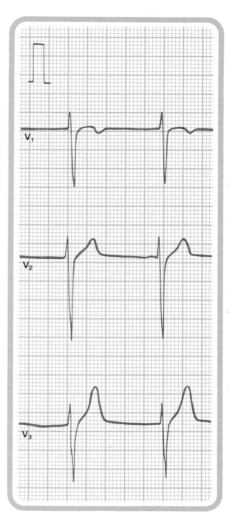

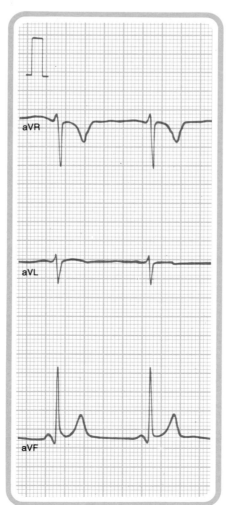

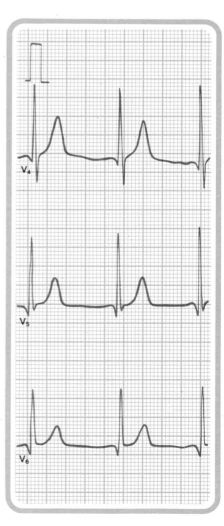

Figure 152

The basic rhythm is of sinus origin. The P-R interval is abnormally short at 0.08 sec. The QRS complexes are normal. The P waves are hardly visible in the precordial leads. This indicates that the P wave vector is directed superiorly and inferiorly and therefore has no major component in the horizontal plane.

The Significance of Ventricular Pre-excitation

Ventricular pre-excitation is relatively uncommon. In terms of its frequency a totally disproportionate amount of space has been devoted to it in this book. This apparently undue emphasis is, however, justifiable in view of the real risk of mistakenly making a diagnosis of serious heart disease when the ECG shows pre-excitation.

The only real clinical consequence of ventricular pre-excitation is episodic supraventricular tachycardia. These attacks may often be a nuisance and can be temporarily disabling but do not usually constitute a risk to the patient unless the rhythm is atrial fibrillation (this is rare – normally it is atrial tachycardia).

The important diagnoses which can be made in error through misinterpretation of an ECG actually showing pre-excitation include the following:-

1. Inferior myocardial infarction (in Types A, B or C).
2. Anterior myocardial infarction (in Types B or C).
3. Left bundle branch block (in Type B).
4. Right bundle branch block (in Types A and C).
5. Right ventricular hypertrophy (in Types A and C).
6. True posterior infarction (in Types A and C).

Also, during an episode of atrial tachycardia in a patient with ventricular pre-excitation, ventricular tachycardia may be mistakenly diagnosed – see Section 3. About 50% of patients with electrocardiographic evidence of ventricular pre-excitation have episodes of paroxysmal tachycardia.

Digitalis – induced Changes in the ECG

Digitalis has complex effects on the heart. It induces both electrical and mechanical changes **directly** by inhibiting the normal active process of sodium ion transport across the membranes of both myocardial and pacemaker cells. This primary interference with sodium ion transport necessarily results in secondary changes in potassium ion movement across the membranes. Digitalis and potassium ions have mutually antagonistic effects on ion-flux across cell membranes (especially flux involving sodium and calcium ions). Digitalis also has **indirect** effects on the heart by increasing the vagal tone.

When a patient is receiving a digitalis preparation in therapeutic doses the electrocardiogram may show recognisable changes, but need not necessarily do so. When such changes are seen they are referred to as "digitalis effect". Digitalis effect does not indicate overdosage and is in no way synonymous with "digitalis toxicity" (*vide infra*).

The possible changes induced by digitalis on the electrocardiogram are:-

1. **Decreased T wave amplitude.**
2. **S-T segment depression.**
3. **Increase in U wave amplitude.**
4. **Shortening of the Q-T interval.**
} "digitalis effect"

5. **Development of various cardiac arrhythmias – arrhythmias due to digitalis are always a sign of toxicity.**
6. **Combinations of the above.**

Whether or not a patient receiving digitalis develops recognisable changes of digitalis effect depends upon a whole variety of factors including the dose of digitalis, the physical size and age of the patient, the general metabolic state (in particular the thyroid function) the serum potassium level and the presence or absence of ventricular hypertrophy.

T Wave Changes

One of the earliest and commonest changes is reduction in the voltage of the T waves. This is, of course, a non-specific change, which has many other possible causes. When it is present it is certainly not possible by inspecting the electrocardiogram to assert that the changes are due to the action of digitalis though the knowledge that the patient is receiving digitalis makes it a possibility (secondary interpretation). The T wave changes are most often seen in leads facing the left ventricle (left precordial leads and those limb leads orientated in the region of the cardiac axis – i.e. aVL and I when the heart is horizontal and II, aVF and III when the heart is vertical). In the presence of right ventricular hypertrophy the T wave changes induced by digitalis may be most pronounced in the right precordial leads. Occasionally the T wave changes may be so pronounced as to give biphasic or even inverted (negative) T waves.

S-T Segment Change

The most frequently recognised finding of digitalis effect is a downward sloping S-T segment depression. This is often associated with T wave flattening and the combined appearance of the sloping S-T segment and flattened T wave has been said to be similar to a reversed tick (or the tick made by a left-handed person) (Figure 153).

Figure 153

This shows the appearances in a left precordial lead in a normal subject (a) in the presence of mild (b) and more pronounced (c) changes of digitalis effect.

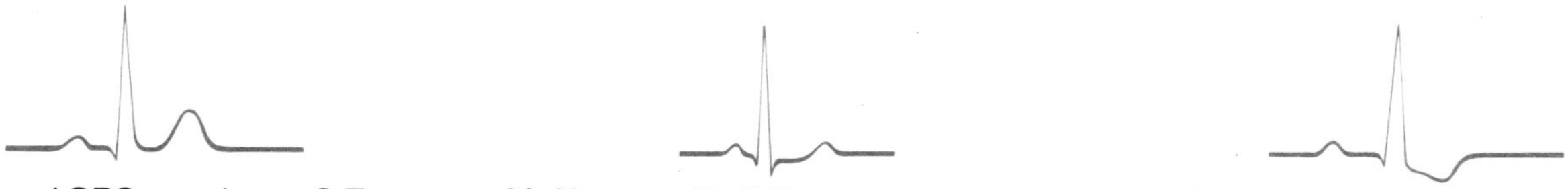

a) Normal QRS complexes, S-T segment and T waves.

b) Non-specific S-T segment depression with reduction in T wave voltage.

c) Downward sloping S-T segment depression with flat T waves – highly typical of, but not diagnostic of, digitalis effect.

Increased U Wave Amplitude

The normal U wave is smaller than the preceding T wave. The U wave becomes more prominent when the patient takes digitalis. The increased U wave height is usually best seen in the mid-precordial leads. The degree of increase in U wave height is usually slight and is less than that found in hypokalaemia or in response to quinidine therapy.

Shortening of the Q-T Interval

The normal Q-T interval bears an inverse relationship to the heart rate. The normality or otherwise of the Q-T interval can only be determined if the Q-T interval measurement is evaluated in relation to the heart rate at the time (see pages 263 and 264). As a rough guide the normal Q-T interval is in the region of 0.36 to 0.44 sec for adults with heart rates in the region of 60-90 per min. As the heart rate increases the Q-T interval falls and vice-versa. The Q-T interval changes in digitalis therapy are slight and rarely recognised unless specifically sought.

The changes in T waves, S-T segments, U waves and Q-T interval described above are the features known as "digitalis effect". An example of "digitalis effect" is shown in Figure 154.

Digitalis Toxicity

The above effects may be found in any patient receiving treatment with digitalis. In the presence of digitalis over-dosage, toxicity occurs. This most frequently presents with gastro-intestinal symptoms such as nausea, anorexia and vomiting and may occasionally present with visual disturbances.

Digitalis-induced arrhythmias are always a manifestation of **toxicity** rather than just digitalis effect. When death occurs as a result of digitalis toxicity, it is always due to ventricular fibrillation.

The common arrhythmias occurring in digitalis toxicity are:-

1. Ventricular premature (ectopic) beats.
2. Coupled ventricular premature beats.
3. Multifocal ventricular premature beats.
4. Nodal (junctional) tachycardia.
5. Sinus bradycardia.
6. Atrial tachycardia with atrio-ventricular block.
7. First-degree heart block (first-degree atrio-ventricular block).
8. Mobitz Type I second-degree atrio-ventricular block (Wenckebach phenomenon).
9. Third-degree atrio-ventricular block.
10. Multifocal atrial premature (ectopic) beats.
11. Ventricular tachycardia.
12. Atrial flutter.
13. Atrial fibrillation.
14. Sino-atrial block.
15. Sinus arrest.
16. Ventricular fibrillation.

The recognition of these arrhythmias will be dealt with in Section 3.

Digitalis toxicity may also occasionally give rise to widening of the QRS complexes even in the absence of arrhythmias.

Figure 154

The rhythm is sinus. The record is normal except for the presence of S-T, T changes. There is S-T segment depression in II, III and aVF and in V_4 to V_6. The T waves are of low voltage in the limb leads and in V_5 and V_6. These changes are non-specific. They are **consistent with** but not **diagnostic of** digitalis effect.

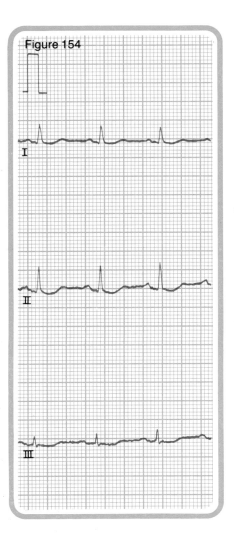

Figure 154

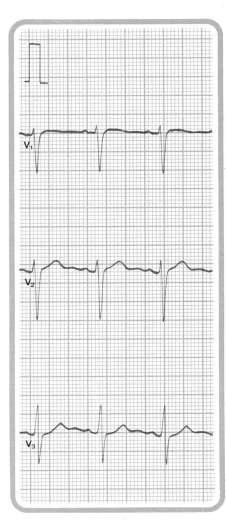

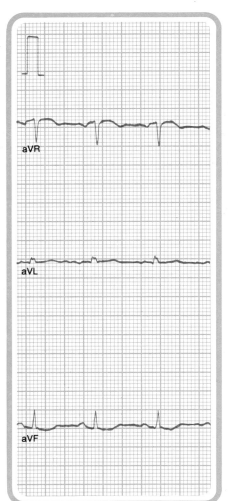

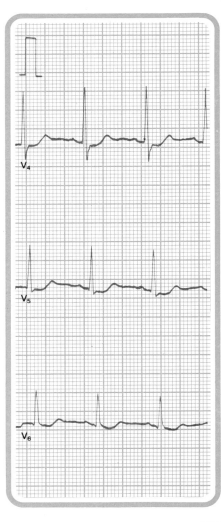

Effects of Other Drugs on the ECG

Numerous drugs produce relatively minor changes in the ECG, some of the commoner, more important ones are listed below:-

Quinidine

1. Low voltage T waves (or T wave inversion).
2. S-T segment depression.
3. Prolongation of the Q-T interval.
4. Increased height of U wave.
5. Widening and notching of P waves.

In toxic doses, quinidine gives rise to widening of the QRS complexes and serious arrhythmias, including heart block, ventricular tachycardia and ventricular fibrillation. Sometimes less severe arrhythmias occur such as sinus bradycardia, sinus arrest or sino-atrial block.

Propranolol (and other beta-blocking drugs)

The most obvious effect is the reduction of the sinus rate. No significant changes in the QRS complexes, S-T segments or T waves occur. Rarely the degree of A-V block may be increased in patients with A-V conduction abnormalities. In patients with atrial fibrillation or atrial flutter, the ventricular rate is reduced.

Phenothiazine drugs and Tricyclic antidepressants

These produce changes similar to those of quinidine.

Lignocaine

In therapeutic doses lignocaine has no recognisable effect on the electrocardiogram. In toxic doses sinus tachycardia, sinus arrest or atrio-ventricular block may occur.

Mexiletine

The actions of this drug are similar to those of lignocaine. In therapeutic doses it has no detectable effect on the electrocardiogram. In toxic doses the central nervous system is primarily affected but sinus bradycardia, nodal rhythm or, rarely, A-V conduction disturbances can occur.

Aprindine, tocainide and lidoflazine are other congeners of lignocaine with similar, minimal effects on the ECG in therapeutic doses. Of the group, lidoflazine has been reported as possibly giving rise to serious ventricular arrhythmias occasionally.

Diphenylhydantoin

In normal doses no noticeable effect on the ECG occurs. Occasionally the P-R interval may be increased and the Q-T interval diminished. In the presence of extensive myocardial disease the intravenous administration of this drug has occasionally been followed by bradycardia, A-V block, asystole or venticular fibrillation.

Procainamide

Therapeutic doses produce only minimal changes. As the dose is increased, prolongation of the P-R interval, QRS duration and Q-T interval occurs. The T wave voltage is reduced and the U wave height increased.

Toxic doses may give rise to gross widening of the QRS complexes, ventricular ectopic beats, ventricular tachycardia, ventricular fibrillation or asystole. These effects are more commonly seen after intravenous administration, than after oral therapy.

Disopyramide

In therapeutic doses the effects are minimal. As the dose is increased, changes similar to those seen with quinidine occur.

Verapamil

This drug acts primarily by inhibiting the slow calcium channel in the myocardial cell membrane. It produces a slowing of the sinus rate and of conduction through the atrio-ventricular node. The latter effect gives rise ultimately to prolongation of the P-R interval. There is no change in the QRS complexes or in the corrected Q-T interval.

The effects of the drug on the sino-atrial and atrio-ventricular nodes are additive with those of beta-blocking drugs and the use of verapamil and beta-blocking drugs simultaneously can give rise to profound and occasionally catastrophic bradycardia.

Nifedipine

This drug is also a slow calcium channel blocker. Its effect on the heart is much less pronounced than that of verapamil, and it has much more effect on the peripheral circulation. No significant changes in the P waves, P-R interval or QRS complexes occur even at doses which produce profound haemodynamic effects.

Perhexilene

This slow calcium channel blocker produces a slowing of the sinus rate, probably by a direct effect on the sino-atrial node. No other significant effects on the electrocardiogram have been noted, but the use of this drug is severely limited by its side effects on liver function and on peripheral nerves.

Amiodarone

Gives rise to prolongation of the Q-T interval and increase in the height of the U waves. This is in keeping with its characteristic electrophysiological effect of prolongation of the action potential.

Electrolyte Disturbances

The normal state of polarisation of cardiac cell membranes is dependent upon the maintenance of normal ionic balance across the membranes. The processes of depolarisation and repolarisation are related to ionic fluxes. It is therefore predictable that disturbance of the normal levels of electrolyte in extracellular or intracellular fluids may give rise to electro-cardiographic changes.

The most important ion in the maintenance of the normal state of polarisation of the membranes is the potassium ion. The resting transmembrane potential is, for all practical purposes, determined by the ratio of intracellular to extracellular potassium ion concentration.* The normal extracellular potassium ion concentration lies in the range 3.5 to 5.0mmol/l. The intracellular concentration is of the order of 140mmol/l. Substantial changes in the extracellular levels may occur in disease states. Changes in intracellular levels in diseases are proportionately much smaller. In view of this difference in the degree to which variations in the intracellular and extracellular absolute levels of potassium concentration can occur, together with the fact that it is the **ratio** of intracellular and extracellular levels which determines membrane stability, it follows that the absolute extracellular level of potassium ion concentration is the single most important factor affecting the cell membranes and therefore also the electrocardiogram. The often repeated assertion that the ECG is a guide to **intracellular** potassium ion levels is false and is the result of confused thinking. It is often also stated that the ECG can be used to monitor the potassium state of the patient. Since the correlation of the degree of ECG changes with the degree of abnormality of the extracellular potassium ion concentration is poor, this is not practicable advice. Indeed none of those who give this advice appear to take it themselves. They always measure the serum potassium ion level when they are concerned about the patient's potassium status (and rightly so!).

* **Note**

$$Em = \frac{RT}{F} \ln \frac{[K^+]_o}{[K^+]_i}$$

where
Em = resting membrane potential
T = absolute temperature
F = Faraday's number
R = Universal gas constant

$[K^+]_o$ = extracellular potassium ion concentration
$[K^+]_i$ = intracellular potassium ion concentration

ECG Changes in Hyperkalaemia

Hyperkalaemia produces changes in the electrocardiogram which are increasingly more severe as the potassium ion level rises. There is, in other words, a **direct** correlation between the degree of increase in the serum potassium ion level and the resulting ECG changes. However, this correlation is **neither precise nor totally consistent.**

If hyperkalaemia is suspected the serum potassium ion level should be measured. If hyperkalaemia is to be "monitored", changes in the serum potassium ion level should be followed. Hyperkalaemia is always a serious problem demanding urgent attention in view of the constant risk of ventricular fibrillation.

An enormous range of possible changes occurs in hyperkalaemia. A few of these are listed in Figure 155.

There are no diagnostic changes of hyperkalaemia. All the changes are non-specific and may be seen in myocardial damage arising from other causes, e.g. infarction and drugs. All parts of the ECG – P waves, QRS complexes, S-T segments, T waves and the cardiac rhythm may be affected in hyperkalaemia.

The typical, progressive changes of hyperkalaemia are as follows:-

Development of tall, pointed narrow T waves.

↓

Reduction in P wave amplitude, reduction in R wave height, widening of QRS complexes, S-T segment change (elevation in some leads, depression in others), development of hemiblock (especially left anterior hemiblock) development of first degree heart block.

↓

More advanced intraventricular block (very wide QRS complexes with right bundle branch block, left bundle branch block, bifascicular or trifascicular block) ventricular ectopic beats.

↓

Absent P waves. Very broad and bizarre QRS complexes (often simulating infarction). Atrio-ventricular block, ventricular tachycardia or fibrillation or ventricular asystole.

In modern clinical practice it is unusual for changes more advanced than the earliest change of tall pointed T waves to be seen. Such tall T waves do not necessarily indicate hyperkalaemia for they may be seen in the precordial leads as a normal variant or in true posterior ischaemia. The diagnosis of or exclusion of hyperkalaemia when there is such a finding is by measurement of the serum level of potassium ions.

Figure 155

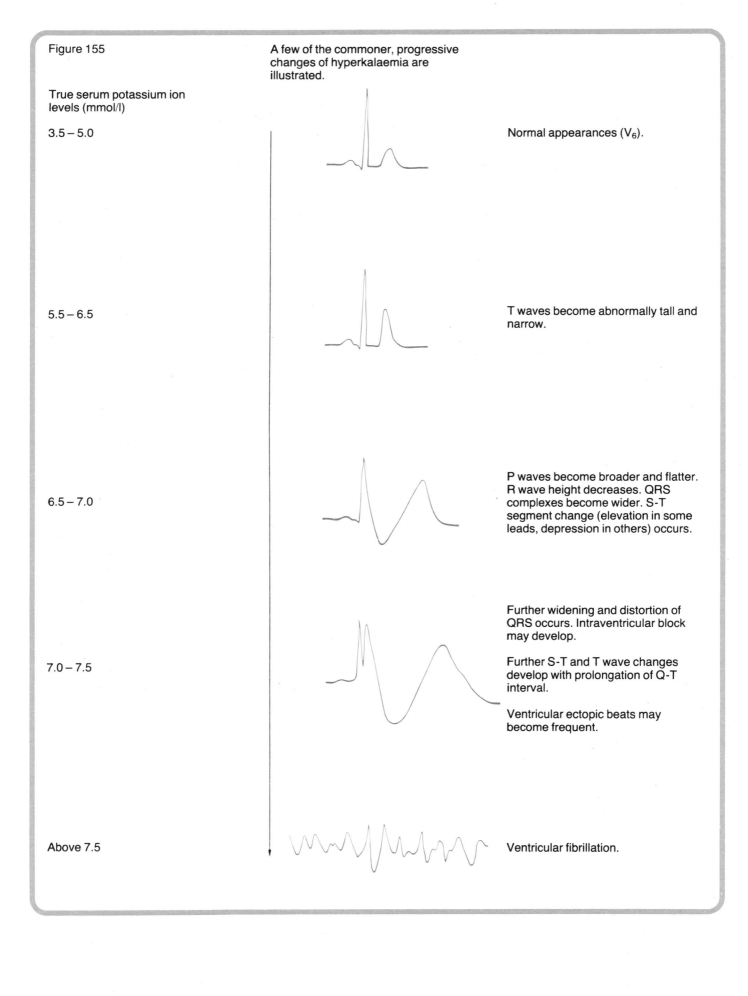

A few of the commoner, progressive changes of hyperkalaemia are illustrated.

True serum potassium ion levels (mmol/l)

3.5 – 5.0 — Normal appearances (V$_6$).

5.5 – 6.5 — T waves become abnormally tall and narrow.

6.5 – 7.0 — P waves become broader and flatter. R wave height decreases. QRS complexes become wider. S-T segment change (elevation in some leads, depression in others) occurs.

7.0 – 7.5 — Further widening and distortion of QRS occurs. Intraventricular block may develop.

Further S-T and T wave changes develop with prolongation of Q-T interval.

Ventricular ectopic beats may become frequent.

Above 7.5 — Ventricular fibrillation.

ECG Changes in Hypokalaemia

Significant hypokalaemia can exist without recognisable changes on the electrocardiogram and when such changes are present, the correlation between the extent of the change and the degree of hypokalaemia is very poor. However, hypokalaemia is encountered much more commonly than hyperkalaemia.

The changes found in hypokalaemia (in descending order of frequency) are:

1. S-T segment depression, decreased amplitude of the T waves, increased U wave height.

2. Cardiac arrhythmias.

3. Prolongation of the QRS duration, increase in P wave amplitude and duration.

Figure 156 shows an example of the most commonly seen changes.

The S-T segment, T wave and U wave changes of hypokalaemia illustrated in Figure 156 are by far the commonest changes seen in hypokalaemia.

Less common changes include minimal (and usually unnoticed) prolongation of the QRS complexes and (rarely) increase in amplitude and duration of the P waves.

Many different types of arrhythmia can occur when the serum potassium ion level falls (since the ratio of extracellular to intracellular potassium ion concentration becomes abnormal and the cell membrane becomes less stable). These arrhythmias include atrial ectopic beats, atrial tachycardia, ventricular ectopic beats, ventricular tachycardia, first, second and third degree heart block and ventricular fibrillation. When unexplained arrhythmias develop, it is worth checking the serum potassium ion level.

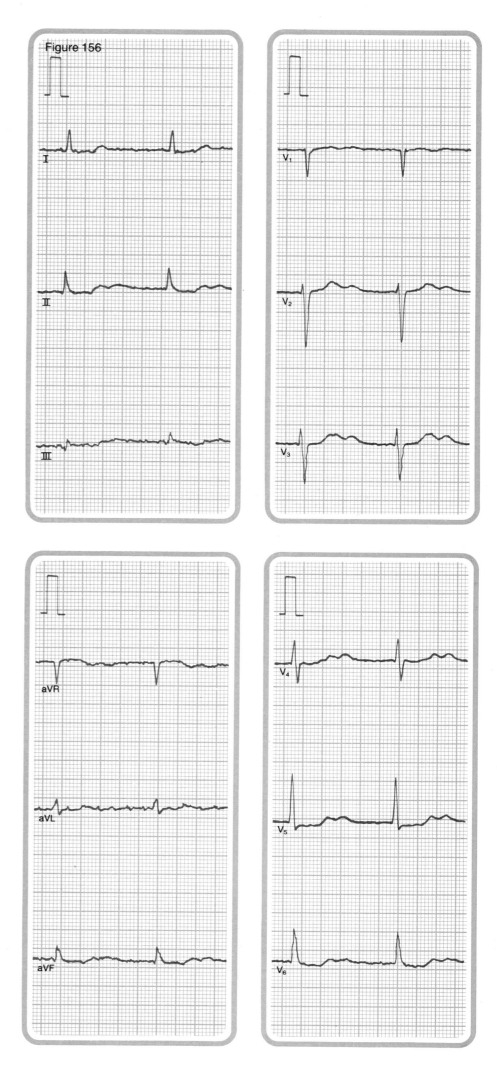

Figure 156

The rhythm is sinus. The T waves are of low voltage in every lead. There is S-T segment depression in I, II, aVF and V_4–V_6. There are abnormally tall U waves seen in II, aVF and V_4–V_6 (in all these leads the U waves are taller than the preceding T waves). The U waves are also prominent in V_1–V_3.

Hypocalcaemia

The main electrocardiographic change in hypocalcaemia is prolongation of the Q-T interval. The duration of the T wave (though it is not usual to measure the T wave duration) is not changed. The S-T segment is prolonged. The degree of prolongation of the Q-T interval is approximately proportional to the degree of lowering of the level of ionic calcium in the serum. It is said that hypocalcaemia is the **only** condition which gives rise to prolongation of the S-T segment without either (i) increased T wave duration or (ii) apparent increased T wave duration due to prominence of the U waves.

Hypothermia may present an exception to this rule.

The ECG changes of hypocalcaemia appear to be of little significance. They are usually unrecognised clinically unless it is known that the serum calcium ion level is low and they are specifically looked for. The P waves, P-R interval and U waves are usually unaltered. The QRS morphology is usually unchanged. The QRS duration may be slightly reduced but it is rare for this to be noticed. Hypocalcaemia does not usually give rise to arrhythmias.

Hypercalcaemia

The main electrocardiographic change in hypercalcaemia is reduction in the Q-T interval. The T wave duration appears unaffected, the reduction being in the duration of the S-T segment. The degree of reduction in the Q-T interval is approximately proportional to the increase in the serum concentration of ionic calcium. At very high levels of serum calcium ions this relationship breaks down because progressive T wave prolongation occurs, offsetting the effect of the reducing S-T duration on the total Q-T interval.

No appreciable change occurs in the P, QRS or T morphology. The dimensions of these deflections are not usually significantly altered except for the above noted tendency for the T wave to become prolonged at very high serum levels of calcium. The U wave amplitude may increase, sometimes contributing to the apparent T wave duration.

Significant cardiac arrhythmias do not often result from hypercalcaemia. However, slight prolongation of the P-R interval and occasionally second or third degree A-V block have been described.

Patients with hypercalcaemia have an increased sensitivity to digitalis. Sinus arrest, sino-atrial block, atrial or ventricular ectopic beats, ventricular tachycardia and ventricular fibrillation have all been described in hypercalcaemic patients taking digitalis. It is said that the intravenous administration of calcium to a fully digitalised patient is potentially dangerous. Fatalities have been recorded in this situation.

Hypo- and Hyper-magnesaemia

Minor electrocardiographic changes are described in both of these electrolyte disturbances. Since there are often simultaneous abnormalities of other electrolytes their specificity is uncertain.

In hypomagnesaemia, changes resembling those of hypokalaemia occur with flattening of the T waves, S-T segment depression, prominence of the U waves and occasionally prolongation of the P-R interval. Like hypokalaemia and hypercalcaemia, hypomagnesaemia aggravates digitalis toxicity. A whole variety of arrhythmias including ventricular fibrillation has been described in association with hypomagnesaemia, but there is frequently associated hypokalaemia and digitalis is often also implicated. Significant arrhythmias induced solely by hypomagnesaemia must be very rare.

The electrocardiographic changes associated with hypermagnesaemia are similar to those in hyperkalaemia. There may be prolongation of the P-R interval and widening of the QRS complexes.

Hypo- and Hyper-natraemia

No significant changes appear in the electrocardiogram in response to changes in the serum level of sodium ions.

Hypothyroidism

Biochemical and clinical hypothyroidism can exist without any recognisable ECG changes. However, when hypothyroidism is severe or prolonged, generalised ECG changes occur. These are the result of interstitial myocardial oedema and often also of the additional presence of a pericardial effusion.

The changes of hypothyroidism are:-
1. **Sinus bradycardia.**
2. **Low voltages of P waves, QRS complexes and T waves.**
3. **Slight S-T segment depression.**
4. **Prolongation of the P-R interval.**
5. **Atrio-ventricular block (occasionally).**
6. **Prominent U waves may occur.**
7. **The Q-Tc interval may be prolonged but measurement of this may be difficult or impossible since the T wave amplitude is diminished and the U wave height may be increased.**

An example is shown in Figure 157.

The changes of hypothyroidism usually resolve within the first few weeks of thyroid replacement therapy. Occasionally improvement may even be apparent within the first few days of treatment.

Arrhythmias are not especially common in hypothyroidism (except for sinus bradycardia) but atrial tachycardia, A-V junctional escape rhythm, A-V block of various degrees and right or left bundle branch block occasionally occur.

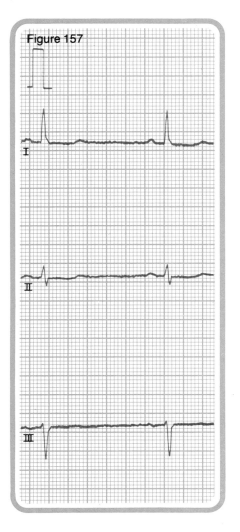

Figure 157

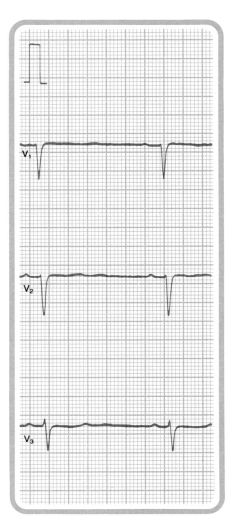

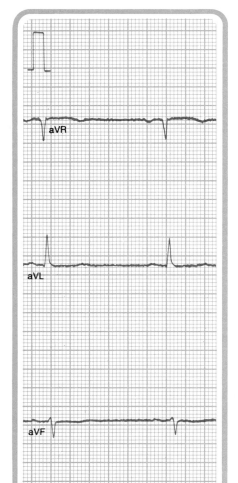

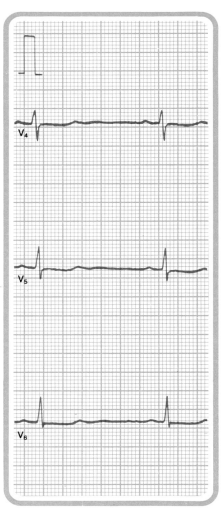

Figure 157

The rhythm is sinus bradycardia. The T waves are of low voltage in every lead. The P waves are of low voltage. The tallest R wave in the precordial leads is 8mm (V_6) – the precordial QRS complexes are therefore of abnormally low voltage (at least one R wave in the precordial series should **exceed** 8mm). There is S-T segment depression in II and V_4–V_6. Prominent U waves (not large but larger than the corresponding T waves) are seen in V_2–V_6.

230

Hyperthyroidism

This produces no morphological change in the electrocardiogram but arrhythmias may occur. Sinus tachycardia is the rule and atrial tachycardia, atrial fibrillation or atrial flutter may occur.

Pericarditis

Acute pericarditis almost always gives rise to transient ECG changes – of which by far the **most typical and most common is generalised S-T segment elevation.** It is thought that this change is due to inflammation of the myocardium in the sub-epicardial region (adjacent to the inflamed pericardium). The only other common cause of S-T elevation is acute myocardial ischaemic damage. It is widely taught that the main difference between the S-T segment elevation of acute pericarditis and the S-T segment of acute myocardial ischaemic damage lies in the configuration of the S-T segments (which are convex upwards in acute myocardial ischaemic damage, and concave upwards in acute pericarditis). However, a more obvious and reliable discriminator is the fact that the S-T segment change in ischaemic damage is **localised** whereas the S-T segment change in pericarditis is **generalised.** This is simply because acute pericarditis is usually a generalised inflammatory process involving the whole of the pericardium, whereas myocardial ischaemic damage is typically localised to one area. The only form of myocardial ischaemic damage which is generalised is sub-endocardial ischaemia and this usually gives rise to S-T segment depression or to T wave inversion.

In pericarditis, there is S-T segment elevation in all the precordial leads and in all the limb leads except those facing the cavity of the ventricles (i.e. aVR (always), aVL (in vertical hearts), and III (in horizontal hearts)). In limb leads facing the cavity of the heart in this way there will be S-T segment depression. In any limb lead at right angles to the frontal plane axis, there will be no significant S-T segment deviation since there will only be a tiny QRS deviation. An example of the changes in acute pericarditis is shown in Figure 158.

If there is a pericardial effusion associated with the acute pericarditis there may be reduction in the P, QRS and T voltages in all leads, but this is relatively uncommon.

The changes in acute pericarditis are transient. After the acute illness is over the ECG usually returns completely to normal. In a small proportion of cases chronic constrictive pericarditis may develop. The changes associated with chronic pericarditis are non-specific. These include:-

1. Abnormal P waves – notched or abnormally wide.

2. S-T segment depression (in most leads).

3. Low voltage T waves or T wave inversion (in most leads).

4. Atrial arrhythmias (atrial ectopic beats, atrial tachycardia, atrial flutter, atrial fibrillation).

5. Abnormal right axis deviation.

6. Generalised low voltage QRS complexes.

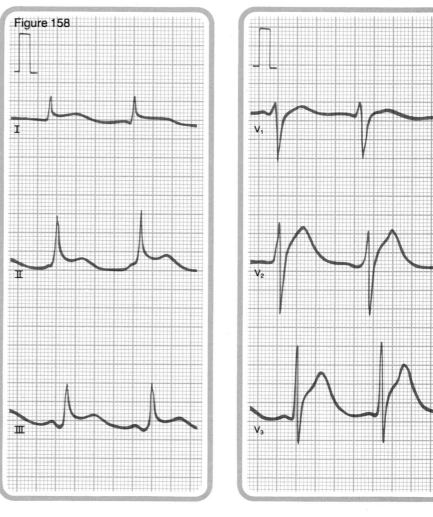

Figure 158

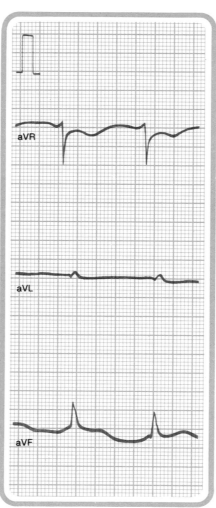

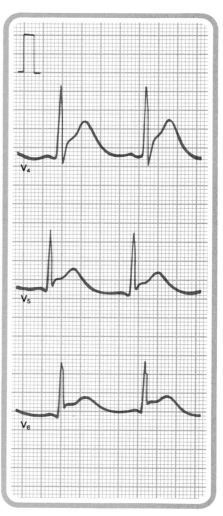

Figure 158

The rhythm is sinus tachycardia. The QRS complexes are normal. There is S-T segment elevation in Leads I, II, III, aVF, and V_1–V_6. The S-T elevation is concave upwards. There is no S-T segment shift in aVL since this lead is at right angles to the frontal plane axis. The only lead in which there is S-T depression is aVR which is a **cavity** lead. The S-T segment deflection in this lead is opposite to that in the surface leads because, and only because, the lead is looking into the cavity of the heart. It is therefore **not** a reciprocal change. Reciprocal changes in myocardial infarction are seen in leads "reciprocal to" the primary changes but the reciprocal leads and the primary leads are both looking at the external surface of the heart (see page 182).

ECG Changes in Acute Disorders of the Central Nervous System

For reasons which are not adequately understood, several types of acute disturbance in the central nervous system give rise to electrocardiographic changes. ECG changes can be seen in relation to infections or tumours in the central nervous system, after head injuries and after neurosurgery, but are most commonly seen in association with subarachnoid haemorrhage and intracranial haemorrhage.

Subarachnoid Haemorrhage

More than 50% of patients with subarachnoid or intracranial haemorrhage develop transient ECG changes.

The most common changes in central nervous system disease are:-

1. **Deep T wave inversion.**
2. **Abnormally tall T waves.**
3. **Prominent U waves.**
4. **S-T segment elevation or depression.**
5. **Prolongation of the Q-T interval.**
6. **Arrhythmias (sinus tachycardia, sinus bradycardia, nodal rhythm, atrial fibrillation, ventricular tachycardia).**

The changes are non-specific but this does not mean that they are necessarily minor or that they are non-significant. The changes can be very impressive indeed. Where there is S-T segment elevation, pericarditis can be wrongly suspected. Where there is extensive, deep, symmetrical T wave inversion, subendocardial infarction can be wrongly suspected. (Occasionally, even abnormal Q waves may develop).

The most generally accepted explanation of the pathogenesis of ECG changes in central nervous system disease is that the changes occur as a result of sympathetic or parasympathetic activity resulting from damage in central areas rich in autonomic connections, but some pathological studies have suggested that subendocardial haemorrhage may occur in acute central nervous system disturbances and that these cardiac effects cause the ECG abnormalities.

Figure 159 shows the appearances in a patient with acute subarachnoid haemorrhage. The patient had no evidence of primary cardiac disease. The record was taken within 24 hours of the onset of symptoms. There was no clinical evidence of pericarditis.

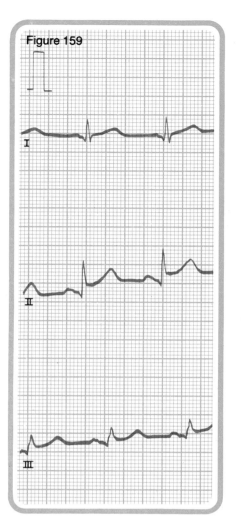

Figure 159

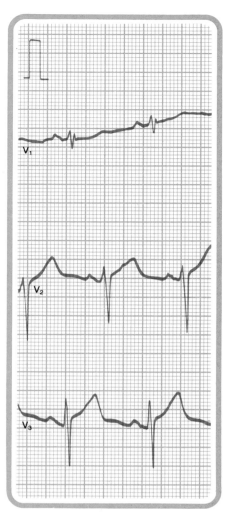

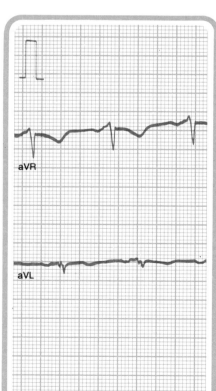

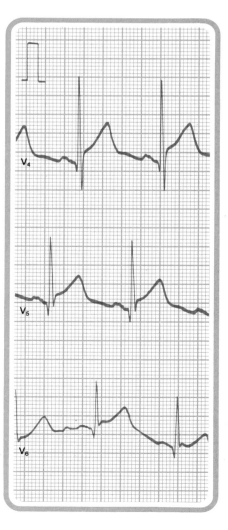

Figure 159

The rhythm is sinus. The mean frontal
plane QRS axis is +75°. Since the heart
is therefore vertical, the appearance in
aVL (with prominent q waves and
T wave inversion) is within normal limits.
There are prominent but not abnormal q
waves in the left precordial leads. There
is a small secondary r wave in V_1
(incomplete right bundle branch block –
see page 119). The striking abnormality
is S-T elevation in I, II, III, aVF and V_2-V_6.
The changes resemble those of acute
pericarditis (compare Figure 158).
Figure 160 shows the appearances in the
electrocardiogram taken from the same
patient, one week later.

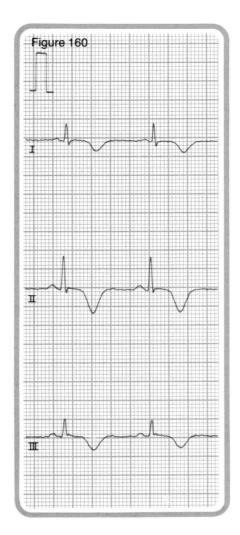

Figure 160

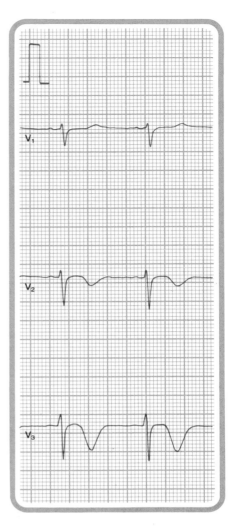

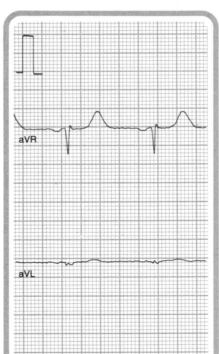

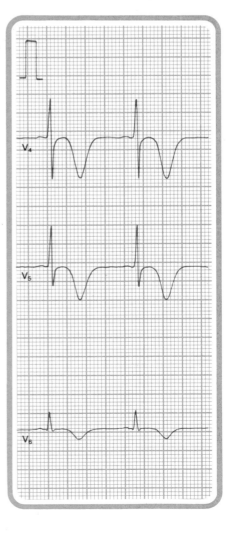

Figure 160

The rhythm is sinus. The mean frontal plane QRS axis is +60°. The QRS complexes are within normal limits (the differences in QRS complexes between this record and the previous one may not be significant – the earlier record was taken on a machine with an inferior frequency response, under adverse conditions when the patient was acutely distressed.) The S-T segments are normal.

The striking abnormality is the deep symmetrical T wave inversion in I, II, III, aVF and V$_2$–V$_6$. (The tall T waves in aVR are part of the same pattern – the T waves are upright in this lead because it is a cavity lead).

Note that these records could easily be misinterpreted as indicating ischaemic heart disease. **Primary interpretation** of the record of Figure 159 might be as follows:-

"Sinus rhythm. The mean frontal plane QRS axis is +75°. There are prominent but not definitely abnormal q waves in the left precordial leads. There is a small secondary r wave in V_1 suggesting incomplete right bundle branch block. There is significant S-T segment elevation in I, II, III, aVF and V_2–V_6. This is frankly abnormal. The changes are non-specific but raise the possibility of pericarditis".

In the light of the clinical information that the patient had acute subarachnoid haemorrhage the **secondary interpretation** would acknowledge that the findings are **consistent with** subarachnoid haemorrhage and do not prove the presence of pericarditis (equally, of course, they do not prove the presence of subarachnoid haemorrhage!).

Likewise, the **primary interpretation** of the record of Figure 160 might be as follows:-

"Sinus rhythm. The mean frontal plane QRS axis is +60°. The QRS complexes are within normal limits. There is deep, symmetrical T wave inversion in I, II, III, aVF and V_2–V_6. The record is frankly abnormal. Changes of this type may be seen in subendocardial ischaemia or infarction and in pericarditis, but other causes cannot be excluded."

In the light of the clinical diagnosis of subarachnoid haemorrhage, the **secondary interpretation** would acknowledge that the findings are **consistent** with subarachnoid haemorrhage.

At no time was there any clinical evidence that the patient (a 25-year-old woman) had any cardiac abnormality. The changes occurring with subarachnoid haemorrhage may persist for weeks after the acute event.

Hypothermia

A drop in the body temperature is associated with a reduction in the sinus rate and with prolongation of the P-R and Q-T intervals. When the temperature falls below 25°C an additional and highly characteristic change occurs. This is the development of an extra deflection occurring at the end of the QRS complex and just overlapping the beginning of the S-T segment. This deflection is called the "J wave". It is usually upright in the leads facing the left ventricle and it increases in size as the temperature falls. It is often mistakenly interpreted as a prolongation of the QRS duration. The broad, second part of the QRS complex (which, in V_1, may superficially resemble right bundle branch block) is also known as the "camel hump sign" and it is accompanied by S-T segment depression and low voltage T waves or T wave inversion. Atrial fibrillation may develop. The Q-T interval may be prolonged. The signs usually reverse as the patient is warmed up. An example of a case of profound hypothermia (from an elderly patient exposed to the cold) is shown in Figure 161.

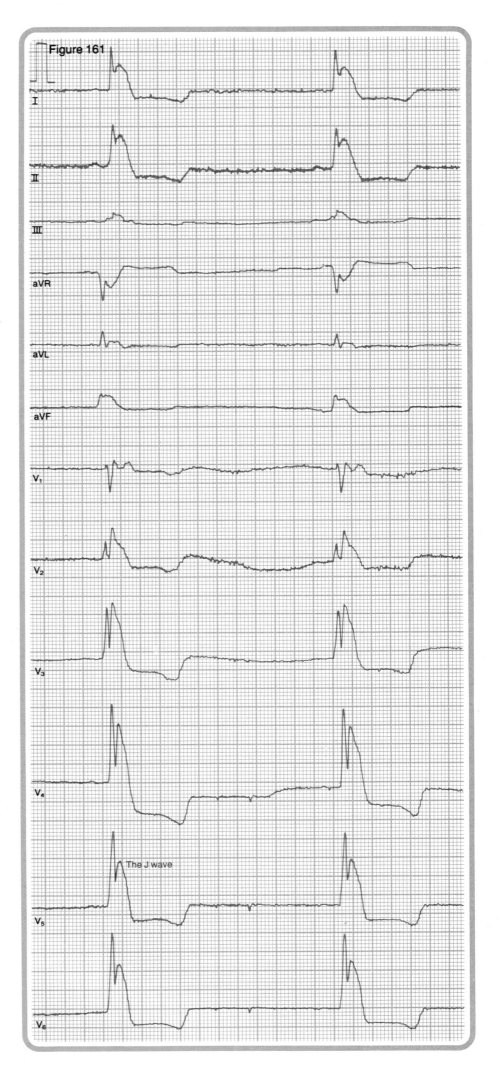

Figure 161

The rhythm is sinus bradycardia. The rate is 28 per min. The P-R interval is 0.20 sec (best seen in Lead II). Broad, slurred J waves are seen adjacent to the initial QRS deflection in all leads, but most obviously in Leads I, II and V₂–V₆. There is pronounced S-T segment depression and T wave inversion.

The Electrocardiogram Associated with Artificial Pacing of the Heart

The commonest indications for cardiac pacing currently are (a) Stokes-Adams syndrome associated with chronic atrio-ventricular block and (b) the sick sinus syndrome (the "brady-tachy syndrome"). There are now many different systems available for temporary or for permanent artificial pacing of the heart. The heart may be paced regularly irrespective of whether or not there is any spontaneous excitation ("fixed rate pacing") or the heart may receive pacing stimuli only when spontaneous activity does not occur ("demand pacing"). Usually, pacing is achieved by stimulation of the ventricle (**ventricular fixed rate** or **ventricular demand pacing).** Occasionally (if atrio-ventricular conduction is known to be normal) **atrial fixed rate** or **atrial demand pacing** may be used. Occasionally, **atrio-ventricular sequential pacing** may be used – the atrium being paced initially, and the ventricles some 0.2 sec later – the delay approximating to the normal atrio-ventricular conduction delay. A more sophisticated system still uses the spontaneous atrial depolarisation (the P wave) to initiate (after a suitable delay) ventricular depolarisation. This is called **atrial synchronous pacing.** These various types of pacing systems and the ECG appearances associated with their normal and with their faulty functioning will be discussed in Section 3, but it will be helpful at this stage to review the appearances of the 12-lead electrocardiogram during sustained ventricular pacing.

During ventricular pacing, depolarisation of the ventricular myocardium is initiated by an artificial stimulus applied directly to the ventricular myocardium from the pacemaker box via the pacing electrode.

Although the electrode may occasionally be stitched onto the surface of the heart, it is much more usual for it to be passed via a proximal vein through the superior vena cava and right atrium into the right ventricle.

During artificial ventricular pacing, a "pacemaker spike" is seen initially, followed immediately by an abnormally wide and abnormally shaped QRS complex. When (as is usual) the pacemaker electrode is situated at the apex of the right ventricle, depolarisation of the interventricular septum necessarily passes from right to left as in left bundle branch block. The induced precordial QRS complexes therefore resemble those in left bundle branch block. In addition, since the ventricular depolarisation begins low down in the right side of the interventricular septum, the predominant pathway of left ventricular depolarisation is upwards and to the left, and this gives rise to an abnormal degree of left axis deviation. Since the QRS complexes are abnormal, the S-T segments and T waves are abnormal, as in left bundle branch block.

An example is shown in Figure 162.

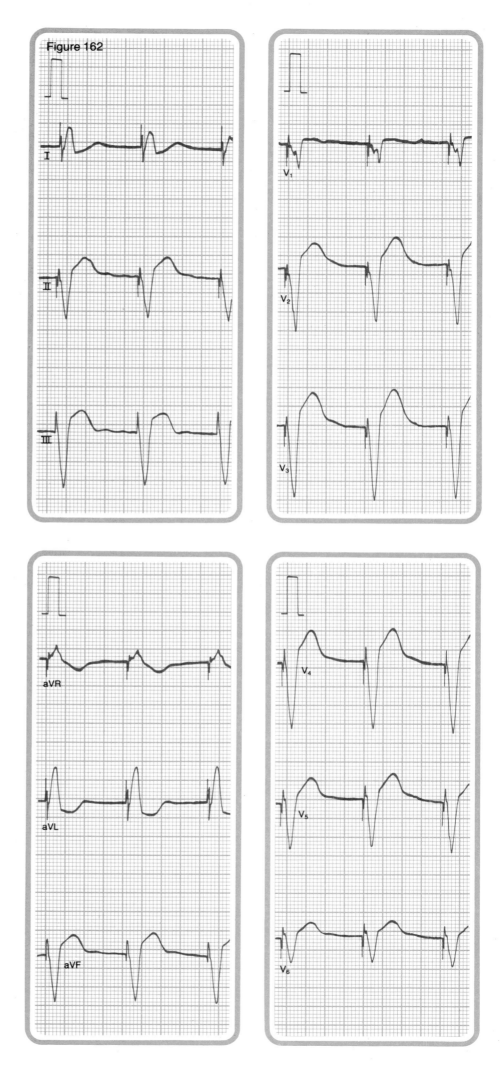

Figure 162

Regular ventricular pacing. The sharp pacemaker spike is seen in all leads preceding the abnormal QRS complexes. The precordial QRS complexes have the left bundle branch block configuration (there is no initial negative (q) wave in V_6 – the initial negative deflection in this lead is part of the pacemaker spike). The mean frontal plane QRS axis is $-75°$, i.e. there is an abnormal degree of left axis deviation.

Pericardial Effusion

The most common electrocardiographic finding in the presence of pericardial effusion is a general reduction in the voltages of all deflections in all leads. Low voltage QRS complexes are also seen in emphysema and in a variety of diffuse myocardial disorders such as haemochromatosis and amyloidosis. The two most common causes of generalised low voltages are hypothyroidism and pericardial effusion. The most obvious electrocardiographic difference between the two is that there is usually a bradycardia with hypothyroidism and a tachycardia with pericardial effusion. However, there are usually very striking clinical differences between the two which render their distinction by electrocardiography superfluous. Occasionally the amplitude of the P, QRS and T waves may be alternately high and low in consecutive beats in patients with large pericardial effusion.

Cor Pulmonale

There are no diagnostic features of cor pulmonale on the electrocardiogram, but **the common findings are a combination of abnormal right axis deviation and clockwise cardiac rotation in the absence of definitive evidence of right ventricular hypertrophy.**

There may, in addition, be evidence of right atrial hypertrophy. Non-specific S-T, T changes may appear, most commonly in the inferior limb leads and there may occasionally be complete right bundle branch block.

Pulmonary Embolism

The electrocardiogram is widely regarded as being a very helpful investigation in the diagnosis of pulmonary embolism, but this is far from the truth. The findings which are most commonly quoted as being very strongly suggestive of pulmonary embolism are the development of the so-called S_1, Q_3, T_3 pattern (i.e. the presence of large S waves in Lead I, large Q waves in V_3 and T wave inversion in Lead III), abnormal right axis deviation, transient right bundle branch block and T wave inversion in the right precordial leads. However, only in a small minority of cases (something of the order of 5%) do these appearances develop in pulmonary embolism. Most cases of pulmonary embolism are unsuspected clinically. Most cases which are suspected clinically either have no electrocardiographic changes at all or only minimal changes. The more massive the pulmonary embolism, the more likely are ECG changes to occur. However, even in massive pulmonary embolism, large-scale studies have shown that the development of the S_1, Q_3, T_3 syndrome, right bundle branch block, right axis deviation and tall pointed P waves in Lead II is seen only in approximately one quarter of the patients. **By far the most common electrocardiographic abnormalities are non-specific T wave changes (which may be found in any of the precordial leads) and non-specific elevation or depression of the S-T segment.** Right axis deviation only occurs in 5-10% of patients with pulmonary embolism, and the development of left axis deviation is actually equally as common. Likewise only a minority of patients with pulmonary embolism develop atrial fibrillation or atrial tachycardia. Occasionally the Q-T interval is prolonged.

The electrocardiogram thus contributes very little to the diagnosis of pulmonary embolism, and normal electrocardiographic findings should never be held to refute the possibility of pulmonary embolism.

Mitral Valve Prolapse

This is an extremely common congenital abnormality, being present in something of the order of 10% of the female population. The patients often have a late systolic click, followed by short systolic murmur and there are characteristic findings on the echocardiogram. **The electrocardiogram often shows non-specific abnormalities. The most common abnormalities are flattening or inversion of the T waves in Leads II, III and aVF. These changes are sometimes accompanied by slight S-T segment depression and they may be wrongly interpreted as evidence of inferior myocardial ischaemia. Sometimes the T waves may be of low voltage in the left precordial leads or there may be shallow T wave inversion in some of the precordial leads. The changes in the precordial leads may be seen either together with, or independently of, changes in the inferior leads. Occasionally prominent U waves may be visible. The Q-T interval may be prolonged. Ventricular pre-excitation is found more commonly in subjects with mitral valve prolapse than in those without. The condition may also be associated with frequent ventricular or atrial premature beats. Supraventricular tachycardia may also occur and occasionally atrial flutter or fibrillation may develop.** In the majority of patients the syndrome is innocent and has no effect on a patient's functional state or his life expectation. A minority of patients may have significant mitral incompetence and occasionally sudden death (thought to be due to paroxysmal ventricular tachycardia or ventricular fibrillation) may occur. **The most important aspect of the electrocardiogram in patients with valve prolapse is that non-specific S-T, T changes in the inferior limb leads may be mistakenly thought to be evidence of inferior myocardial ischaemia if the existence of the mitral valve prolapse syndrome is not recognised.** Of course the presence of mitral valve prolapse does not **prove** that any S-T, T changes are due to the mitral prolapse but at least it admits the possibility.

Heredofamilial Neuromyopathic Disorders

Three major hereditary and familial neuromyopathic disorders are usually associated with cardiac involvement and may give rise to electrocardiographic changes. These conditions are the progressive muscular dystrophies, dystrophia myotonica and Friedreich's ataxia.

Progressive Muscular Dystrophy

There are various different forms of progressive muscular dystrophy and all may show electrocardiographic changes. **Many of them show sinus tachycardia, sometimes with an unusual degree of lability of the heart rate. They may also be associated with the sick sinus syndrome, with atrial ectopic beats, ventricular ectopic beats, atrial flutter, atrial tachycardia, atrial fibrillation, paroxysmal ventricular tachycardia, right or left bundle branch block and various degrees of heart block. In addition the Duchenne type of progressive muscular dystrophy frequently has an abnormal R/S ratio in V_1 (i.e. the R wave is dominant in V_1). There may also be prominent q waves in the limb leads or the left precordial leads and these may simulate infarction.**

Dystrophia Myotonica

In dystrophia myotonica there may be a variety of cardiac arrhythmias including sinus bradycardia, atrial fibrillation, atrial flutter, atrial ectopic beats, ventricular ectopic beats and ventricular tachycardia. There may also be disturbances of conduction with prolongation of the P-R interval, left or right bundle branch block, left anterior hemiblock or complete heart block. The abnormal R/S ratio in the Duchenne type of muscular dystrophy does not appear to occur in dystrophia myotonica.

Friedreich's Ataxia

In Friedreich's ataxia, inappropriate sinus tachycardia, supraventricular or ventricular ectopic beats, atrial tachycardia, atrial fibrillation, atrial flutter and ventricular ectopic beats are the commonest arrhythmias and the commonest abnormalities in morphology are non-specific S-T, T changes (flattening and possible inversion of the T waves and slight S-T segment depression) occasionally the electrocardiogram may satisfy the voltage criteria for left ventricular hypertrophy and rarely bi-ventricular hypretrophy can be found.

Obesity

The most common electro-cardiographic manifestations of obesity are a **generalised reduction in voltages of the P waves, QRS complexes and T waves. Sometimes there is persistent sinus tachycardia.**

Pregnancy

Minor electrocardiographic changes may occur in relation to pregnancy. **Sinus tachycardia is common. As pregnancy advances there is usually a leftward shift of the mean frontal plane QRS axis** (as a result of the shift in the physical position of the heart with the abdominal distension). Prominent q waves may be seen in Lead III in pregnancy (but this should never be taken as an indication of an abnormality in any event, see Section I, pages 53 and 54). In patients subject to paroxysmal supraventricular tachycardia the episodes may be more frequent during pregnancy than in the non-pregnant state. The author does not recommed the diagnosis of pregnancy from the appearance of the electrocardiogram!

Post-myocardial Infarction Syndrome (Dressler's Syndrome)

This is a syndrome in which pleuro-pericarditis occurs within the first 12 weeks following an episode of acute myocardial infarction. The pericarditis is secondary to the myocardial infarction and is induced by an abnormal auto-immune mechanism.

Anti-myocardial antibodies may be present in the serum of the affected patients. **The electrocardiogram shows the typical diffuse S-T segment elevation as in pericarditis of other causes. Later there may be T wave flattening and minor S-T changes.**

Post-cardiotomy Syndrome

This syndrome is very similar to the post-myocardial infarction syndrome. It occurs usually within the first 12 weeks following cardiac surgery and in some degree may be present in 20-30% of patients following cardiac surgery. As in the post-myocardial infarction syndrome the mechanism is thought to be an auto-immune response and there is pleurisy and pericarditis. In addition there may be a fever and a raised erythrocyte sedimentation rate. **The electro-cardiogram shows widespread S-T segment elevation as in acute pericarditis of any origin. Later, low voltage T waves may occur and there may be minor S-T segment changes.**

Connective Tissue Disease

The heart may be involved in any of the connective tissue diseases, the commonest ones to involve the heart are scleroderma and systemic lupus erythematosus. The electrocardiogram is abnormal in about half of patients with scleroderma.

Scleroderma

The commonest abnormalities are non-specific S-T, T changes but evidence of right or of left ventricular hypertrophy may occur. Occasionally bi-ventricular hypertrophy is seen. Sometimes there is generalised reduction in the QRS voltage or the development of abnormal q waves simulating myocardial infarction. Right or left bundle branch block may occur, and **there may be abnormalities of the P wave configuration.**
Various arrhythmias including atrial and ventricular ectopic beats and conduction disturbances may be present.

Systemic Lupus Erythematosus

Similar changes may be apparent in **systemic lupus erythematosus**, but more often the electrocardiographic changes in this condition are confined to **non-specific S-T, T changes with reduction in the T wave voltage and occasionally with S-T segment elevation, indicative of pericarditis. Supraventricular and ventricular ectopic beats and tachycardias may occur.**

Haemochromatosis

In this condition the electro-cardiogram may show **generalised low voltage of the QRS complexes, with low voltage T waves or T wave inversion. Ventricular and** **supraventricular ectopic beats and tachycardia may occur and there may be right bundle branch block, left bundle branch block or first, second or third degree heart block.**

Amyloidosis

This condition is by no means always associated with cardiac involvement, but when there is cardiac involvement the electrocardiogram may well be abnormal. **There may be left axis deviation, right or left bundle** **branch block, complete heart block or absence of initial r waves in V_1-V_3 (simulating antero-septal myocardial infarction). In addition, there may be generalised low voltage of the QRS complexes and T waves.**

Myocarditis

Transient acute myocarditis is very common in systemic viral infections. It occurs in association with influenza, poliomyelitis, mumps, viral hepatitis and infectious mononucleosis.

Viral Myocarditis

In the majority of cases **the electrocardiographic changes involve non-specific flattening of the T waves, minimal S-T segment depression and the occurrence of frequent atrial or ventricular premature beats. Occasionally abnormal q waves, simulating myocardial infarction, may occur.**

Acute Rheumatic Myocarditis

In the myocarditis of acute rheumatic fever the commonest abnormality is **prolongation of the P-R interval, but second degree heart block of the Wenckebach type may occur and minor non-specific S-T changes are also common.**

Cardiomyopathy

In **congestive cardiomyopathy** (which is usually of unknown aetiology) there may be **abnormalities of the P waves, QRS complexes, the S-T segments, the T waves and the cardiac rhythm. In other words, almost any form of electrocardiographic abnormality may occur. The appearances may simulate left or right ventricular hypertrophy or myocardial infarction. Left anterior and left posterior hemiblock may occur and there may also be heart block. The single most characteristic** feature of the ECG in cardiomyopathy is evidence of involvement of all four chambers, e.g. left ventricular hypertrophy plus right atrial abnormality plus right bundle branch block plus ectopic beats arising in the left atrium. Figure 163 shows an electrocardiogram from a patient with congestive cardiomyopathy.
The widespread nature of the changes, involving P waves, QRS complexes, S-T segments, T waves and the cardiac rhythm is typical of the findings in cardiomyopathy.

Similar changes may occur in **hypertrophic obstructive cardiomyopathy.** The earliest changes in this condition are those of **left ventricular hypertrophy and left atrial hypertrophy, but subsequently arrhythmias (atrial or ventricular) left or right bundle branch block and either left anterior or left posterior hemiblock may occur. Not uncommonly in this condition abnormal q waves which, in other circumstances, would suggest myocardial infarction, may be seen.**

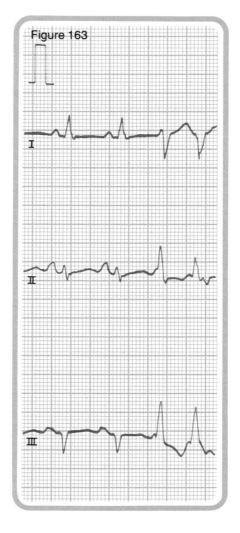

Figure 163

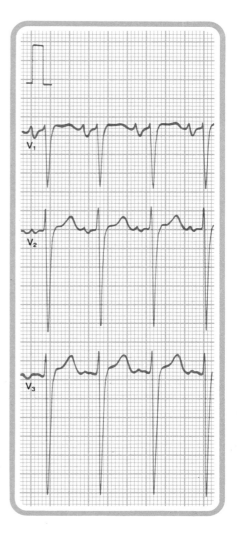

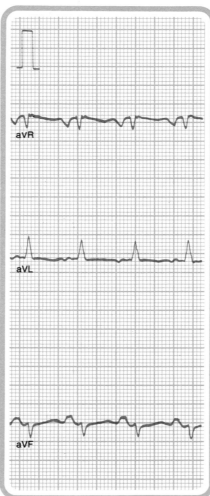

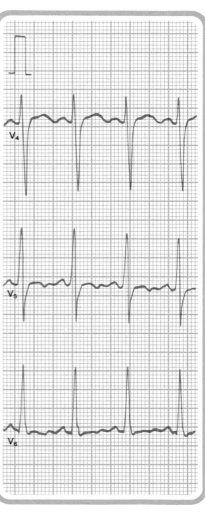

Figure 163

The basic rhythm is sinus tachycardia (the heart rate is often raised in congestive cardiomyopathy owing to the reflex sympathetic drive which occurs consequent upon decreased ventricular output). Two ventricular ectopic beats are seen (the third and fourth beats seen in Leads I, II and III). The P waves show evidence of right atrial abnormality (abnormally tall P waves in II) and of left atrial abnormality (dominant negative component to the P wave in V_1). The precordial QRS complexes satisfy the voltage criteria for left ventricular hypertrophy. There are non-specific S-T, T changes in the limb leads and in the left precordial leads. The mean frontal plane QRS axis is at the extreme left hand side of the normal range at $-30°$.

Dissecting Aneurysm

This may be associated with **non-specific S-T segment depression, low voltage of the T waves and occasionally T wave inversion. It may** actually give rise to myocardial infarction, in which case the usual changes of this condition would be seen.

Chest Deformities

Abnormalities of the anatomy of the thorax may induce secondary changes in the electrocardiogram, usually because of the change in the physical position of the heart. If there is appreciable depression of the sternum the heart may be displaced to the right or to the left.

Pectus Excavatum

Pectus excavatum may be associated with **counter-clockwise or clockwise cardiac rotation.**

Pulmonary Atalectasis

With collapse of the left lung or with the presence of a large right pleural effusion, the mean frontal plane QRS axis may be shifted to the left.

Pleural Effusion

Conversely, in the presence of a large left pleural effusion, the frontal plane axis can be shifted to the right.

Congenital Heart Disease (In the adult)

Atrial Septal Defect

This condition is usually associated with **borderline abnormal right axis deviation and complete or incomplete right bundle branch block**. There may also be **clockwise cardiac rotation** (this applies to the common, ostium secundum type of atrial septal defect. In the case of the less common ostium primum type of atrial septal defect, complete or incomplete right bundle branch block is seen in association with **left** axis deviation).

Ventricular Septal Defect

The electrocardiogram is normal in cases of ventricular septal defect associated with a small shunt. If there is a very large defect with a resulting large left-to-right shunt, the electrocardiogram may shows signs of **left ventricular hypertrophy**. In cases associated with pulmonary hypertension, there may be right ventricular hypertrophy or bi-ventricular hypertrophy.

Patent Ductus Arteriosus

In the majority of cases the electrocardiogram is normal. If the shunt is large there may be evidence of left ventricular hypertrophy and possibly of left atrial hypertrophy. In the presence of pulmonary hypertension, abnormal right axis deviation and ultimately right ventricular hypertrophy may be seen.

Coarctation of the Aorta

The common findings are those of **left ventricular and left atrial hypertrophy**. Occasionally there may be an abnormal degree of left axis deviation. For reasons which are not understood a complete or incomplete right bundle branch block pattern may also be found.

Pulmonary Stenosis

The electrocardiographic changes here are simply those of **right ventricular hypertrophy and right atrial hypertrophy.**

Fallot's Tetralogy

The vast majority of patients with this condition have an abnormal electrocardiogram. There is nearly always evidence of **right ventricular hypertrophy and right atrial hypertrophy**. In addition, a **right bundle branch block pattern is sometimes seen.**

Ebstein's Anomaly

This is a relatively rare congenital abnormality in which the tricuspid valve is displaced downwards from its normal position towards the apex of the right ventricle. The electrocardiogram frequently shows **atrial ectopic beats, atrial tachycardia, atrial flutter, atrial fibrillation or nodal tachycardia.** When the patient is in sinus rhythm, **the P waves are often abnormally tall and abnormally wide and the P-R interval may be prolonged.** Sometimes **second or third degree heart block may be present.** The QRS complexes may show a **right bundle branch block configuration and sometimes ventricular pre-excitation of the Wolff-Parkinson-White variety** (most commonly Type B) **can be found.**

Dextrocardia

"Situs inversus" describes a congenital developmental "abnormality" in which every organ in the body develops as a left-to-right mirror image of the usual pattern. The heart lies in the right side of the chest with the "left", i.e. systemic, ventricle to the right and the "right", i.e. pulmonary, ventricle to the left. When all the organs in the body are transposed in this way the heart is usually normal, apart from its position. The "dextrocardia" is then part of the "situs inversus". Isolated dextrocardia (in which the heart is the **only** organ to be transposed) may also occur. This too can occur with a heart which is, in respects other than its position, normal but complex congenital cardiac abnormalities of great functional significance are much more likely to occur in association with isolated dextrocardia than with dextrocardia which is part of the pattern of "situs inversus".

In the presence of dextrocardia (whether isolated or part of "situs inversus") striking changes are seen in the ECG and if the electrocardiogram is recorded in the normal way (i.e. using the standard recording positions as recommended by the British Cardiac Society and the American Heart Association (Section I, page 27)), then profound "abnormalities" of the electrocardiogram will be seen. These "abnormalities" are in no way indicative of disease. They merely reflect the abnormal anatomical relationship of the heart to the usual recording positions. Figure 164 shows an example of the kind of appearances which may be found.

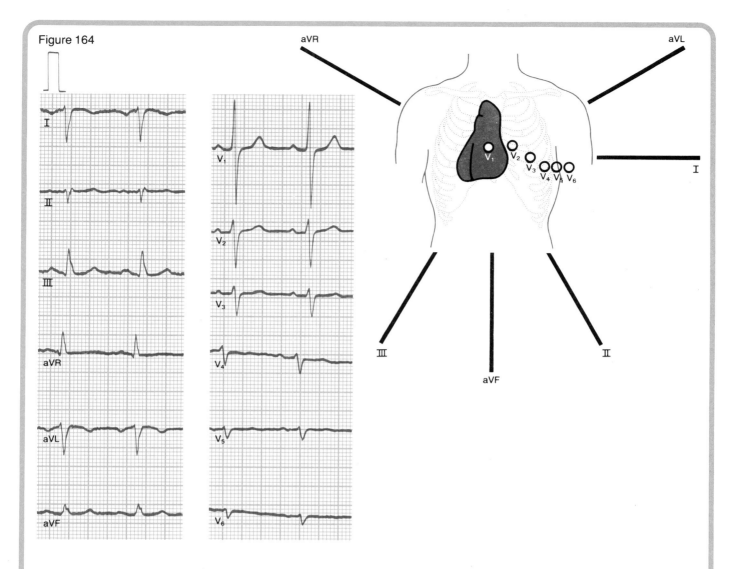

Figure 164

The ECG recording on the left is from a patient with mirror-image dextrocardia. There was no evidence of organic heart disease. The patient was simply born with left/right inversion of the body organs. When the conventional electrocardiographic recording is made (i.e. the precordial electrodes positioned in their conventional sites and the limbs connected according to the normal convention) appearances similar to those in the left-hand side of the figure are seen.

As usual (page 15)

I = +L−R
II = +F−R
III = +F−L

Lead 1 shows an inverted P wave, QRS complex and T wave which is a very unusual finding. The only alternative explanation for this finding is "technical dextrocardia" – see later. The appearances in V_1 are consistent with normality, but from V_2-V_6 the r waves become progressively

smaller rather than larger and there is T wave inversion. These are very abnormal findings. These abnormal findings do not indicate structural abnormality within the heart for the conventional electrode positions are not suitable for obtaining an electrocardiogram when the heart is mirror-image inverted. The diagram on the right shows the position of the heart (in dextrocardia) in relation to the position of the recording electrodes.

The conventional positions for the recording electrodes are therefore inappropriate for patients with dextrocardia. For this reason the recording system used in Figure 165 is chosen. In this system the right and left arm connections are deliberately reversed and the precordial connections are also right/left inverted.

Thus:
(inverted commas are used to indicate the lead achieved by the deliberately "false" connections. The corresponding conventional connections are expressed without quotation marks).

$$\text{"L"} = R$$
$$\text{"R"} = L$$
$$\text{"F"} = F$$

Since $\quad$ "I" $\quad = + \text{"L"} - \text{"R"}$
therefore $\quad$ "I" $\quad = + R - L$
$\qquad\qquad\quad = I \text{ turned upside down}$
Similarly $\quad$ "II" $\quad = + \text{"F"} - \text{"R"}$
$\qquad\qquad\quad = + F - L$
$\qquad\qquad\quad = III$
and $\qquad$ "III" $\quad = + \text{"F"} - \text{"L"}$
$\qquad\qquad\quad = + F - R$
$\qquad\qquad\quad = II$

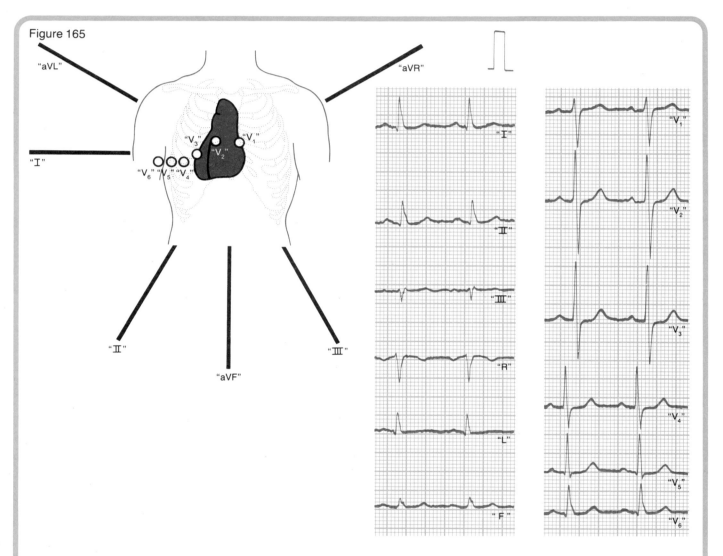

Figure 165

This figure shows the position of the heart in the patient with mirror-image dextrocardia as in Figure 164, however, a "mirror-image" recording system is used in which the precordial leads are left/right inverted (they are sited exactly as quoted in Figure 34, page 27, except that all right-sided positions become left, and all left-sided positions become right). The limb lead connections are mirror-image inverted simply by reversing the right and left arm connections. The foot lead connection is a central connection and does not need to be inverted. Leads recorded in this way are shown between inverted commas to distinguish them from the conventional recording system.

Note that the appearances in "V₁" (Figure 165) are identical to those in V₂ (Figure 164) and the appearances in "V₂" (Figure 165) are identical to those in V₁ (Figure 164).

The remainder of the precordial leads in Figure 165 have no counterpart in Figure 164 for the leads in Figure 164 are inappropriately placed, distant from the heart.

In the limb leads "I" (Figure 165) is the same as I (Figure 164) upside down, "II" (Figure 165) is identical with III (Figure 164) and "III" (Figure 165) is the same as II (Figure 164). Likewise "L" (Figure 165) equals R (Figure 164) and "R" (Figure 165) equals L (Figure 164). "F" (Figure 165) equals F (Figure 164).

It should be noted that the electrocardiogram in dextrocardia looks very abnormal if recorded in the conventional way. **The great clue to its presence is the fact that the P waves, the QRS complexes and T waves are all negative in Lead 1 and that the precordial leads show a completely abnormal R wave progression with the R wave voltages getting** **progressively smaller from V_1-V_6 for** these electrodes are progressively further and further away from the heart. **The greatest clue lies in the negative P wave in I.** This is very rarely seen in the presence of sinus rhythm except in dextrocardia. The only condition with which it is likely to be confused is technical dextrocardia.

Technical Dextrocardia

Technical dextrocardia refers to the electrocardiographic appearances which are obtained as a result of an **error** in the ECG recording technique. The error involves the accidental connection of the right arm to the left arm lead, and the left arm to the right arm lead. Thus the appearances in aVR and in aVL are interchanged, and those in aVF are unchanged. The appearances in Leads II and III are also interchanged and the appearances in Lead I are inverted. The result is that in the **limb leads** the appearances are identical to those in true dextrocardia. However, the appearances in the **precordial leads** are entirely normal. An example is shown in Figure 166.

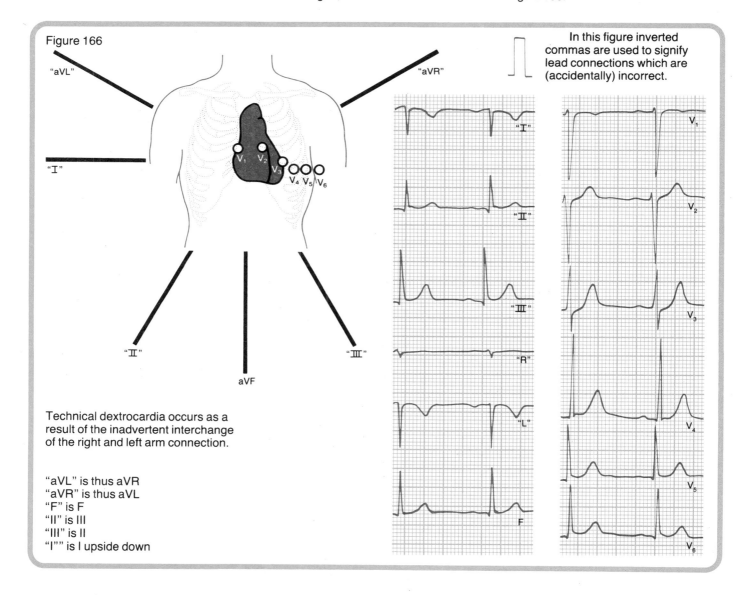

Figure 166

In this figure inverted commas are used to signify lead connections which are (accidentally) incorrect.

Technical dextrocardia occurs as a result of the inadvertent interchange of the right and left arm connection.

"aVL" is thus aVR
"aVR" is thus aVL
"F" is F
"II" is III
"III" is II
"I"" is I upside down

The Recognition of Dextrocardia

When the P wave is inverted in Lead I in the presence of sinus rhythm the only likely explanations are dextrocardia or technical dextrocardia. The latter is considerably more common than the former. **When the precordial R wave progression is normal the explanation is technical dextrocardia.** The true appearances of the record are then already shown in the precordial leads. The true appearances in the limb leads can be ascertained by interchanging aVL and aVR, interchanging II and III, turning I upside down and leaving aVF as it is. **When the R wave voltage progressively decreases from V_1 to V_6 there is true dextrocardia.** The true appearances can be assessed in the limb leads by interchanging aVR and aVL, interchanging II and III, turning I upside down and leaving F alone. The true appearances in V_1 and V_2 can be determined by interchanging them but the true appearances in V_3-V_6 can only be determined by recording again using right-sided V_3-V_6 placements. By far the simplest approach in true dextrocardia is to obtain a record using **appropriate** electrode placings, i.e. deliberately to interchange the R and L connections and to use right-sided precordial leads as indicated in Figure 165.

Multiple and Complex Abnormalities

In this book, as in most other text books of electrocardiography, abnormalities have been explained and demonstrated individually – and this is necessary in the interests of clarity. However, in real life, abnormalities of the electrocardiogram are not necessarily conveniently "packaged" into individual types. Combinations of abnormalities may occur by coincidence (for example, if a patient with right ventricular hypertrophy due to congenital pulmonary stenosis develops acute viral pericarditis) but much more commonly combinations of abnormalities may occur because of common aetiology (e.g. when there is left ventricular hypertrophy on the basis of hypertension and the patient develops either acute myocardial infarction or atrial fibrillation). Some combinations of abnormalities are virtually inevitable, for the development of one abnormality gives rise to the development of a second abnormality. The most obvious example in this category is that in the presence of ventricular hypertrophy, hypertrophy of the corresponding atrium is inevitable. Thus **left ventricular hypertrophy** is **usually** accompanied by **left atrial hypertrophy** (left atrial hypertrophy can only be recognised if the rhythm is sinus) – an example is shown in Figure 104 – and **right ventricular hypertrophy** is **usually** accompanied by **right atrial hypertrophy** (which latter can likewise only be recognised if the rhythm is sinus). An example is shown in Figure 108.

Other combinations of abnormalities, whilst by no means inevitable, are nevertheless common – for the disease process may involve more than one area. Examples include:-

1. Right bundle branch block with left anterior hemiblock – for degenerative disease commonly affects these two fascicles of the conductive system. An example is shown in Figure 100.

2. Left atrial hypertrophy with right ventricular hypertrophy. This combination (in the absence of left ventricular hypertrophy) usually implies obstruction at the mitral valve orifice (most commonly due to mitral stenosis, and rarely due to atrial myxoma).

3. Anterior myocardial infarction and right bundle branch block. When the infarct involves the myocardium of the interventricular septum carrying the bundle branches, block of either bundle branch may occur. Anterior myocardial infarction and right bundle branch block can both be diagnosed from the same electrocardiogram since neither interferes with the diagnostic processes involved in the other (Figure 169).

4. Anterior myocardial infarction with left bundle branch block. If left bundle branch block and myocardial infarction co-exist, usually only the left bundle branch block is apparent for this so distorts the electrocardiogram that the normal criteria for infarction cannot be applied (see page 125). It is **sometimes** possible to diagnose myocardial infarction in the presence of left bundle branch block but this is **always** difficult and is **never** completely reliable.

Diagnosis of Myocardial Infarction in the Presence of Left Bundle Branch Block

It must be repeated that (a) it may prove impossible to diagnose myocardial infarction in the presence of left bundle branch block, and (b) when the diagnosis is attempted, subsequent autopsy examination indicates that the diagnosis may be in error in a significant number of cases (i.e. the specificity of the criteria for myocardial infarction in the presence of left bundle branch block is very low).

The criteria which have been applied by various authors are:-

1. Abnormal Q waves in I, aVL, V_4–V_6
(i.e. a q wave of 0.04 sec or more in duration or more than ¼ of the height of the ensuing R wave). This is probably the most reliable indicator of infarction in the presence of left bundle branch block, but it will immediately be seen that this defies one of the two "essential" criteria for the diagnosis of left bundle branch block in the first place! The diagnosis of left bundle branch block is then dependent upon (a) a prolonged QRS duration of 0.12 sec or more (b) dominant positive waves in V_6, and (c) displacement of the S-T segment and T waves in a direction opposite to the dominant deflection of the QRS complex in any lead, and (d) absence of a secondary R wave in the right precordial leads (thus demonstrating that there is no right bundle branch block).

The form of the QRS complex in V_6 in the presence of left bundle branch block, complicated by anteroseptal infarction, is shown in Figure 167.

2. QS or W-shaped deflection in II, III and aVF
This is usually an indication of inferior infarction, but it is not a totally reliable criterion. The criteria for LBBB listed (a) to (d) in 1 above must still obtain.

3. Primary S-T or T wave changes
In uncomplicated left bundle branch block the S-T segments and T waves are usually opposite in sign to the dominant QRS deflection. These are the expected "secondary" changes (i.e. they are secondary to the QRS abnormality, page 124). When, in leads with upright QRS complexes, there is S-T segment elevation and the T waves are tall and upright, infarction is possible. These are "primary" S-T or T changes, i.e. they are changes not induced inevitably by the QRS abnormality. S-T depression or T inversion in leads in which the dominant QRS deflection is negative have the same significance.

Several examples of combined abnormalities are now shown.

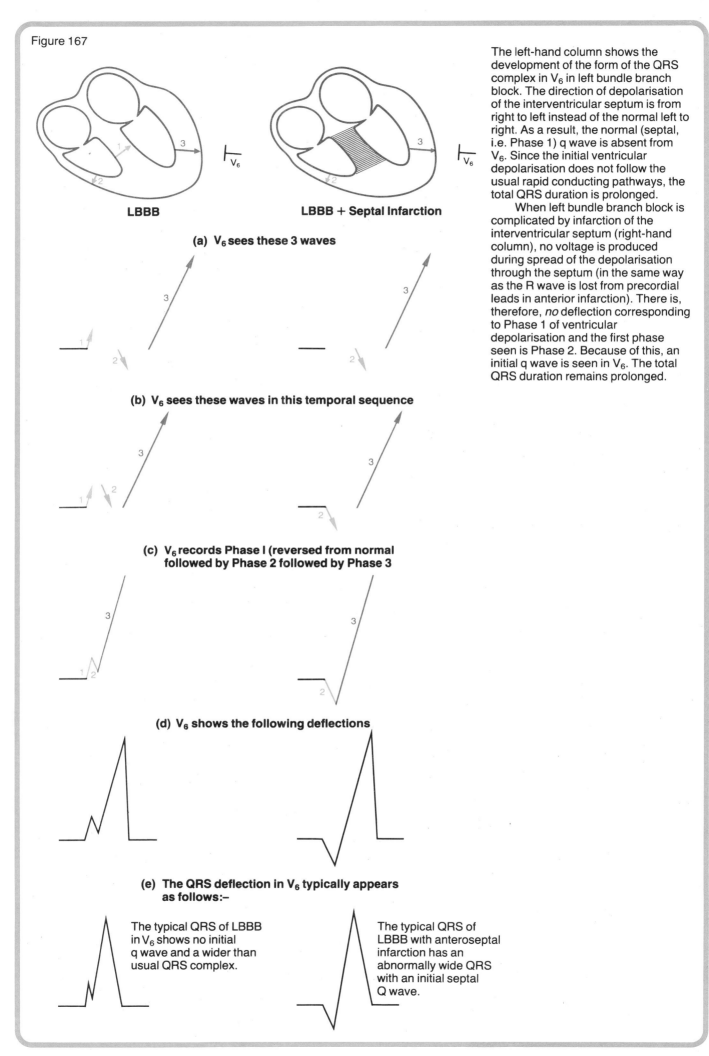

Figure 167

LBBB

LBBB + Septal Infarction

The left-hand column shows the development of the form of the QRS complex in V₆ in left bundle branch block. The direction of depolarisation of the interventricular septum is from right to left instead of the normal left to right. As a result, the normal (septal, i.e. Phase 1) q wave is absent from V₆. Since the initial ventricular depolarisation does not follow the usual rapid conducting pathways, the total QRS duration is prolonged.

When left bundle branch block is complicated by infarction of the interventricular septum (right-hand column), no voltage is produced during spread of the depolarisation through the septum (in the same way as the R wave is lost from precordial leads in anterior infarction). There is, therefore, *no* deflection corresponding to Phase 1 of ventricular depolarisation and the first phase seen is Phase 2. Because of this, an initial q wave is seen in V₆. The total QRS duration remains prolonged.

(a) V₆ sees these 3 waves

(b) V₆ sees these waves in this temporal sequence

(c) V₆ records Phase I (reversed from normal followed by Phase 2 followed by Phase 3

(d) V₆ shows the following deflections

(e) The QRS deflection in V₆ typically appears as follows:–

The typical QRS of LBBB in V₆ shows no initial q wave and a wider than usual QRS complex.

The typical QRS of LBBB with anteroseptal infarction has an abnormally wide QRS with an initial septal Q wave.

1. Left Bundle Branch Block, with Left Atrial Hypertrophy and Left Anterior Hemiblock (Figure 168)

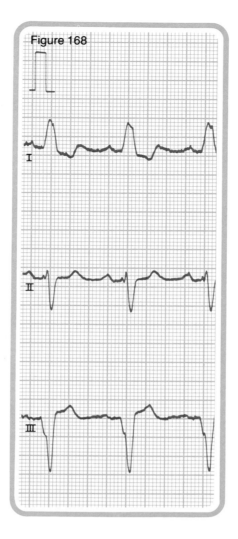

Figure 168

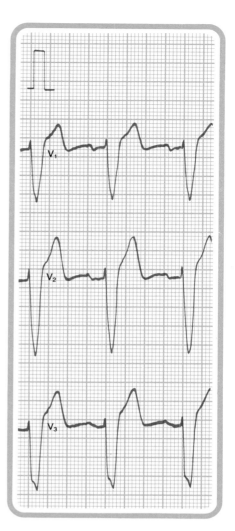

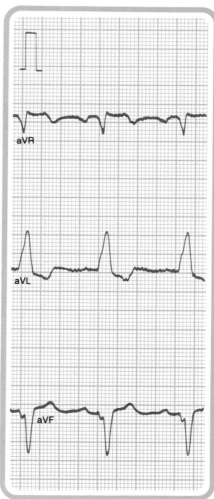

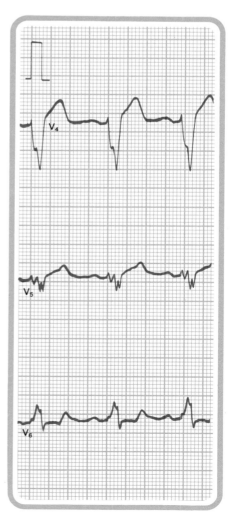

Figure 168

The rhythm is sinus. The total QRS duration is abnormal at 0.16 sec. There is no secondary R wave in V_1 to indicate right bundle branch block. There is no initial q wave in V_6, I or aVL and there is therefore **left bundle branch block**. The mean frontal plane QRS axis is abnormal at $-75°$. The two common causes of such an axis are inferior infarction and left anterior hemiblock. The former cannot be confidently diagnosed in the presence of left bundle branch block. There may well be distal disease in the anterior division of the left bundle branch as well as a proximal lesion in the main left bundle branch and the **probability** is that there is **left anterior hemiblock** as well as left bundle branch block (left bundle branch block alone **does not** cause left axis deviation). The form of the P waves in V_1 suggests left atrial hypertrophy.

A suitable report on this record would be:-

"Sinus rhythm. There is complete left bundle branch block. There is an abnormal degree of left axis deviation ($-75°$) suggesting additional left anterior hemiblock. The form of the P waves in V_1 suggests left atrial hypertrophy."

This patient had hypertrophic obstructive cardiomyopathy.

2. Anterior Myocardial Infarction, Inferior Myocardial Infarction and Right Bundle Branch Block (Figure 169)

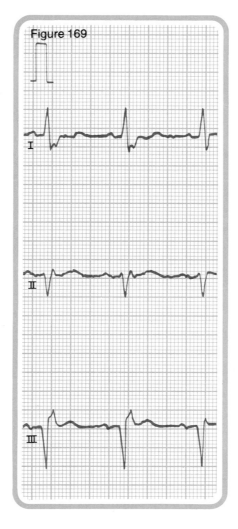

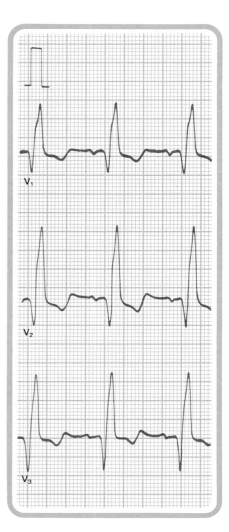

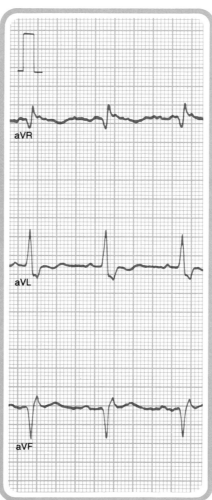

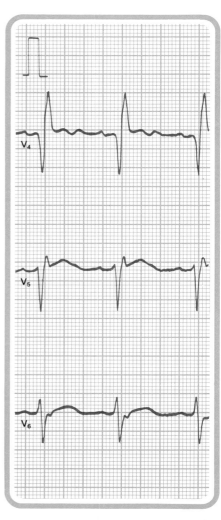

Figure 169

The rhythm is sinus. There are abnormal Q waves in aVF, indicative of inferior infarction. There are abnormal Q waves from V₁–V₄ indicating anteroseptal infarction. The frontal plane QRS axis is abnormal at $-60°$ (due to the inferior infarction). The total QRS duration is prolonged indicating bundle branch block. There is a large, "secondary" R wave in V₁ to indicate the presence of right bundle branch block. (Even though there is no initial q wave in V₆, this does not indicate *left* bundle branch block (page 124)). The "secondary" r wave is visible but the "primary" r wave is lost because of the anteroseptal infarction (remember, the initial part of the QRS complex is normal in all leads in right bundle branch block and the criteria for infarction can be applied – page 118, Figure 82).

A suitable report on this record would be:-

"*Sinus rhythm. Inferior myocardial infarction (resulting in abnormal degree of left axis deviation). There is anteroseptal infarction and complete right bundle branch block.*".

This patient had unequivocal clinical evidence of ischaemic heart disease.

3. Left Ventricular Hypertrophy, Left Atrial Hypertrophy, Right Atrial Hypertrophy (Figure 170)

Figure 170

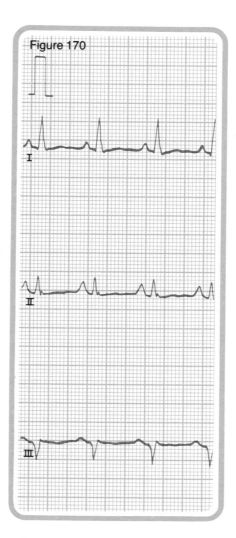

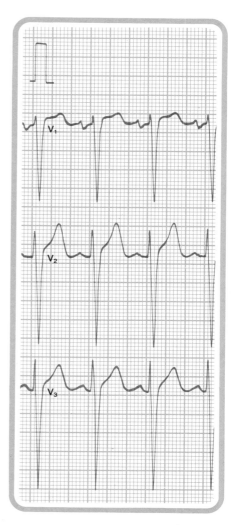

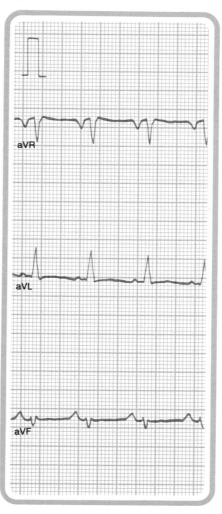

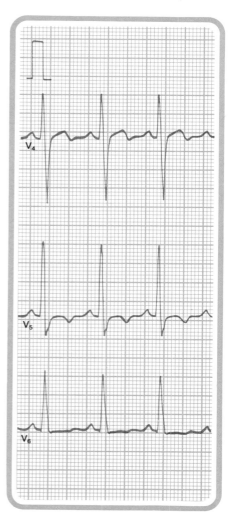

Figure 170

The rhythm is sinus (at about 100/min). The precordial QRS complexes satisfy the voltage criteria for left ventricular hypertrophy. There is T wave inversion in V_5 and S-T segment depression in V_6. These are non-specific changes which could well be secondary to the QRS abnormalities. The P waves in V_1 have a dominant negative component indicative of left atrial hypertrophy (strictly "abnormality"). The P waves in II are abnormally tall and pointed and indicate right atrial hypertrophy (strictly "abnormality"). The mean frontal plane QRS axis is $-15°$. The frontal plane T wave axis is indeterminate. Since the QRS axis is determinate and the T wave axis indeterminate, the frontal plane T waves are abnormal (page 58).
A suitable report for this record would be as follows:-
"Sinus tachycardia. The mean frontal plane QRS axis is $-15°$, but the frontal plane T wave axis is indeterminate indicating that the frontal plane T waves are abnormal. This is a non-specific abnormality. There is evidence of left and right atrial abnormality and of left ventricular hypertrophy. There are non-specific S-T, T changes in the left precordial leads".
This patient had a congestive cardiomyopathy, thought to be due to excessive alcohol consumption.

4. Anteroseptal Infarction with Left Anterior Hemiblock (Figure 171)

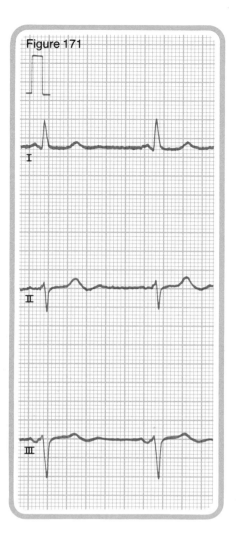

Figure 171

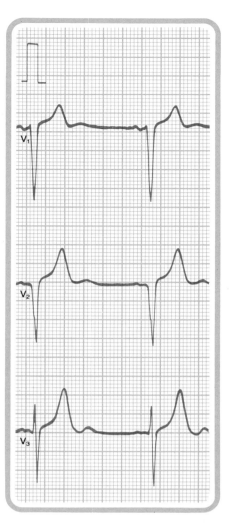

Figure 171

The rhythm is sinus. The r wave in V_1 is small. There is no r wave at all in V_2 (there are deep QS complexes) and the appearances are those of an old anteroseptal infarction. The mean frontal plane QRS axis is $-45°$. This is an abnormal degree of left axis deviation. Abnormal left axis deviation is not a feature of anteroseptal infarction. There is no evidence of inferior infarction (initial r waves are seen aVF) and the likely cause is therefore left anterior hemiblock, which may indicate that the infarct involves the anterior division of the left bundle branch in the interventricular septum. There are prominent, but not abnormal (see page 195) U waves in II, III, aVF and V_1-V_6.

A suitable report for this record would be as follows:-

"*Sinus bradycardia. The form of the QRS complexes in V_1 and V_2 is very strongly suggestive of an old anteroseptal infarction. There is an abnormal degree of left axis deviation ($-45°$) indicative of left anterior hemiblock. The U waves are prominent, but not definitely abnormal, in most leads. The possibility of hypokalaemia should be considered*".

The patient had clear clinical evidence of ischaemic heart disease. The serum potassium ion level was 3.2 mmol/l.

Note

This serum potassium ion level is abnormally low but it does not follow that the prominent U waves were necessarily related to this.

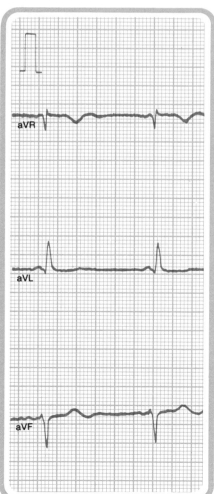

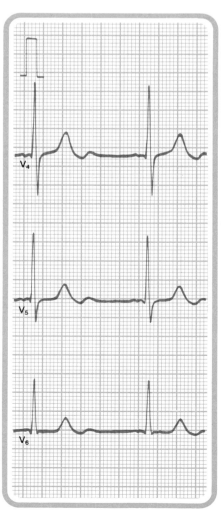

5. Right Bundle Branch Block with Lateral Infarction (Figure 172)

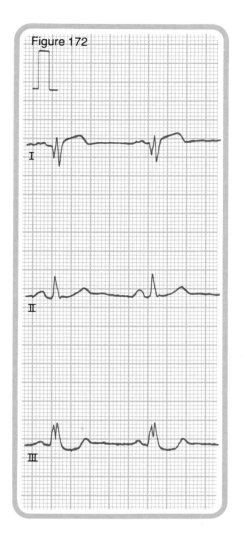
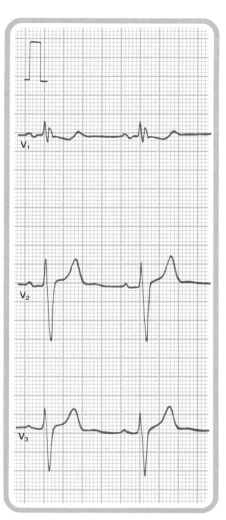

Figure 172

There is an Rsr' complex in V_1 with a total QRS duration of 0.13 sec (well seen in V_2 and V_3). There is therefore complete right bundle branch block. There are abnormal Q waves in I and aVL (more than one quarter of the height of the ensuing R wave and also more than 0.04 sec in duration).

Since the mean frontal plane QRS axis is $+105°$, the abnormal Q waves in aVL could simply be related to the heart position (i.e. aVL is a cavity lead). However, this cannot explain the abnormal Q waves in I, which indicates a lateral infarction. No evidence of infarction is seen in the precordial leads but some evidence might be found if high lateral leads were used (Table 4, page 180). There is S-T segment elevation and terminal T wave inversion in I and aVL suggesting **recent** infarction. The S-T segments and T waves in V_6 are minimally abnormal. The abnormal degree of right axis deviation could be due to right inferior hemiblock, but abnormal right axis deviation has many causes including anterolateral infarction without involvement of the inferior division of the left bundle. In this case there is actually probably a different reason altogether – see below[*].

A suitable report for this record would be as follows:-

"Sinus rhythm. The mean frontal plane QRS axis is abnormal at $+105°$. There is complete right bundle branch block. There are abnormal q waves in I and aVL, indicating lateral myocardial infarction. The form of the S-T segments and T waves in these leads and in V_6 suggest that the infarct is recent".

Note

[*]This patient had just suffered acute myocardial infarction. The physical signs suggested the presence of an atrial septal defect. The latter – a congenital lesion unrelated to the infarction and previously unsuspected – was subsequently confirmed by cardiac catheterisation. Coronary angiography revealed occlusive disease in the diagonal branch of the left coronary artery.

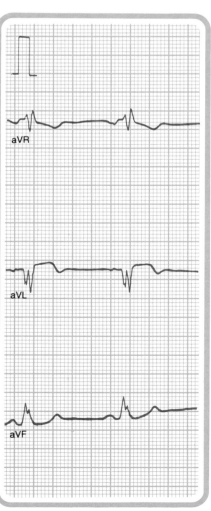
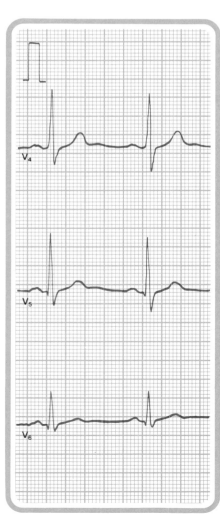

6. Right Ventricular Hypertrophy with Acute Pericarditis (Figure 173)

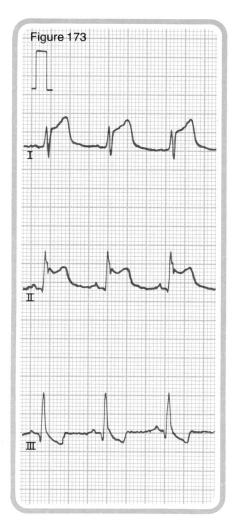

Figure 173

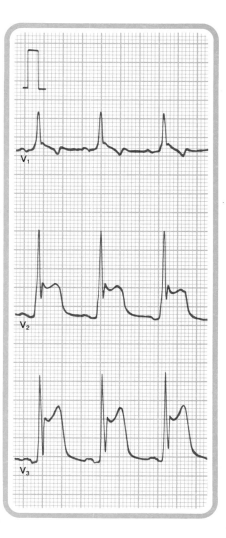

Figure 173

The rhythm is sinus. There is striking S-T segment elevation in virtually all leads (aVR, being a cavity lead, naturally shows S-T segment depression. This is **not** a reciprocal change). Such widespread S-T elevation is usually indicative of acute pericarditis. The S-T elevation is concave upwards which is also typical. The R wave in V_1 is dominant and the total QRS duration is normal. This is powerfully suggestive of right ventricular hypertrophy. One would expect right ventricular hypertrophy to be associated with S-T segment depression in V_1 and the apparently neutral S-T segment in this lead may be the result of the cancelling out of opposite effects – S-T segment depression, anticipated due to the right ventricular hypertrophy and S-T segment elevation anticipated due to the pericarditis.

A suitable report for this record would be as follows:-

"Sinus rhythm. There is widespread S-T segment elevation indicative of acute pericarditis. The form of the QRS complexes in V_1 is indicative of right ventricular hypertrophy."

The patient had an atrial septal defect. The record was taken in the immediate post-operative period. The pericarditis was a reaction to the operation.

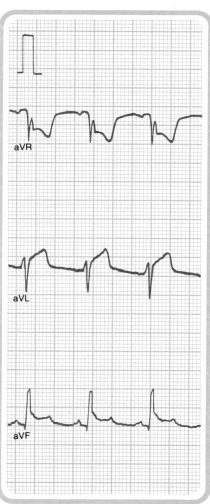

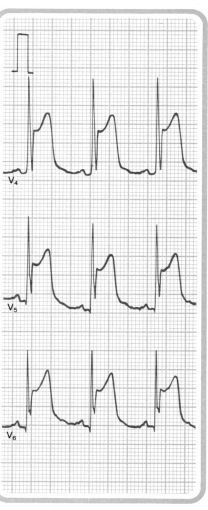

7. Non-specific T Wave Changes with Left Anterior Hemiblock and Technical Dextrocardia (Figure 174a)

Figure 174a

The P wave is negative in I and the QRS deflection is dominantly negative in this lead. This raises the suspicion that the right and left arm leads have been inadvertently interposed. When this happens the T wave in I is usually also inverted so the present appearances are not typical. However, the reason for this will emerge later. This record is actually an example of accidental right/left arm lead interposition, i.e. of technical dextrocardia. Figure 174b shows a further record, taken within minutes of the first one with the right and left arm leads correctly arranged. Comparison between 174a and 174b shows the effects of technical dextrocardia and how the two appearances can be judged without retaking the record:-

Technical Dextrocardia	
Incorrect Lead	**Relation of Observed to True Deflection**
I	Invert appearances to show true Lead I
II	Actually shows the true appearances of Lead III
III	Actually shows the true appearances of Lead II
aVR	Actually shows the true appearances of aVL
aVL	Actually shows the true appearances of aVR
aVF	Actually shows the true appearances of aVF

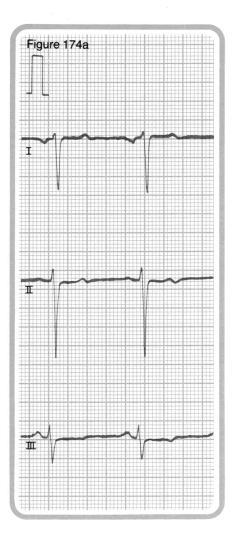

Figure 174a

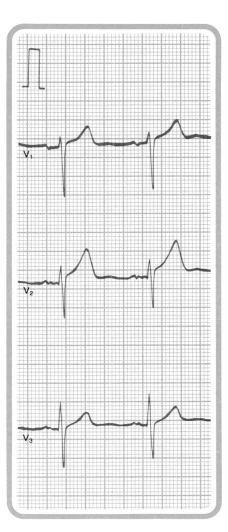

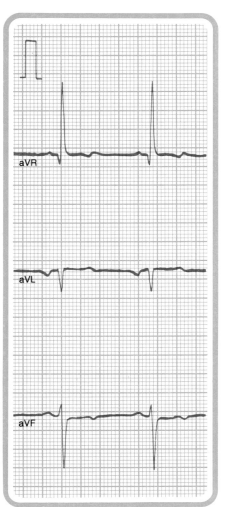

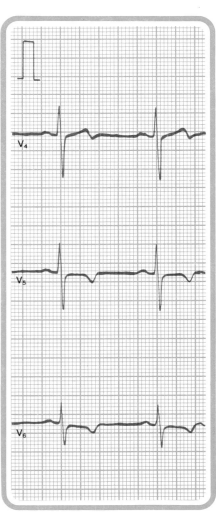

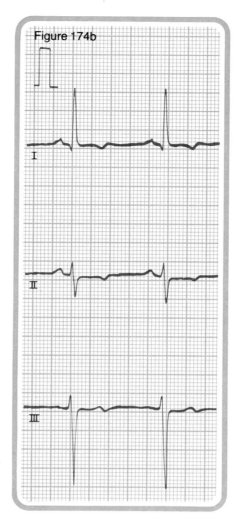

Figure 174b

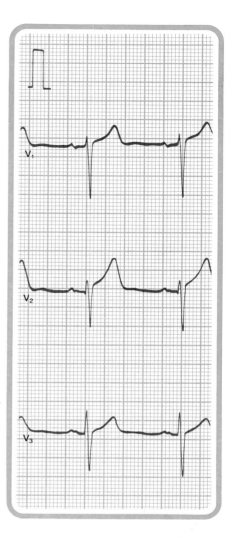

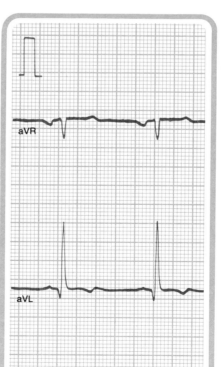

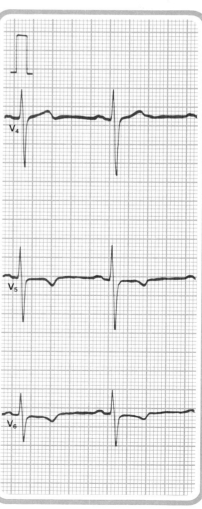

Figure 174b

Figure 174b shows why the T waves were not negative in I when there was technical dextrocardia – because the T wave is actually abnormal (inverted) in I. Record 174b might be reported as follows:-

"Sinus rhythm. The mean frontal plane QRS axis is −45° indicating left anterior hemiblock. The frontal plane T axis is −150°. The angle between the frontal plane QRS and T wave axes is therefore abnormal, indicating that the frontal plane T waves are abnormal. There is T wave inversion in V₅ and V₆ which is frankly abnormal. The T wave changes are non-specific. There is pronounced clockwise cardiac rotation."

8. Arrhythmias together with Morphological Abnormalities

Such combinations are extremely common. They will be dealt with in Section 3.

Practical Aids in ECG Interpretation

This section does not present a systematic approach to a single topic – rather it points to several useful topics which are helpful to bear in mind during ECG interpretation. In most aspects of medicine, there are diagnostic possibilities which are easily forgotten – perhaps because the signs are subtle or because the condition is relatively uncommon. Examples of such syndromes in clinical medicine in the author's experience include, for example, amyloidosis and haemochromatosis. To consider these possibilities when presented with a clinically obscure problem takes little time and may occasionally be very rewarding. These examples are not necessarily optimal for everyone. Each has blind spots or weak spots in his own diagnostic approach and it is useful to recognise when this has happened and to add this diagnosis to one's list of such possibilities so that subsequently, at each diagnostic level, the contents of the list may be considered in the diagnostic process. The same principle applies in electrocardiography and it is in this spirit that this section is presented.

Causes of QS Complexes in the Right Precordial Leads

1. Clockwise cardiac rotation (V_1 only).
2. Anteroseptal myocardial infarction.
3. Left bundle branch block.
4. Ventricular pre-excitation.

Causes of Dominant R Waves in V_1

1. Right ventricular hypertrophy.
2. True posterior myocardial infarction.
3. Ventricular pre-excitation.
4. Duchenne-type muscular dystrophy.
5. Pronounced counter-clockwise cardiac rotation (very occasionally). (Dominant R waves may also be seen as part of the RBBB pattern but this should not cause confusion since the presence of the secondary R wave and of prolongation of the total QRS duration is easily recognised).

Conditions which may give rise to an Incorrect Diagnosis of Myocardial Infarction

1. Ventricular pre-excitation.
2. Left bundle branch block.
3. Left anterior hemiblock.
4. Hypertrophic obstructive cardiomyopathy (abnormal q waves may occur in this condition without infarction).
5. Congestive cardiomyopathy (abnormal q waves may occur in this condition without infarction).
6. Extreme clockwise cardiac rotation.
7. Left ventricular hypertrophy (occasionally the r wave in the right precordial lead may be so small as to suggest infarction).
8. Pulmonary embolism.
9. Hyperkalaemia.
10. Intracranial haemorrhage.

Useful Advice

Remember
It is **always difficult, often impossible,** and **sometimes dangerous** to diagnose myocardial infarction in the presence of left bundle branch block.

Remember
Ventricular pre-excitation is easily missed and can give rise to a false diagnosis of left bundle branch block or of myocardial infarction.

Causes of a Mean Frontal Plane QRS Axis more positive than +90°

1. Right ventricular hypertrophy
2. Anterolateral infarction
3. Left posterior hemiblock
4. Normal finding in infants and children (90° to 120°)
5. Normal finding occasionally in tall slim adults (90° to 105°)
6. Chronic lung disease
7. Pulmonary embolism
8. Atrial septal defect (ostium secundum type)
9. During coronary angiography (injection of contrast into right coronary artery)

Causes of a Mean Frontal Plane QRS Axis more negative than −30°

Common Causes

1. Left anterior hemiblock
2. Inferior myocardial infarction

Rare Causes

3. Ventricular pre-excitation
4. Hyperkalaemia
5. Tricuspid atresia

6. Atrial septal defect (ostium primum type)
7. Artificial cardiac pacing from apex of right or left ventricles

Easily Recognisable Cause

8. During coronary angiography (injection of contrast into left coronary artery)

Conditions giving rise to Prominent U Waves

1. Hypokalaemia.
2. Hypomagnesaemia.
3. Hypercalcaemia.
4. Bradycardia.
5. Following exercise.
6. Left ventricular hypertrophy.
7. Mitral valve prolapse.
8. Central nervous system disorders.
9. Hyperthyroidism.
10. During treatment with digitalis, quinidine, procainamide or phenothiazines.

Conditions giving rise to U Wave Inversion

1. Left ventricular hypertrophy.
2. Myocardial ischaemia.

Conditions giving rise to Prolongation of the Q-Tc Interval

Ischaemic heart disease.
Myocarditis.
Cardiomyopathy.
Hypocalcaemia.
Hypothermia.
Mitral valve prolapse.
Intracranial haemorrhage.
Drugs (quinidine, disopyramide, procainamide, amiodarone, tricyclic antidepressants, phenothiazines).
Hypothyroidism (but see page 229).

Acute cor pulmonale.
Post Stokes-Adams seizures.
Long Q-T syndrome.
(This is a syndrome consisting of a long Q-Tc interval, episodes of syncope and sudden death. It is often referred to as the Romano-Ward syndrome. When there is also congenital deafness it is referred to as the Jarvell and Lange-Nielsen syndrome).

Conditions giving rise to Shortening of the Q-Tc Interval

Hypercalcaemia.
Digitalis therapy.

Evaluation of the Q-T Interval

The Q-T interval is the time interval from the first recognisable part of the QRS complex to the final recognisable part of the T wave in the same lead. Since the QRS deflections are usually sharp the onset of the Q-T interval is usually easy to measure. However, the terminal part of the T wave is often a rather gentle slope and the precise position of the final part of the T wave may be difficult or even impossible to determine with total confidence. In the presence of a prominent U wave the difficulty is increased. The Q-T interval is therefore a relatively difficult measurement to make.

In addition to the difficulties in making the **measurement** of the Q-T interval there are considerable difficulties in **interpreting** the significance of measurement. This is because the Q-T interval varies inversely with the heart rate. There are two ways of overcoming this problem. The first is to consult a table of known values for the upper and lower limits of the Q-T duration at various heart rates. Several such tables are available in the literature. A second approach is to "correct" the measured Q-T interval at the observed heart rate to that which would be predicted for the same electrocardiogram if the heart rate were the "standard" rate of 60/minute. This corrected heart rate, or Q-Tc, can be obtained from nomograms which show Q-Tc in terms of observed heart rate and observed Q-T interval or can be obtained by the application of Bazett's formula (described in 1920):-

$$Q\text{-}Tc = \frac{\text{Measured Q-T interval}}{\sqrt{R\text{-}R \text{ interval}}}$$

[The units of the variable "Q-Tc" are usually expressed as "seconds", whereas strictly speaking they should be "seconds$^{1/2}$" i.e. "$\sqrt{\text{seconds}}$"].

There is some disagreement among various authorities on the range of normality of Q-Tc. The values are less for men than for women and are less for children than for adults.

Table 9 shows the predicted upper limits of normal for the Q-T intervals in men and women at various heart rates. The heart rate values are chosen on the basis of there being an integral number of 0.04 sec intervals (and therefore a precise number of small squares of the ECG graticule) in each chosen R-R interval. The maximum Q-T interval is that predicted by the Bazett formula using a maximum Q-Tc for men of 0.42 sec and for women of 0.43 sec. In practice it is more convenient to count the number of small squares (on the ECG graticule) between consecutive R waves (the "cycle time") and to use this to obtain the upper limit of normal for the Q-T duration rather than to work out the heart rate itself.

Table 9

Heart rate (per min)	Cycle time (number of 0.04 sec units)	Maximum Q-T (sec) (Males)	(Females)
300	5	.19	.19
250	6	.21	.21
214	7	.22	.23
187	8	.24	.24
166	9	.25	.26
150	10	.27	.27
136	11	.28	.29
125	12	.29	.3
115	13	.3	.31
107	14	.31	.32
100	15	.33	.33
93	16	.34	.34
88	17	.35	.35
83	18	.36	.36
78	19	.37	.37
75	20	.38	.38
71	21	.38	.39
68	22	.39	.4
65	23	.4	.41
62	24	.41	.42
60	25	.42	.43
57	26	.43	.44
55	27	.44	.45
52	28	.44	.46
51	29	.45	.46
50	30	.46	.47
48	31	.47	.48
46	32	.48	.49
45	33	.48	.49
43	34	.49	.5
42	35	.5	.51
41	36	.5	.52
40	37	.51	.52
39	38	.52	.53
38	39	.52	.54
37	40	.53	.54
36	41	.54	.55
35	42	.54	.56
35	43	.55	.56
34	44	.56	.57
33	45	.56	.58
32	46	.57	.58
32	47	.58	.59
31	48	.58	.6
30	49	.59	.6
30	50	.59	.61

The majority of conditions which alter the Q-T interval do so by causing Q-T prolongation. For that reason the upper limits of normality are more often required in detail than the lower limits. Significant shortening of the Q-T interval is less common and such a detailed table for the lower limits of normality is unnecessary. The following simple Table (10) gives the lower limits of normal for the Q-T interval at various ranges of heart rate.

Table 10

Heart Rates (per min)	Minimum 'Q-T interval' (sec)
45–55	.39
55–65	.36
65–75	.34
75–85	.32
85–105	.30

A Systematic Approach to the Interpretation of the ECG ("Updated")

We are now in a position to re-formulate the systematic approach to ECG interpretation which was first presented in Section I (pages 62–69). The basic approach is unchanged, but we can now graft on to it some additions and refinements as a result of our understanding of some electrocardiographic abnormalities.

Documentation and Recording Quality

It remains obligatory to ensure that the record **documentation** is satisfactory, i.e. that the **patient's name**, the **date** (and preferably also **time**) of the recording and the **lead labelling** and **gain calibration** are correctly entered on the record.

It remains obligatory also to ensure that the recording **quality** is adequate. In particular, baseline drift, skeletal muscle interference and mains frequency interference should be absent or minimal and the frequency response of the machine should be adequate (and preferably up to American Heart Association standards).

Provided the above preliminary requirements have been satisfactorily fulfilled, interpretation may proceed.

It is useful at this stage to review the systematic approach to ECG interpretation and to repeat the more important guidelines to the commoner and more significant abnormalities. The contents of the next four pages are repeated on the pull-out card in the flap at the back of this book.

Preliminary Assessment of Record Quality

Check
Name, date, lead labelling, normal gain calibration, paper recording speed.
Ensure
Minimal baseline drift, skeletal muscle interference, and muscle frequency interference and adequate machine frequency response.

Systematic Interpretation of ECG and Normal Criteria for Adults

1A. Determine Cardiac Rhythm

Criteria for normality of P waves only apply if rhythm is of sinus origin. Criteria for normality of QRS complexes, S-T segments and T waves only apply if rhythm is of supraventricular origin.

1B. Check P-R Interval

If 0.11 sec or less, consider pre-excitation. If pre-excitation is present (defined by (a) P-R interval is 0.11 sec or less, plus (b) total QRS duration is 0.11 sec or more, plus (c) slurring of initial 0.03 to 0.05 sec of QRS complex) **normal criteria for QRS complexes, S-T segments and T waves do not apply.**

2. Assess QRS Morphology in Precordial Leads

a) V_1 should have rS;

rS

V_6 should have qR but may have R, Rs or qRs.

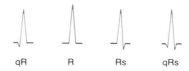

qR   R   Rs   qRs

(In the presence of clockwise rotation there may be no initial q in V_6 but a normal initial q may be seen in leads farther to left, i.e. I and aVL).

b) r wave should progressively increase in size from V_1 to V_6. However, it is quite normal for the R wave in V_6 to be smaller than that in V_5 and it is also normal for the R wave in V_5 to be less than that in V_4 provided the R wave in V_6 is also less than that in V_5 (compare Figure 42).
c) Transition (from right ventricular to left ventricular complexes) zone in precordial leads marked either by change from initial r to initial q (e.g. V_3-V_4 below) or by development of dominant R wave (V_3 below).

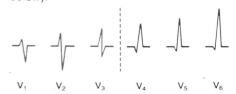

V_1 V_2 V_3 V_4 V_5 V_6

3. Check QRS Dimensions in Precordial Leads

a) Total QRS duration should not exceed 0.10 sec (2½ small squares).

> If QRS duration is 0.12 sec or more and there is no initial q wave in V_6, I and aVL and there is no secondary R wave in V_1 (and assuming the rhythm is supraventricular), there is left bundle branch block. In this situation the normal criteria for the QRS complexes, S-T segments and T waves do not apply.

b) At least one R wave should exceed 8 mm.

c) The tallest R wave should not exceed 27 mm.
d) The deepest S wave should not exceed 30 mm.
e) The sum of the tallest R and deepest S should not exceed 40 mm.
f) The ventricular activation time should not exceed 0.04 sec.
g) Any q wave seen should not have a depth exceeding ¼ of the height of the ensuing R wave.
h) Any q waves seen should not equal or exceed 0.04 sec in duration.

4A. Assess Precordial T Waves

a) The T wave in V_1 may be upright, flat or inverted. If upright in earlier records, it must be still upright.
b) The T wave in V_2 may be upright, flat or inverted. If upright in earlier records or

if upright in V_1, it must be upright.
c) The T wave in V_3–V_5 must be upright.
In general the T wave should be more than ⅛ but less than ⅔ of the R wave height.

4B. Assess the U Waves

The normal U wave is upright in all leads in which the T wave is upright. It should also be upright in the right precordial leads, even if the T waves are inverted here. Its average amplitude is less than 0.5mm. It tends to be largest in V_2 and V_3 where it may occasionally reach 2mm in height. In general it is less than 25% of the height of the preceding T wave. It is definitely abnormal when it is taller than the preceding T wave. Some authorities regard U waves taller than 1.5mm as abnormal. U wave inversion is abnormal.

5. Assess Precordial S-T Segments

The S-T segments must not deviate from the iso-electric line by more than ±1mm. Note that this should not be rigidly applied in V_1 and V_2. Caution should also be exercised in the presence of a tachycardia which may render assessment of the iso-electric position difficult or impossible.

6. Assess QRS Complexes in Limb Leads

a) A q wave in aVL*,I, II or aVF should not equal or exceed 0.04 sec in duration.
b) A q wave in aVL*,I, II or aVF should not have a depth greater than ¼ of the height of the ensuing R wave.

Note
*q waves exceeding this criterion are acceptable in aVL if the frontal plane axis is more positive than +60° (i.e. +75° or more).

c) The R wave in aVL should not exceed 13 mm and that in aVF should not exceed 20 mm.
d) The frontal plane axis should not lie outside the range −30° to +90°.

7A. Assess T Waves in Limb Leads

a) The mean frontal plane T wave axis should not differ from the frontal plane QRS axis by more than ±45°.

b) In the presence of abnormal q waves in II, III, and aVF, T wave inversion in these leads is abnormal even if the above criterion is not fulfilled.

7B. Assess the U Waves

The U waves should be upright where the T waves are upright. The criterion for U wave size is as given in 4B above.

8. Assess S-T Segment in Limb Leads

These should not deviate by more than 1 mm above or below iso-electric line (see precautions under 5 above).

9. Assess P Waves

a) The P waves should not exceed 0.12 sec in duration in II.
b) The P waves should not exceed 2.5mm in height in II.

c) Any negative component to the P wave in V_1 should not have a greater area than the positive component.

10. *Measure Q-T Interval

Make sure not to include a U wave. The number of 0.04 sec intervals (i.e. small squares on the ECG graticule) between consecutive R waves should be counted and the normality or otherwise of the measured Q-T interval in relation to the observed R-R interval determined by reference to Tables 9 and 10 on page 264.

Note
*Q-T interval measurement is a difficult measurement to make and is often unrewarding. In the author's experience most abnormalities of Q-T duration are discovered in retrospect when the primary abnormality (e.g. hypocalcaemia) is already apparent.

Criteria for some of the Commoner or More Important Abnormalities

Ventricular Pre-excitation (WPW type)	**a)** P-R interval of 0.11 sec or less **plus** **b)** QRS duration of 0.11 sec or more **plus** **c)** Slurring of initial 0.03–0.05 sec of QRS complex.	In the presence of ventricular pre-excitation the normal criteria for QRS complexes, S-T segments and T waves do not apply. TAKE CARE NOT TO MAKE AN INCORRECT DIAGNOSIS OF LEFT BUNDLE BRANCH BLOCK OR MYOCARDIAL INFARCTION.
Left Bundle Branch Block (LBBB)	**a)** Total QRS duration of 0.12 sec or more **plus** **b)** Absence of initial q wave in V_5, V_6 I and aVL **plus** **c)** Absence of secondary R wave in V_1 to indicate RBBB.	In the presence of LBBB the normal criteria for QRS complexes, S-T segments and T waves do not apply. The normal criterion for the frontal plane axis does apply. TAKE CARE NOT TO MAKE AN INCORRECT DIAGNOSIS OF MYOCARDIAL INFARCTION OR LEFT VENTRICULAR HYPERTROPHY
Right Bundle Branch Block (RBBB)	**a)** Total QRS duration of 0.12 sec or more **plus** **b)** Secondary R wave in V_1.	In the presence of RBBB the normal criteria for the QRS complexes and for the frontal plane axis apply.
Left Anterior Hemiblock (LAH)	**a)** Mean frontal plane QRS axis more negative than $-30°$ **plus** **b)** Absence of q wave evidence of inferior infarction (i.e. initial r waves are visible in II and aVF).	Left anterior hemiblock and inferior infarction are the two commonest causes of left axis deviation. The criteria for LAH are based on this. Other less common causes of left axis deviation include ventricular pre-excitation, hyperkalaemia, tricuspid atresia, ostium primum atrial septal defect and artificial cardiac pacing.
Left Ventricular Hypertrophy (LVH) One or more of:-	**a)** R in V_4, V_5 or V_6 exceeds 27mm **b)** S in V_1, V_2 or V_3 exceeds 30mm **c)** R in V_4, V_5 or V_6 plus S in V_1, V_2 or V_3 exceeds 40mm **d)** R in aVL exceeds 13mm **e)** R in aVF exceeds 20mm **f)** Ventricular activation time exceeds 0.04 sec **g)** S-T segment depression, T wave flattening, T wave inversion in leads facing left ventricle.	The reliability of the electrocardiographic diagnosis of left ventricular hypertrophy is directly related to the number of criteria fulfilled. Abnormal left axis deviation is not an expected finding in LVH.
Right Ventricular Hypertrophy (RVH)	**a)** Dominant R in V_1 (i.e. R, Rs, RR', qR or qRs) **plus** **b)** Frontal plane axis more positive than $+90°$	Dominant R in V_1 can occur in true posterior infarction, ventricular pre-excitation and Duchenne-type muscular dystrophy.

Left Atrial "Hypertrophy"

(Strictly "abnormality")

a) P duration longer than 0.12 sec or P wave bifid in I, II, aVF and aVL
or
b) P wave in V_1 has negative component with area greater than that of positive component.

Right Atrial "Hypertrophy"

(Strictly "abnormality")

a) P wave height 3.0mm or more in II, III or aVF.

Myocardial Infarction

a) q waves 0.04 sec or more in duration (excluding always Leads aVR and III, and, when the frontal plane QRS axis +75° or more positive, excluding also aVL).
or
b) q waves more than ¼ the height of the ensuing R wave (excluding always Leads aVR and III and, when the frontal plane QRS axis is +75° or more positive, excluding also aVL).
or
c) qs or QS complexes (excluding always Leads aVR and III and, when the frontal plane QRS axis is +75° or more positive excluding also aVL).
or
d) Inappropriately low R wave voltage in local area (when the facts can confidently be ascertained).

The concomitant presence of significant S-T elevation suggests that the infarct is not more than days old. If the S-T segments are normal but there is still T inversion, it suggests that the infarct is not more than several weeks old.
IT IS ALWAYS DIFFICULT, OFTEN IMPOSSIBLE, AND SOMETIMES DANGEROUS TO DIAGNOSE INFARCTION IN THE PRESENCE OF LBBB OR VENTRICULAR PRE-EXCITATION.

Note

The above "diagnostic criteria" for myocardial infarction can occasionally be fulfilled in certain particular conditions which gives rise to "pseudo-infarction" patterns (pages 198 and 242). The most likely such condition is cardiomyopathy. The diagnosis of myocardial infarction is extremely unlikely to be incorrect if the full **sequence** of changes (S-T elevation, QRS changes, T wave changes and restoration of normality to the S-T segments) is seen.

Conditions in which "Normal" Criteria do not apply

In the presence of supraventricular arrhythmias the normal criteria for P waves do no apply.

In supraventricular arrhythmias atrial depolarisation begins from an abnormal site. The normal pathway for atrial myocardial depolarisation cannot therefore be followed and the P waves are, in consequence, abnormal. Assuming there is normal intraventricular conduction the normal criteria for QRS complexes, S-T segments and T waves continue to apply.

In the presence of ventricular arrhythmias or of ventricular pre-excitation the normal criteria for the QRS complexes do not apply.

In ventricular arrhythmias ventricular depolarisation begins from an abnormal site and the normal pathway for ventricular myocardial depolarisation cannot be followed. In consequence the QRS complexes are abnormal. The S-T segments and T waves are usually also abnormal in this situation for primary depolarisation (QRS) abnormalities often result in secondary repolarisation (S-T segments and T wave) abnormalities.

The 12-Lead ECG : Annotated Records

This final chapter will review a series of 40 12-lead electrocardiograms. These are referred to as "Records" rather than figures for they may be used either for instruction or for audit. A similar approach was used at the end of Section 1, where 30 "records" were presented. To prevent confusion the first record described here in Section 2 will be labelled "Record 31". For each of the first 10 records, each detailed step of the systematic interpretation originally described on pages 66–69 and subsequently modified on pages 266 to 268 will be followed and described using the same numbering for the paragraphs. Abnormalities will be shown in **heavy type**. Records 41 to 70 then appear without any supporting text. On page 321 each of these last 30 records will be defined as being normal or abnormal. For those records which are abnormal, a list of the abnormal features will appear on pages 322 to 326. This list will use the paragraph headings corresponding to the systematic approach described on pages 266 to 268 (as modified from the list which originally appeared in Section I on pages 67 to 69). The student may use this section either for further systematic tuition or for self-evaluation. Finally, an interpretation of Records 1-30 from Section I will be given on pages 327 to 329. Abnormalities will be expressed in **heavy type**.

Record 31

Normal Record

1. Sinus rhythm. The P-R interval is normal at 0.12 sec (well seen in II).

2. a) V_1 has an rS complex. V_6 has a qR complex.

b) V_1–V_6 shows normal r wave progression from V_1–V_4, with the slight fall-off between V_4 and V_5, and again between V_5 and V_6 which is entirely normal.

c) The transition zone is between V_2 and V_3 (using criterion of dominant R wave, or between V_4 and V_5 using criterion of development of q wave).

3. a) Total QRS duration equals 0.07 sec.

b) The r waves in V_3, V_4, V_5 and V_6 all exceed 8mm.

c) The tallest r wave in the left precordial lead (V_4) measures 17mm.

d) The deepest S wave in the right precordial leads (V_2) measures 13mm.

e) $S_{V_2} + R_{V_4} = 30$mm.

f) Ventricular activation time (well seen in V_5) = 0.03 sec.

g) q waves are seen in V_5 and V_6. They are obviously less than one quarter of the height of the ensuing r waves in the same lead.

h) q waves in V_5 and V_6 are clearly less than 0.04 sec in duration.

4A. The T waves are upright and of normal voltage throughout the precordial leads. The tallest T waves in this case are seen in V_2 and V_3 which is usually the case in normal records and the T wave height in the left precordial leads is not less than $\frac{1}{8}$th and not more than $\frac{2}{3}$rds of the height of the preceding R wave.
4B. Normal (low voltage but upright) U waves are seen in V_1–V_5.

5. The precordial S-T segments are iso-electric. Note that it is easier to see discrete S-T segments in V_4, V_5 and V_6 than it is in V_1 and V_2. This is usually the case.

6. a) Small q waves are seen in Leads I, II and aVF. They are less than 0.04 sec in duration.

b) The q waves seen in I and II are not greater than one quarter of the height of the ensuing R wave. The q wave in aVF is at the extreme upper end of the normal range in depth, but is not definitively abnormal. (q waves in Lead III which are broader or deeper than the normally accepted criteria are not significant unless abnormal q waves are also present in Lead II or aVF).

c) The R wave in aVL does not exceed 13mm and the R wave in aVF does not exceed 20mm.

d) The mean frontal plane QRS axis is +60°. This is within normal limits.

7A. The mean frontal plane T wave axis is +45°. The difference from the QRS axis is 15°, which is within the normal range.
7B. No U waves are visible in the limb leads. This is quite normal.

8. The S-T segments in the limb leads are iso-electric.

9. a) The P wave duration in II is 0.10 sec.

b) The P wave height in II is 1.5mm.

c) There is no dominant negative component to the P wave in V_1.

10. The Q-T interval is 0.42 sec. The heart rate is 57 per min but it is unnecessary to work this out. The "cycle time" (see page 263) is 26 (i.e. there are 26 small squares (on the ECG graticule) between consecutive R waves. Table 9 (page 264) shows that the upper limit of normal of the Q-T interval appropriate to this heart rate (or cycle time) is 0.43 sec for men or 0.44 sec for women. The Q-T interval is therefore normal.

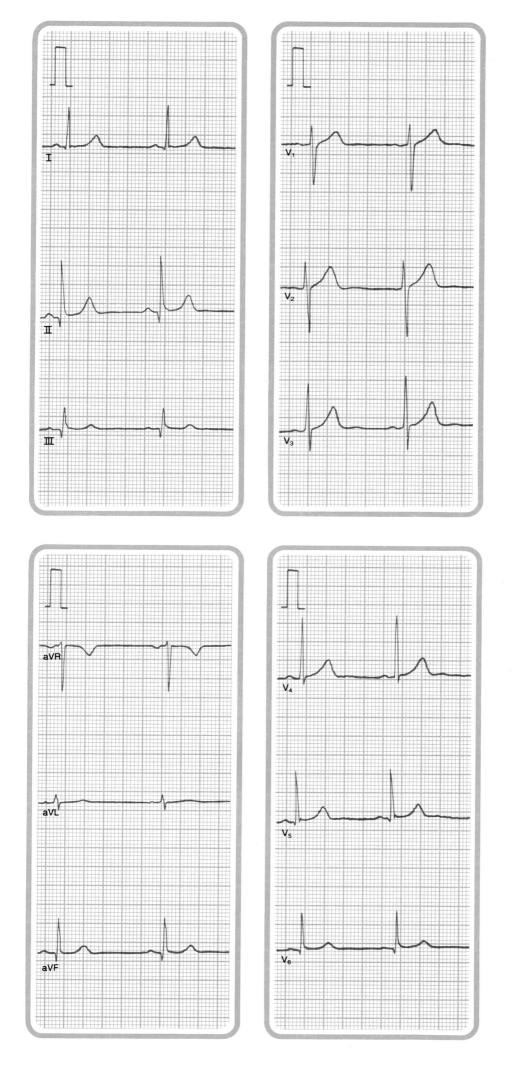

272

Record 32

Abnormal Record

1. Sinus rhythm. The P-R interval is normal at 0.18 sec.

2. a) **V₁ has a qR complex**. This is frankly abnormal. V₆ has a qRS complex. The S wave is much larger than one would normally expect, but this does not constitute a definite abnormality in its own right. (It is the result of the pronounced clockwise cardiac rotation which obtains in this record).

b) The r wave progression from V₁–V₆ is completely abnormal, but this is due entirely to the fact that the R waves are abnormally tall in the right precordial leads, i.e. it does not constitute an additional abnormality over and above that indicated by the abnormal R wave height in V₁.

c) **The transition zone is beyond (i.e. further to the left than) V₆. This indicates extreme clockwise cardiac rotation.**

3. a) The total QRS duration is within the normal range at 0.09 sec (well seen in V₆).

b) All the R waves in the precordial leads exceed 8mm.

c) The tallest R wave in the left precordial lead (V₄) is within the normal range at 18mm.

d) The S waves in the right precordial leads are much smaller than are usually seen and they certainly are not abnormally deep.

e) The sum of the deepest S waves (V₃) and the tallest R waves (V₄) is 37mm. This is within the normal range.

f) No true estimate of the ventricular activation time can be obtained since no true left ventricular complexes are possible in the precordial series (again due to the pronounced clockwise cardiac rotation).

g) The q waves in V₆ are manifestly not deeper than ¼ of the height of the following r wave.

h) The q waves in V₆ are certainly less than 0.04 sec in duration.

4A. The T waves are inverted from V₁-V₅. This is definitely abnormal. **The T waves are iso-electric in V₆.** This is also abnormal.
4B. No definite U waves are visible in the precordial leads. This is not an abnormality.

5. The S-T segments are depressed from V₁-V₅. This is frankly abnormal.

6. a) Small q waves are visible in aVF. They are less than one quarter of the height of the following r wave.

b) The q waves in aVF are less than one small square in duration (i.e. less than 0.04 sec).

c) The R wave in aVL does not exceed 13mm nor does that in aVF exceed 20mm.

d) **The mean frontal plane QRS axis is +120°.** This is frankly abnormal.

7A. The mean frontal plane T wave axis is +90°. The difference between the frontal plane QRS and T wave axes is within the normal range at 30°. The limb lead T waves are therefore within normal limits.
7B. No definite U waves are visible. This is not abnormal.

8. There is minimal S-T segment depression in Lead III and the foot-lead, but this is not beyond the normal permitted limits of ± 1mm from the iso-electric line.

9. a) The P wave duration in Lead II is 0.11 sec.

b) The P wave height in Lead II is 2mm.

c) **The negative component of the P waves in V₁ is larger than the positive component, indicating left atrial abnormality.**

10. The Q-T interval is 0.38 sec. The cycle time (page 263) is 20 (i.e. heart rate 75) and the Q-T interval is therefore normal.

The combination of a dominant R wave in V₁ with abnormal right axis deviation indicates **right ventricular hypertrophy**. *The S-T segment depression and T wave inversion in the precordial leads and the pronounced clockwise cardiac rotation are frequent accompaniments of right ventricular hypertrophy. In addition there is* **left atrial abnormality**.

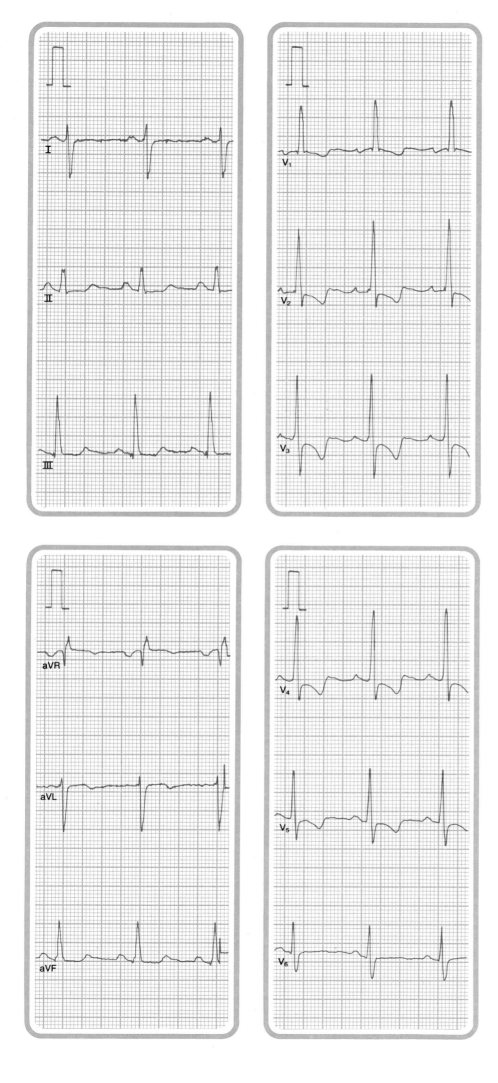

274

Record 33

Abnormal Record

1. Sinus rhythm. The P-R interval is 0.16 sec.

2. a) V_1 has a rS complex. V_6 has a qR complex.

b) V_1–V_6 has a **relatively** normal R wave progression, but the R waves in the left precordial leads are not as tall as one would expect, i.e. the R wave progression does not appear to have developed as well as usual.

c) The transition zone is between V_4 and V_5.

3. a) The total QRS duration is 0.07 sec.

b) The r wave in V_3 is 9mm, i.e. it just exceeds the minimum requirement of 8mm.

c) The tallest R wave is well within the normal range at 9mm (in V_3).

d) The deepest S wave is seen in V_2 and this is within the normal range of 7mm.

e) The sum of the S in V_2 and the R in V_3 is well within the normal range at 15mm.

f) The ventricular activation time is of the order of 0.02 sec.

g) q waves are seen in V_6, and these are clearly less than one quarter of the height of the ensuing r wave in the same lead.

h) q waves in V_6 are clearly less than 0.04 sec in duration.

4A. T waves in V_1, V_2 and V_3 are normal. **The T waves in V_4, V_5 and V_6 are of abnormally low voltage (they are almost iso-electric).**
4B. Prominent U waves are seen in these leads and **in V_5 the U wave is bigger than the P wave which precedes it, which is definitely abnormal.**

5. The S-T segments from V_1 to V_4 are iso-electric. The S-T segments in V_5 and V_6 are minimally depressed but not beyond the normal permitted range of $\pm$ 1mm.

6. a) q waves are seen in Leads I, II and aVL. In all cases they are less than 0.04 sec in duration.

b) **The q wave in Lead II has a depth which is greater than one quarter of the height of the R wave following it, which is abnormal.**

c). The R wave in aVL does not exceed 13mm and the r wave in aVF does not exceed 20mm.

d) The mean frontal plane QRS axis is $-15°$, which is within the normal range.

7A. The mean frontal plane T wave axis is $-45°$. **Although the angle between the mean frontal plane QRS axis and T wave axes is within the normal range, the negative T waves in Leads II, III and the foot-lead should be regarded as being abnormal since there is an abnormal q wave in Lead II, indicative of inferior myocardial infarction** (pages 60 and 178).
7B. Small upright (normal) U waves are seen in I and aVL.

8. The S-T segments in the limb leads are iso-electric.

9. a) The P wave duration is within the normal range at 0.10 sec.

b) The P wave height is within the normal range in Lead II at 1.5mm.

c) The negative component of the P wave in V_1 is about equal to that of the positive component. This is not abnormal.

10. The Q-T interval is 0.44 sec. For a cycle time of 27 (heart rate 55) this is within normal limits.

There is unequivocal evidence of inferior myocardial infarction of intermediate age. It has not occurred within the last few days since there is no residual S-T segment elevation. It is not more than a few weeks old since there is still T wave inversion. The low voltage T waves in the left precordial leads and the prominent U waves there, are non-specific abnormalities. The probability is that they are related to ischaemia in the lateral wall of the ventricle, but one cannot be dogmatic on this point.
Note that aVF shows rS complexes. Even though the r waves are very small, they preclude the diagnosis of inferior infarction from the QRS configuration in this lead. It is possible that these small r waves have "regenerated" (page 179), i.e. that QS complexes were formerly apparent in this lead.

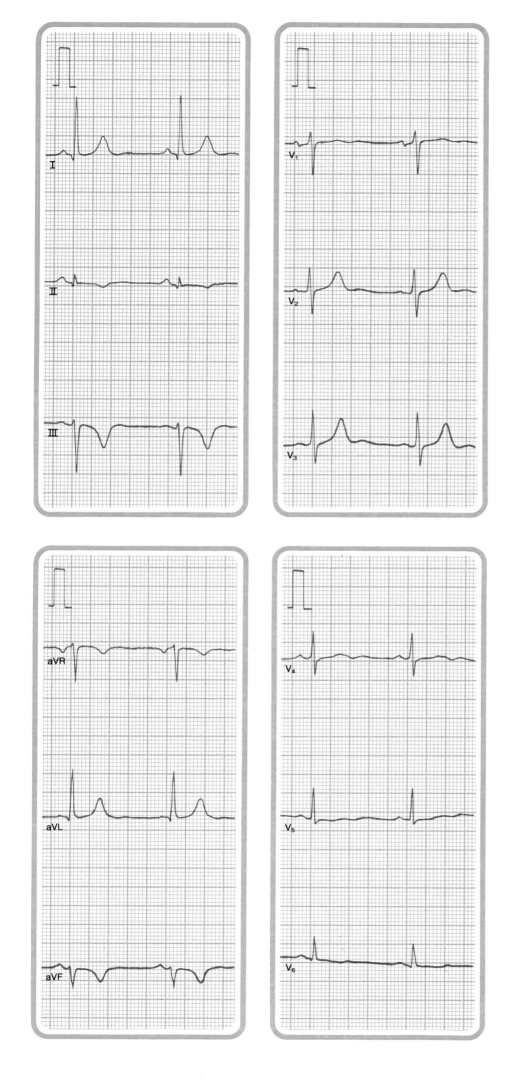

276

Record 34

Abnormal Record

1. The rhythm is sinus. The P-R interval is within the normal range at 0.12 sec (well seen in V_2).

2. a) V_1 has a rS complex. The r wave is very small indeed and it might be thought that there is a QS complex in this lead, however, there is a definite r wave in V_2 and even if there were no initial r wave in V_1, it would not actually constitute an abnormality*.
V_6 shows a qR complex. The q wave is again very small and is perhaps best seen in the second QRS complex of V_6.
  b) The r wave progression from V_1–V_6 is normal.
  c) The transition zone is between V_3 and V_4.

3. a) The total QRS duration is normal at 0.09 sec (well seen in the third QRS complex in V_2).
  b) The R waves in the left precordial leads all exceed 8mm.
  c) The tallest R wave (V_5) is within the normal range at 18mm.
  d) The deepest S wave (V_2) is abnormal at 34mm.
  e) The sum of S in V_2 and R in V_5 is abnormal at 52mm.
  f) The ventricular activation time is 0.04 sec (well seen in V_5).
  g) The q waves in V_6 are not deeper than one quarter of the height of the ensuing r waves.
  h) The q waves in V_6 are less than 0.04 sec in duration.

4A. The T waves are inverted from V_4–V_6. This is frankly abnormal.
4B. Small, upright (normal) U waves are seen in V_2 and V_3.

5. The S-T segments are depressed in V_4, V_5 and V_6. This is frankly abnormal. The S-T depression is sloping rather than flat. It is therefore non-specific.

6. a) Small q waves are seen in aVF. They are less than 0.04 sec in duration.
  b) The q waves in aVF are not deeper than a quarter of the height of the ensuing r wave.
  c) The R wave in aVL does not exceed 13mm and the R wave in aVF does not exceed 20mm.
  d) The mean frontal plane QRS is $+45°$.

7A. The mean frontal plane T wave axis is indeterminate. Since the mean frontal plane QRS axis is highly determinate, the T waves in the limb leads are abnormal.
7B. No significant U waves are seen in the limb leads.

8. There is S-T segment depression in Lead II and the foot-lead. This is beyond the acceptable limit of one millimetre (well seen in both of these leads) compared with the T-P interval.

9. a) The P wave duration in Lead II is within normal limits at 0.10 sec.
  b) The P wave height is normal at 1.5mm.
  c) The negative component of the P wave in V_1 does not exceed the positive component.

10. The Q-T interval is 0.32 sec. The cycle time is 16 (heart rate 93) for which the upper limit of normal for the Q-T interval is 0.34 sec.

The changes are those of left ventricular hypertrophy. The voltage criteria for left ventricular hypertrophy are fulfilled in the precordial leads. The S-T, T changes in the left precordial leads are probably secondary to the primary QRS abnormality. The S-T, T changes in the limb leads are non-specific, but the probability is that these too are secondary to the abnormal QRS complexes. Note the superficial similarities of the morphology of the QRS complexes to that in left bundle branch block. However, there is no left bundle branch block since:-
a) the total QRS duration is well within the normal range, and
b) the small initial q waves are seen in V_6.

Note
*Occasionally the normal ECG has no recognisable r waves in V_1 (page 45).

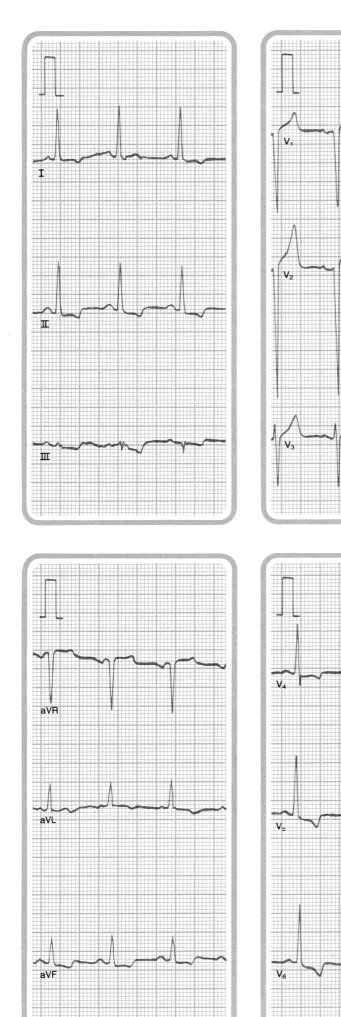

Record 35

Abnormal Record

1. The rhythm is sinus. The P-R interval is within the normal range at 0.12 sec (well seen in Lead II). The P-R interval in the left precordial lead looks to be abnormally short on casual inspection (especially in V_5). However, note that the P waves are bifid and that the true origin of the P waves is earlier than initially suspected. The P waves in Lead II are also bifid and the normal length of the P-R interval is readily visible in this lead.

2. a) V_1 has an rS complex. V_6 has a qR complex.
b) **The r wave progression from V_1–V_6 is not normal.**
There is a normal r wave in V_1, **but V_2 shows a QS complex (i.e. complete absence of the r wave) and V_3 shows a qrS complex. The r wave progression in V_2 and V_3 is therefore frankly abnormal.**
c) The transition zone is in the region of V_4.

3. a) The total QRS duration is within the normal range at 0.10 sec (well seen in V_3).
b) The R waves in the left precordial leads clearly exceed 8mm.
c) The tallest R wave in the left precordial leads (V_5) is within the normal range at 19mm.
d) The deepest precordial S wave (V_1) is 22mm.
e) $S_{V_1} + R_{V_5}$ is 41mm, which is strictly speaking just beyond the normal range.
f) The ventricular activation time is 0.04 sec.
g) **There are QS complexes in V_2. This is frankly abnormal.** (By definition, the q waves in a QS complex exceed ¼ of the ensuing R wave since there is no r wave).
The q wave in V_3 is clearly much larger than one quarter of the height of the ensuing r wave, and these q waves are therefore abnormal.
h) **The q waves in V_2 and V_3 are also abnormal in terms of their duration, which exceeds 0.04 sec.**

4A. The T waves are normal from V_1 to V_5. T waves in V_6 are upright, but are of rather lower voltage than one would expect. It is possible (but not certain) that this is an abnormality.
4B. Small, but upright (i.e. normal) U waves are seen in V_2–V_5.

5. The precordial S-T segments are within normal limits. The slight degree of S-T segment elevation seen in the right precordial leads, whilst possibly consistent with the presence of anteroseptal infarction, is also quite possibly within the normal range. Minimal degrees of S-T segment elevation are frequently seen in these leads.

6. a) Initial q waves are seen in Lead I and aVL. In neither case are the q waves 0.04 sec or more in duration.
b) The q waves seen in I and aVL do not have a depth exceeding one quarter of the height of the ensuing r wave.
c) The R wave in aVL does not exceed 13mm and the r wave in aVF does not exceed 20mm.
d) The mean frontal plane QRS axis is −30°. This is at the extreme left hand end of the normal range. There is therefore borderline abnormal left axis deviation.

7A. The mean frontal plane T wave axis is of the order of +90°. It is not highly determinate, but is certainly in this region. The T waves in the limb leads are therefore abnormal either because the angle between the frontal plane T and QRS axes is beyond the normal range, or because the frontal plane T wave axis is not highly determinate whilst the frontal plane QRS axis is highly determinate.
7B. Small (normal U waves are seen in II, III and aVF.

8. The S-T segments are depressed in Leads I and aVL. The degree of **depression is minimal but probably abnormal.** It may well be that this S-T segment depression has developed as a result of the presence of ischaemic heart disease but one cannot, from the electrocardiogram, with total confidence say that the S-T segment depression is abnormal since it is not beyond the normally accepted range.

9. a) The P wave duration in II is 0.12 sec which is at the extreme upper end of the normal range.
b) The P wave height in II is normal at 1 mm.
c) The P wave in V_1 does not have a dominant negative component.

10. The Q-T interval is 0.46 sec. The cycle time is 31 (heart rate 48) for which the normal upper limit for the Q-T interval is 0.47 sec.

The electrocardiogram shows a definite abnormality of the QRS complexes in V_1 - V_3. This abnormality is indicative of loss of viable myocardium in this area. The most likely cause is an old anteroseptal infarction but other causes (pseudo-infarction patterns) can occur in various cardiomyopathies or infiltrative lesions. In addition there are non-specific S-T, T changes in the limb leads and in V_6. These could well be related to the same basic cause as the abnormal QRS complexes in the precordial leads, but one cannot be totally confident of this. The precordial QRS complexes just satisfy the voltage criteria for left ventricular hypertrophy but it is unwise to make this diagnosis when these criteria are only just fulfilled and there are no additional criteria for the condition fulfilled.

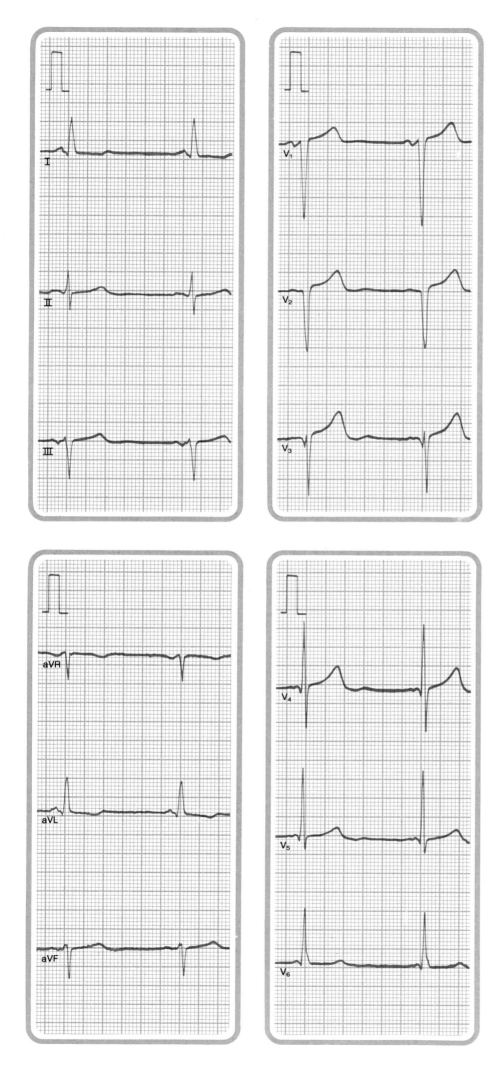

280

Abnormal Record

1. The rhythm is sinus. The P-R interval is 0.19 sec (well seen in Lead II).

2. a) V$_1$ has an rS complex. V$_6$ does not have a qR complex. No initial q wave is seen in V$_6$. **It is obvious also at this stage that the total QRS duration is prolonged. The total QRS duration is 0.18 sec (well seen in V$_6$). Since there is no initial septal q wave in V$_6$ the total QRS duration is prolonged and there is no secondary r wave in the right precordial leads, there is therefore left bundle branch block. In view of this, there is no point in making any further assessment of the precordial QRS complexes, S-T segments or T waves. The deep S waves in V$_1$ and the deep QS complexes in V$_2$ and V$_3$ are all part of the left bundle branch block pattern. The depressed S-T segments in V$_6$ and T wave inversion in this lead and the elevated S-T segments in the right precordial leads are also part of the left bundle branch block pattern.**

Once left bundle branch block has been diagnosed, no further diagnostic processes should be applied to the QRS complexes, the S-T segments or the T waves in the precordial leads. In the limb leads the only diagnostic process which should be applied is the determination of the mean frontal plane QRS axis.

6. d) This is seen to be abnormal at −45°. There is therefore an abnormal degree of left axis deviation and this might imply peripheral disease in the anterior division of the left bundle branch system in addition to the proximal lesion causing complete left bundle branch block.

9. The normal criteria can be applied to the P waves and it can be seen that the **P wave in V$_1$ has a dominant negative component. This indicates left atrial abnormality.**

The only other feature for comment is the presence of a small initial q wave in aVL. This is unusual in left bundle branch block and indeed is normally part of the criteria that initial q waves should be absent not only in V$_5$ and V$_6$, but also in Leads I and aVL. This raises the possibility of myocardial infarction as well as left bundle branch block, but as stressed in the text this diagnosis can only rarely be made with confidence and should always be applied with very great caution.

This record is best considered as showing complete left bundle branch block, an abnormal degree of left axis deviation and abnormal P waves indicating left atrial abnormality. (The patient was actually suffering from congestive cardiomyopathy).

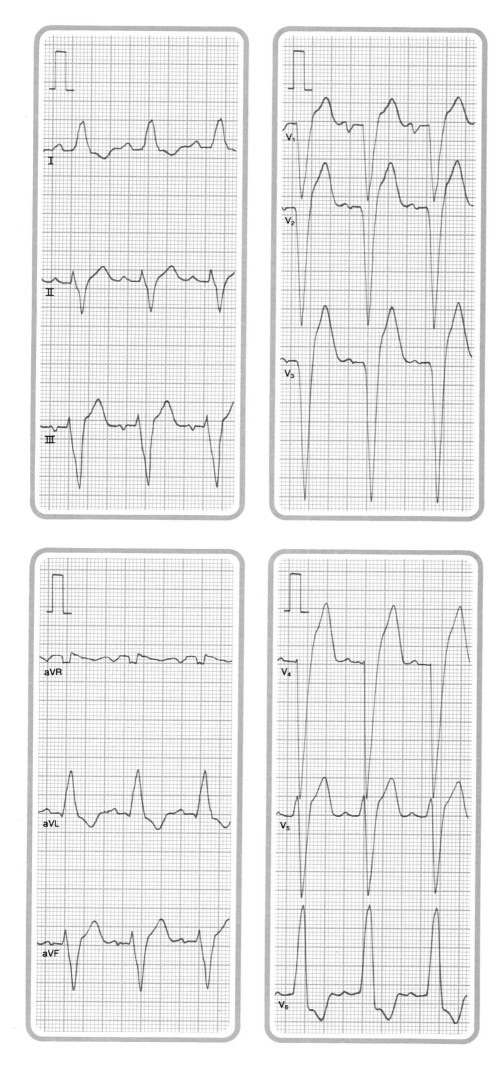

282

Record 37

Abnormal Record

1. The rhythm is sinus. The P-R interval is 0.14 sec.

2. a) There is no initial r wave in V_1 which shows a QS complex. There is no initial q wave in V_6. This leads one to consider the possibility that the interventricular septum might be depolarising in the wrong direction (complete or incomplete left bundle branch block). There is clearly no complete left bundle branch block since the total QRS duration can be seen to be normal. When no initial q wave is seen in V_6, one should inspect other leads looking at the left ventricle. When the heart is horizontal, as is usually the case, this will be Leads I and aVL. In this case the heart is almost vertical (with, as we shall see later, a frontal plane QRS axis of $+75°$) and the left ventricular facing limb leads are therefore Leads II and aVF. These both show small initial q waves and we may therefore conclude that the interventricular septum is depolarising in the normal direction. The absence of a q wave in V_6 is therefore not abnormal.

b) **The r wave progression in the precordial leads is clearly abnormal. No r wave is visible from V_1–V_4. Normal R waves "suddenly" appear in V_5 and V_6.**

c) The transition zone is between V_4 and V_5. Since the R wave progression is abnormal the transition zone has little meaning.

3. a) The total QRS duration is within the normal range at 0.08 sec.

b) The R waves in V_5 and V_6 both satisfy the minimal voltage criterion of 8mm.

c) The tallest precordial R wave (V_5) is well below the maximum permitted normal at 11mm.

d) The deepest S wave is actually seen in V_5. (The negative waves from V_1 to V_4 are not S waves, they are QS complexes and the S wave criteria do not apply to these). The S wave in V_5 is not abnormally deep.

e) $S_{V_5} + R_{V_5} = 14$, which is well within the permitted range.

f) The ventricular activation time cannot be determined since no qR complex is visible in the left precordial leads.

g) **The q waves from V_1 to V_4 are clearly abnormal. In each case they are QS complexes and they are clearly therefore more than a quarter of the height of the ensuing r wave.**

h) **The q waves from V_1 to V_4 are also abnormally long. They are well in excess of the permitted maximum of 0.03 sec*. This criterion would itself be sufficient to indicate the presence of infarction.**

4A. There is terminal T wave inversion in V_2, V_3 and V_4, and low voltage T waves in V_5.

4B. Small, upright (normal) U waves are seen in V_5.

5. There is clear-cut, definitive S-T segment elevation from V_1–V_4 and minimal S-T segment elevation in V_5.

6. a) Small q waves are seen in Leads II and aVF. In no case is their depth more than one quarter of the height of the ensuing R wave.

b) Likewise the q waves in II and aVF do not equal or exceed 0.04 sec in duration.

c) The r wave in aVL does not exceed 13mm and the R wave in aVF does not exceed 20mm.

d) The mean frontal plane QRS axis is $+75°$ (it could be interpreted as being $+60°$. It depends whether or not one thinks that the algebraic sum of QRS deflections in aVL is actually zero or slightly negative).

7A. The mean frontal plane T wave axis is $+75°$. The frontal plane T waves are therefore normal.

The T waves in Lead I are flat and those who interpret the electrocardiogram via pattern recognition approach would probably regard them as abnormal. However, they do not actually fulfil the criteria for abnormality. The T waves are flat in Lead I simply because the repolarisation vector is almost at right angles to this lead.

7B. No significant U waves are seen in the limb leads.

8. The S-T segments in the limb leads are iso-electric.

9. a) The P wave duration is normal at 0.10 sec.

b) The P wave height is normal at 1mm.

c) The P waves in V_1 do not have a dominant negative component.

10. The Q-T interval is 0.34 sec (well seen in aVF). The cycle time is 16 (heart rate 93) and the maximum Q-T interval at this heart rate is 0.34 sec.

The record shows unequivocal evidence of recent anteroseptal myocardial infarction.

The record shows relatively recent anterior myocardial infarction. The QS complexes from V_1 - V_4 indicate "through and through" (transmural) infarction. The presence of S-T elevation from V_1 - V_4 (with, in addition, minimal S-T elevation in V_5) indicates that the infarct is relatively recent – probably less than one week old. The terminal T wave inversion in V_2, V_3 and V_4 and the low voltage waves in V_5 are also consistent with the diagnosis of recent anterior infarction.

Note

* To say that a "q wave is in excess of 0.03 sec" is the same as saying that its "duration is 0.04 sec or more" since the best temporal resolution in the ECG is 0.01 sec.

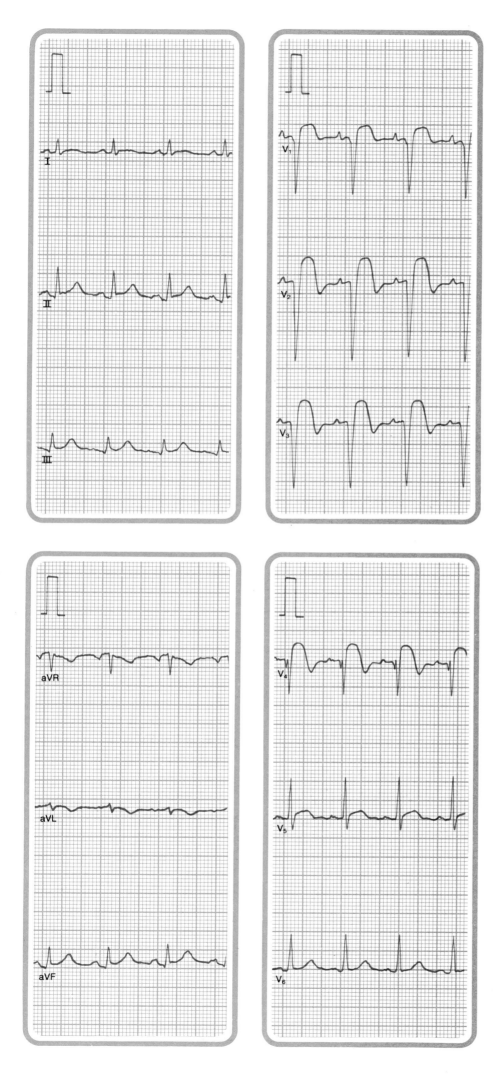

284

Record 38

Abnormal Record

1. The rhythm is sinus. The P-R interval is 0.14 sec.

2. a) **V_1 has an rsR' complex. This is abnormal.** V_6 has a qRs complex.

b) The progression from V_1–V_6 of the initial r waves in each lead is normal.

c) The transition zone is between V_4 and V_5 (assessed by development of initial q waves).

3. a) **The total QRS duration is abnormal at 0.18 sec (well seen in V_1). The combination of the rsR' pattern in V_1 with an increase in the total QRS duration indicates right bundle branch block.**

b) The R waves in V_4, V_5 and V_6 all satisfy the minimal voltage criterion of 8mm.

c) The maximum R waves in the left precordial leads (V_4) are within the normal range at 17mm (V_4).

d) The deepest S wave is seen in V_4 and in this lead it is 7mm.

e) $S_{V_4} + R_{V_4} = 24$mm, which is well within the normal maximum of 40mm.

f) The ventricular activation time is seen in V_6 to be 0.03 sec.

g) The q waves in V_5 and V_6 are not deeper than one quarter of the height of the r waves in the same lead.

h) The q waves in V_5 and V_6 are less than 0.04 sec in duration.

4A. The T waves in the precordial leads are within normal limits.
4B. No significant U waves are seen in the precordial leads.

5. There is S-T segment depression in V_1, but in the other precordial leads the S-T segments are within the normal range. The S-T segment depression in V_1 is almost certainly secondary to the QRS abnormality (right bundle branch block).

6. a) Small q waves are seen in aVL. Their depth does not exceed a quarter of the height of the ensuing r wave.

b) The q waves in aVL are less than 0.04 sec in duration.

c) The R wave in aVL does not exceed 13mm and that in aVF does not exceed 20mm.

d) The mean frontal plane QRS axis is indeterminate. (This is not abnormal).

7A. The mean frontal plane T wave axis is +30°. **Since the frontal plane QRS axis is indeterminate and the frontal plane T wave axis is determinate, the T waves are abnormal in the frontal plane leads. This abnormality is almost certainly also secondary to the right bundle branch block.**
7B. No significant U waves are visible in the limb leads.

8. The S-T segments in the limb leads are iso-electric.

9. a) The P wave duration in Lead II is 0.12 sec.

b) The P wave height is 0.5mm.

c) The negative component of the P wave in V_1 does not exceed the positive component in area.

10. The Q-T interval is 0.41 sec. The cycle time is 24 (heart rate 62) and the maximum Q-T interval corresponding to this rate is 0.41 sec.

The appearances are those of straightforward, uncomplicated, complete right bundle branch block.

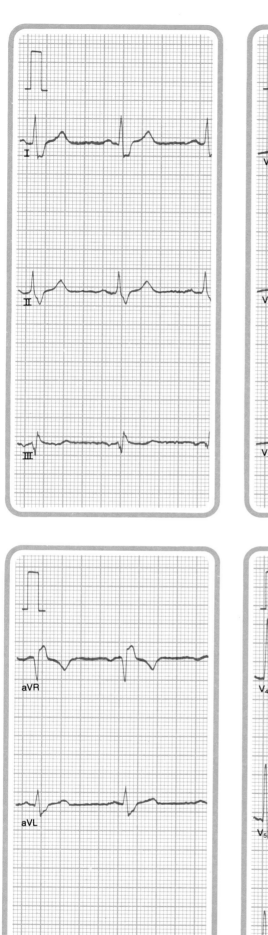
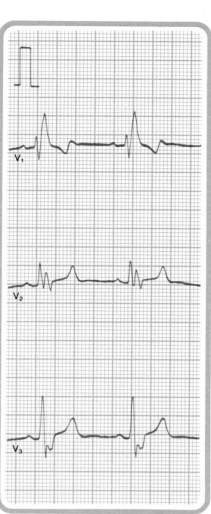
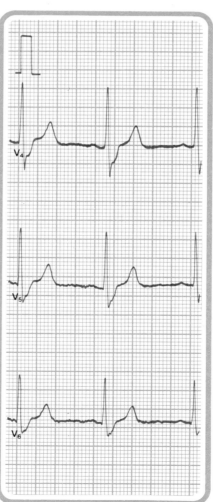

Record 39

Abnormal Record

1. The rhythm is sinus tachycardia. The P-R interval is 0.14 sec.

2. a) The QRS morphology in V_1 is normal (rS). The morphology in V_6 is also normal (qR).

b) The r wave progression appears normal from V_1–V_3, but the R waves in V_4, V_5 and V_6 are smaller than would be expected. (The minimal voltage criterion for the precordial r waves is not in fact satisfied, see 3b below).

c) The transition zone is between V_4 and V_5.

3. a) The total QRS duration is normal at 0.10 sec.

b) **The tallest R wave in the precordial leads is in V_3, where it is 8 mm. The criterion for normality is that at least one r wave should exceed 8 mm. This is therefore an abnormality.**

c) The tallest precordial r wave certainly does not exceed the maximal permitted level for normality (27 mm).

d) The deepest precordial S wave is seen in V_2 and is 26 mm. This is well below the maximum normal of 30 mm.

e) The sum of the tallest R and deepest S waves is well below the maximum of 40 mm.

f) The ventricular activation time is seen in V_6 to be 0.04 sec.

g) q waves are seen in V_5 and V_6. In neither case do they have depth exceeding one quarter of the height of the ensuing r wave.

h) The q waves in V_5 and V_6 do not equal or exceed 0.04 sec in duration.

4A. The T waves in V_1, V_2 and V_3 are normal. **The T waves in V_4, V_5 and V_6 are of low voltage. This is a non-specific abnormality.**
4B. Normal, (low voltage and positive) U waves are seen in V_1–V_4.

5. The S-T segments are normal from V_1–V_4. **There is minimal, but significant S-T segment depression in V_5 and V_6. This is just beyond the normal accepted limit of 1 mm below the iso-electric line.**

6. a) Initial q waves are seen in Leads II and aVF. Their duration is less than 0.04 sec.

b) The depth of the q waves in II and aVF is less than one quarter of the height of the ensuing r wave.

c) The r wave in aVL does not exceed 13 mm and the R wave in aVF is at the extreme upper end of the normal range at 20 mm.

d) The mean frontal plane QRS axis is +90°. This is at the extreme right hand end of the normal range.

7A. The T wave axis in the frontal plane leads is indeterminate. Since the frontal plane QRS axis is highly determinate, the frontal plane T waves are abnormal.
7B. No significant U waves are seen in the limb leads.

8. The S-T segments in the limb leads appear to be depressed in Leads II, III and aVF. However, closer inspection indicates that the apparent S-T segment depression begins before the QRS complex (i.e. immediately after the P wave). These appearances in Leads II, III and aVF are actually due to a prominent atrial repolarisation wave. This is a normal accompaniment of sinus tachycardia.

9. a) The P wave duration is 0.13 sec.

b) **The P wave height in Lead II is 3 mm. This is abnormal and suggests right atrial hypertrophy.**

c) No significant negative component to the P wave in V_1, is visible.

10. The Q-T interval is 0.33 sec. (The Q-T interval is only really measurable in the right precordial leads). The cycle time is 15 (heart rate 100). The maximum Q-T interval corresponding to this rate is 0.33 sec.

The record shows sinus tachycardia, right atrial hypertrophy with a prominent atrial repolarisation wave and borderline abnormal right axis deviation. These features are non-specific but suggest the possibility of chronic lung disease. There are non-specific S-T, T changes in the left precordial leads. The QRS complexes are low voltage in the left precordial leads. This could be due to obesity, emphysema or pronounced clockwise cardiac rotation.

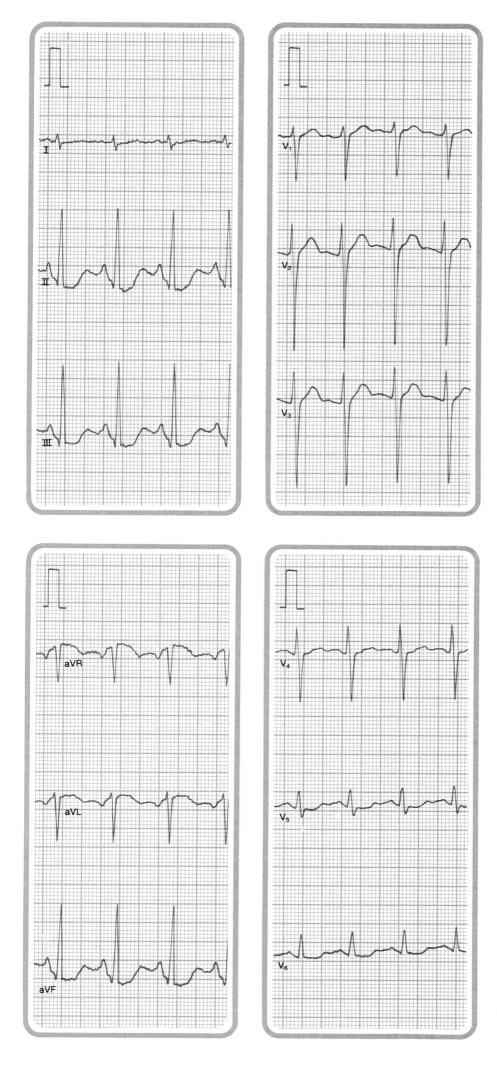

288

Record 40

Abnormal Record

1. Sinus rhythm. The P-R interval is 0.12 sec.

2. a) **The QRS waveform is abnormal in V_1. Instead of having rS there is an Rs complex. The QRS waveform is also abnormal in V_6 in that instead of having qR, there is Qr.**

   b) **The r wave progression from V_1–V_6 is abnormal. After V_2 the R wave disappears completely and this is frankly abnormal.**

   c) Since the R wave progression is so abnormal, the term "transition zone" has no meaning.

3. a) The total QRS duration is within the normal range at 0.10 sec (well seen in V_6).

   b) **No precordial r wave exceeds the minimum voltage of 8 mm. This is abnormal.**

   c) The tallest r wave obviously does not therefore exceed 27 mm.

   d) The deepest S wave (V_2) is 15 mm (the negative wave in V_3 is not an S wave, it is a QS complex).

   e) The sum of the tallest r and deepest S waves certainly does not exceed 40 mm.

   f) The ventricular activation time cannot be measured since this is dependent upon the presence of a normal configuration qR complex in the left precordial leads.

   g) **q waves are seen V_3–V_6. In V_3 and V_4 these are actually QS complexes. From V_2–V_6 the q waves in all cases grossly exceed in depth one quarter of the height of the ensuing r wave. This is abnormal and indicates infarction in the myocardium underlying the electrodes.**

   h) **From V_4–V_6 the q waves are more than 0.03 sec in duration. This is frankly abnormal and indicates infarction of the subjacent myocardium.**

4A. The T waves are normal from V_1–V_3, but **from V_4–V_6 the T waves are abnormally flat. This is a non-specific abnormality.** It is probably secondary to the extensive QRS abnormalities in the precordial leads which indicate extensive anterior myocardial infarction extending from V_1–V_6.

4B. Small, upright (normal) U waves are seen in V_2 and V_3.

5. The precordial S-T segments are within normal limits, indicating that the infarct is not less than a week old.

6. q waves are seen in Leads I, II and aVF.

   a) **The q waves in Leads I and II are greater than one quarter of the height of the ensuing r wave and this is probably also true of the q waves in the foot-lead.**

   b) **The q waves in I are certainly in excess of 0.03 sec. The abnormal q waves in Lead I are part of the anterolateral infarction which is also shown in the precordial leads. The q waves in Lead II and also the q waves in aVF (if the latter are actually abnormal), almost certainly indicate additional inferior myocardial infarction.**

   c) The r waves in aVL and aVF certainly do not exceed the maximum permissible voltage of 13 and 20 mm respectively.

   d) **The mean frontal plane QRS axis is very abnormal at +150°. This is due to the extensive anterolateral infarction which removes electrical forces directed upwards and to the left leaving the predominant direction of ventricular depolarisation as downwards and to the right. It is therefore not necessarily indicative of left posterior hemiblock.**

7A. The mean frontal plane T wave axis is indeterminate. Since the frontal plane QRS axis is hightly determinate, the T waves in the frontal plane leads are abnormal.

7B. No significant U waves are seen in the limb leads.

8. The S-T segments in the frontal plane leads are normal.

9. a) The P waves in Lead II have a normal duration of 0.10 sec.

   b) The P wave height in Lead II is within the normal range at 1.5 mm.

   c) **The P waves in V_1, have a dominant negative component indicative of left atrial hypertrophy.**

10. The Q-T interval is 0.35 sec. The cycle time is 19 (heart rate 78) which is associated with a maximum Q-T interval of 0.37 sec.

The abnormal q waves from V_3–V_6 and also in Lead I indicate extensive anterolateral myocardial infarction. The abnormal q waves in Leads II and the foot-lead indicate inferior infarction. In this context the dominant r wave in V_1 probably indicates true posterior infarction. The abnormal P waves in V_1 indicate left atrial abnormality. This could be the result of left atrial hypertrophy or of left atrial ischaemia.

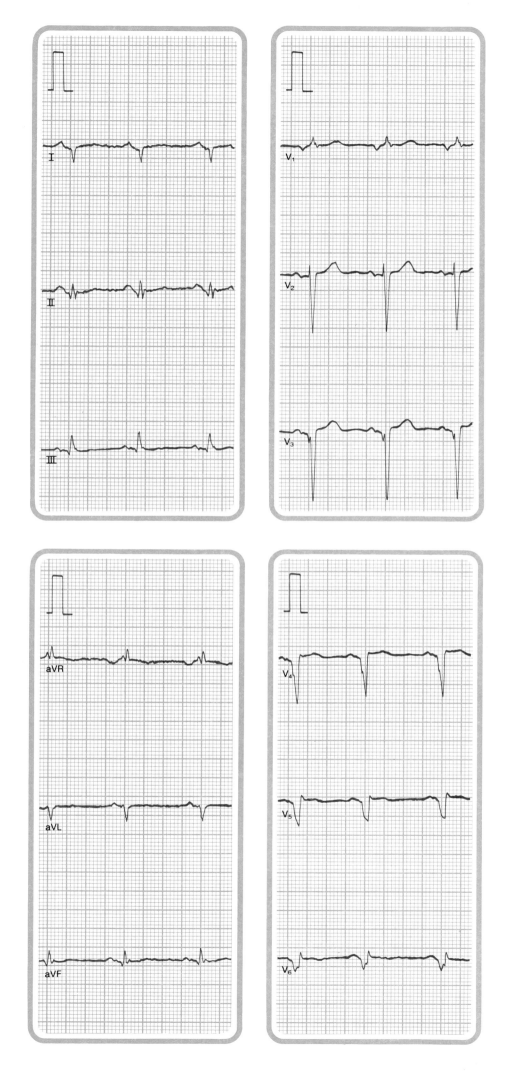

290

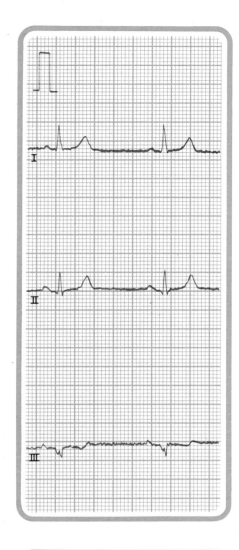

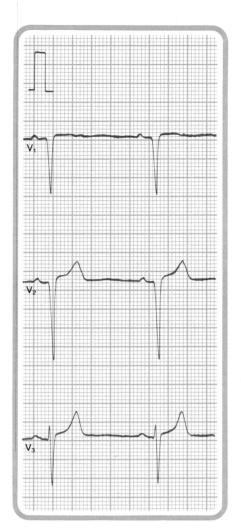

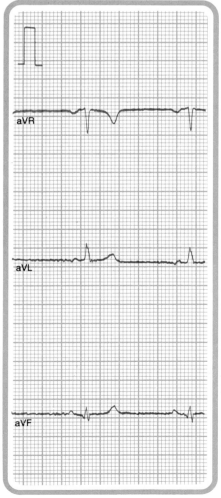

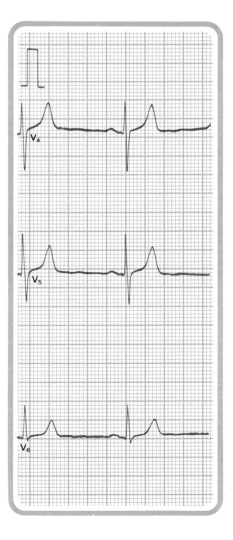

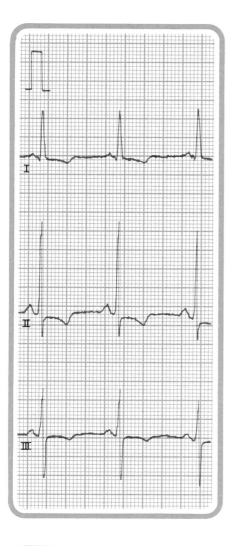

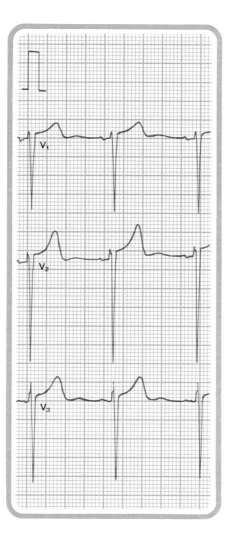

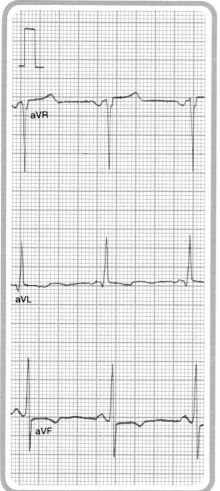

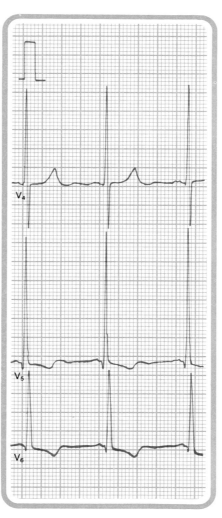

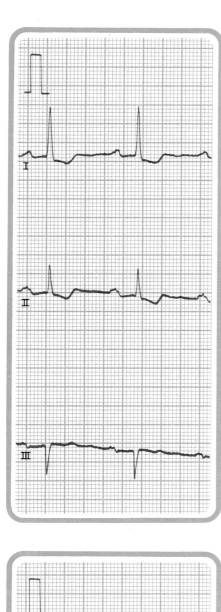

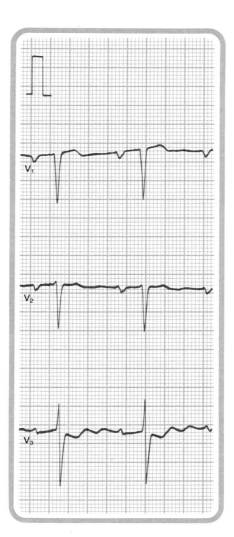

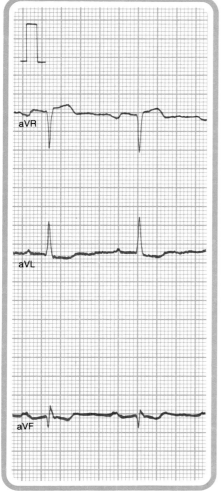

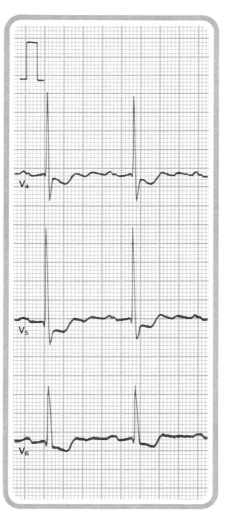

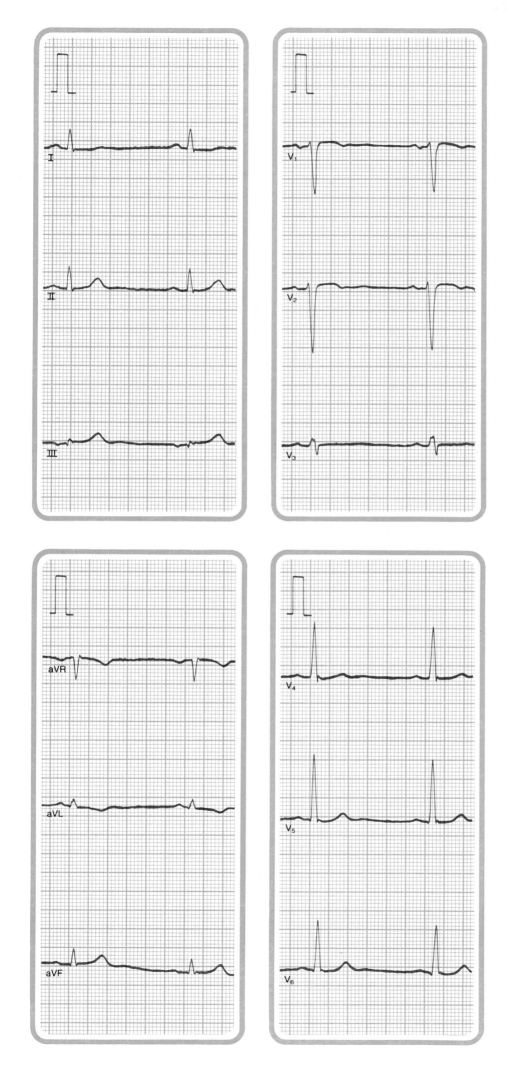

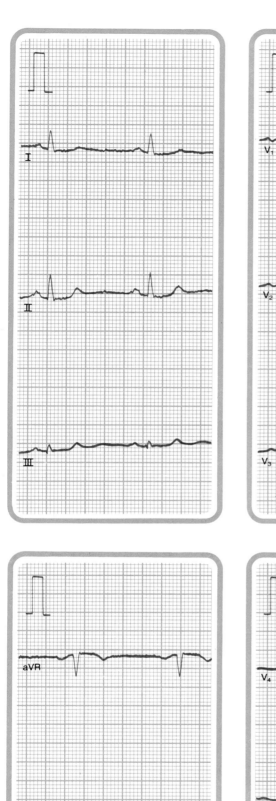

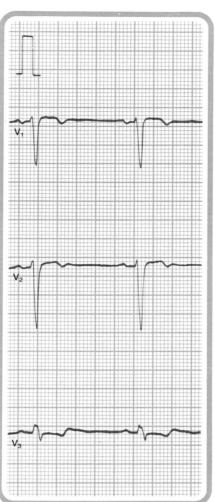

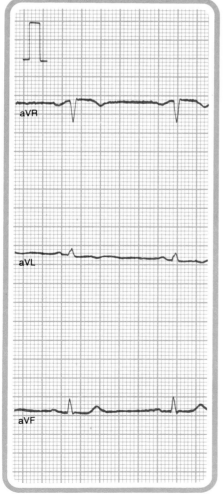

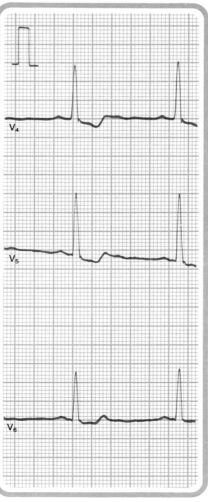

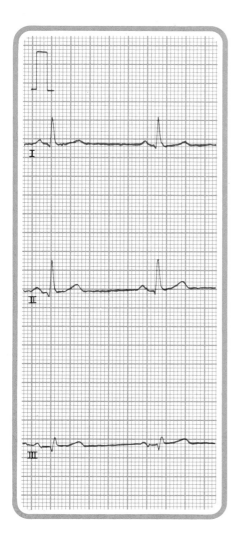

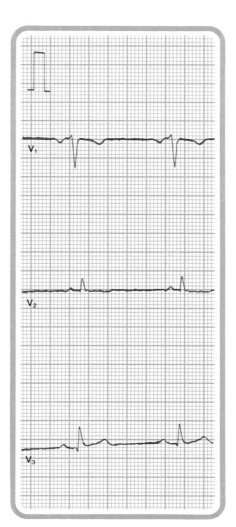

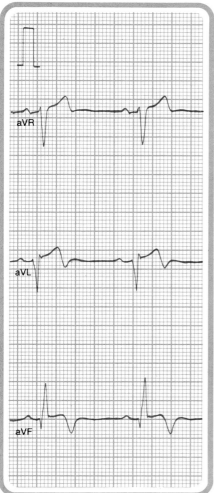

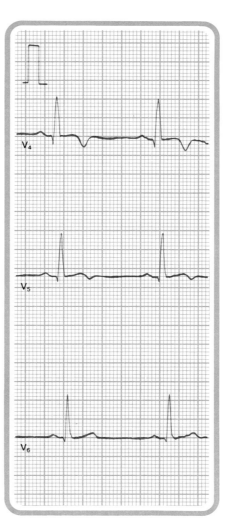

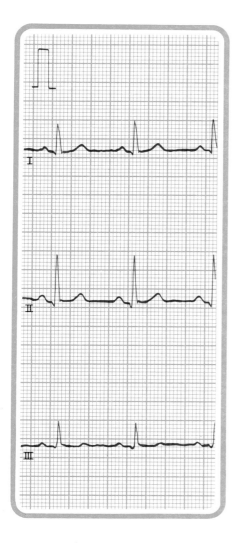

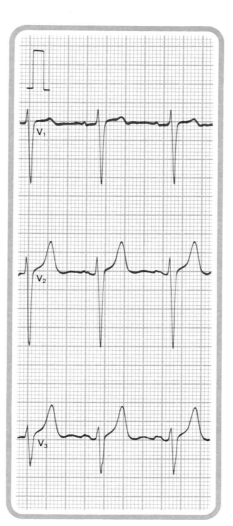

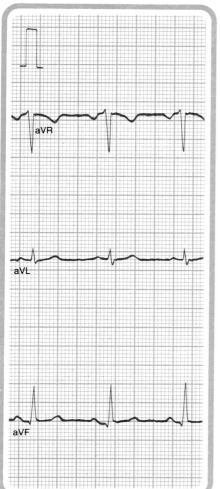

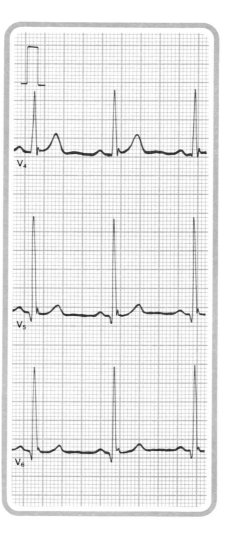

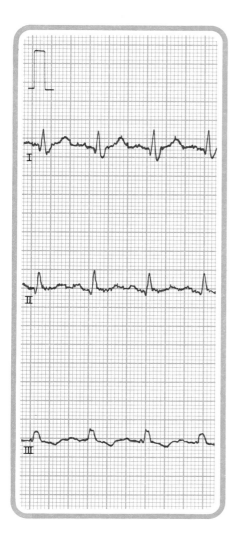

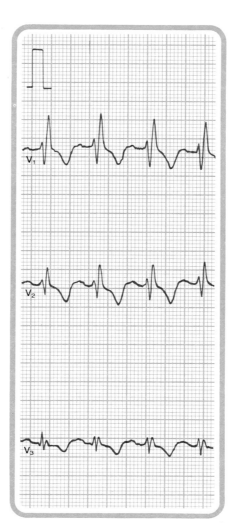

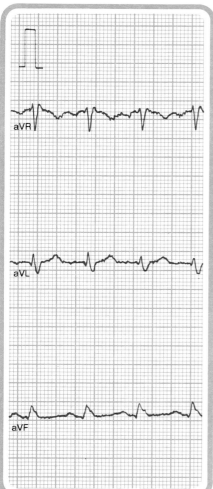

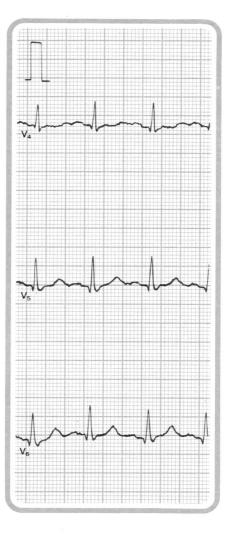

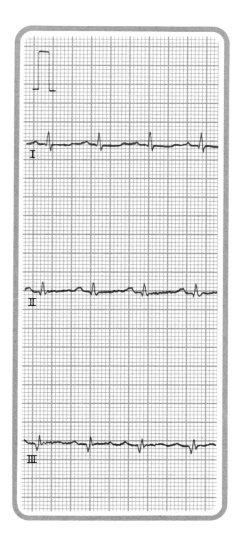

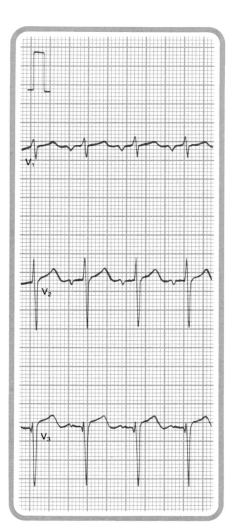

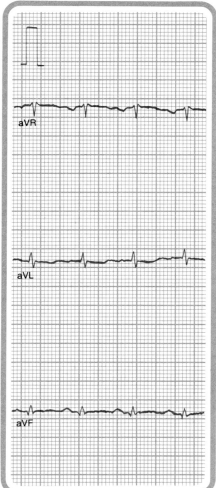

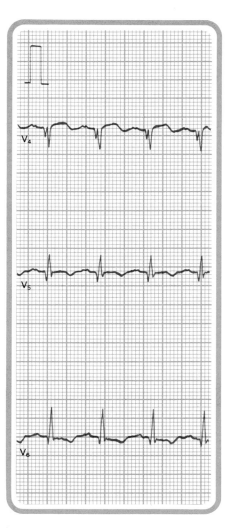

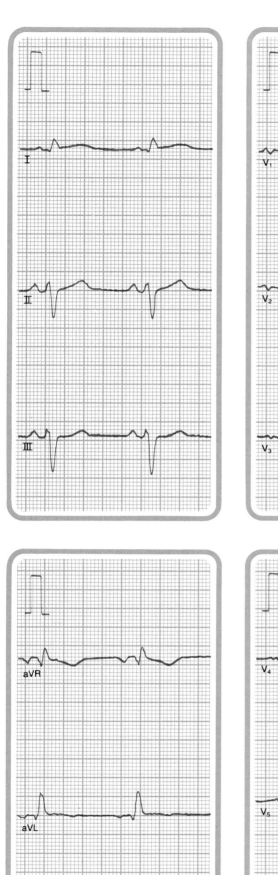
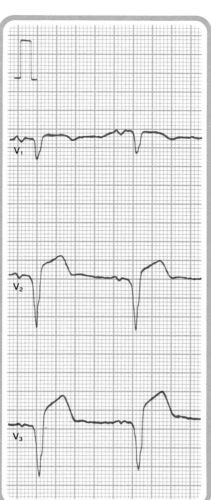
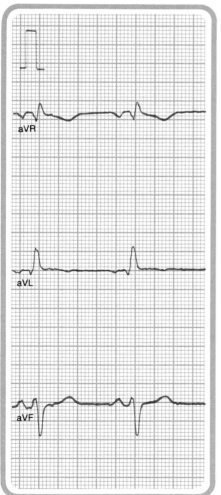
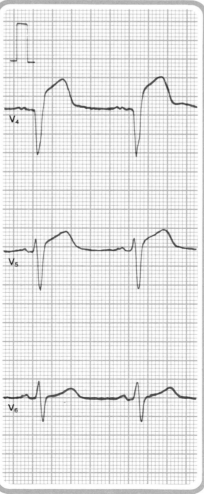

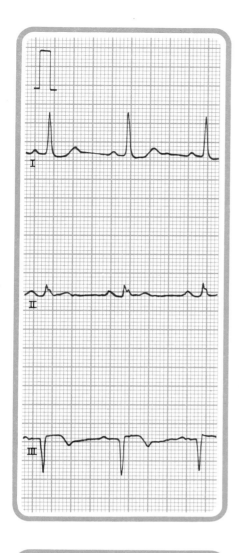

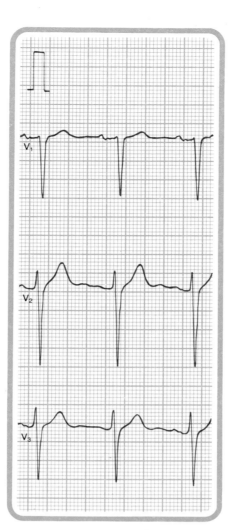

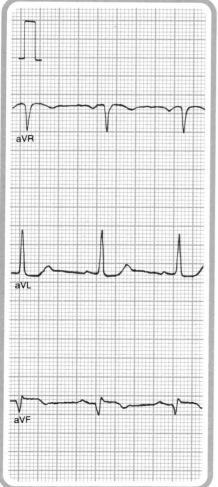

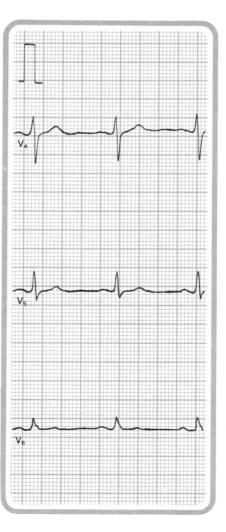

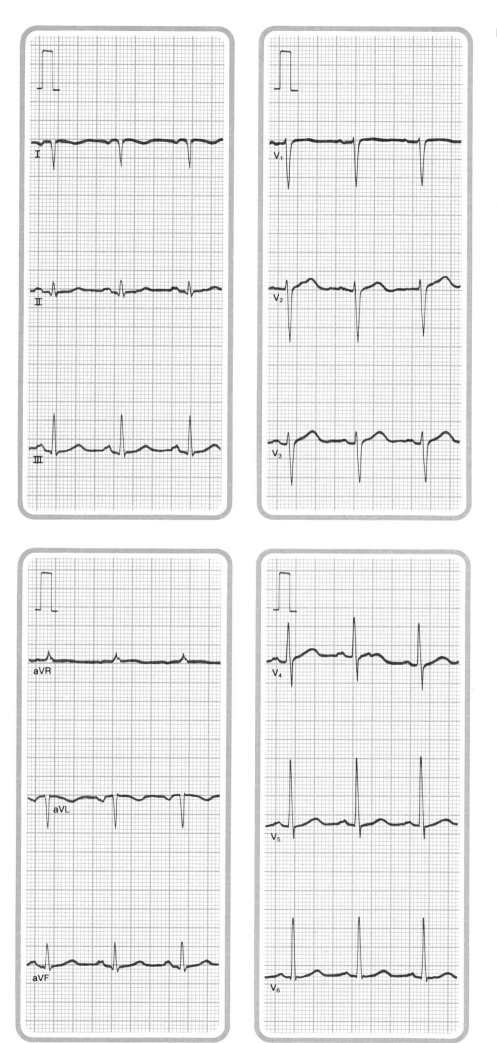

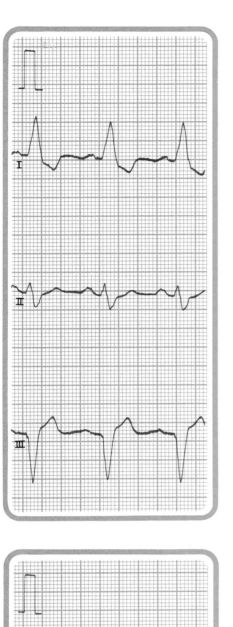

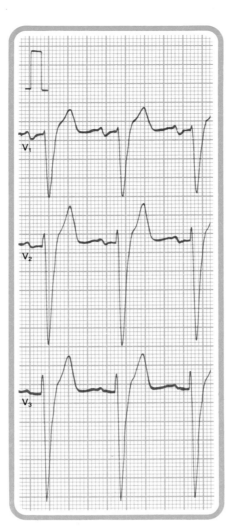

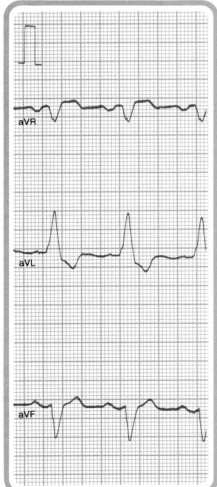

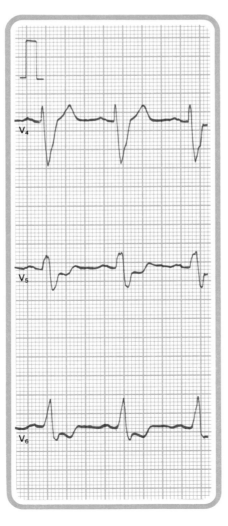

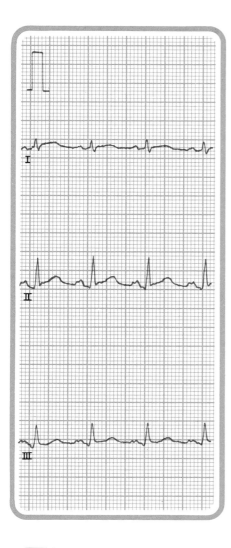

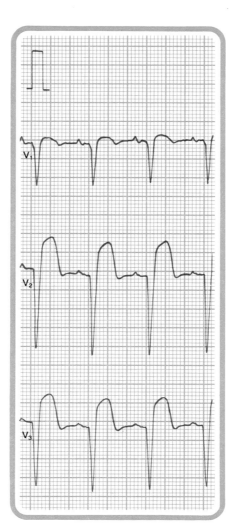

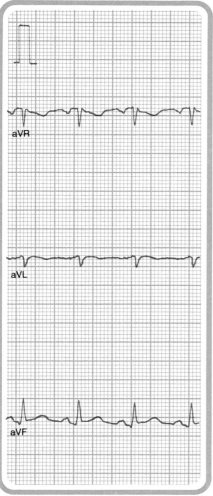

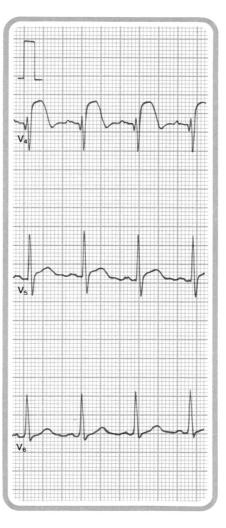

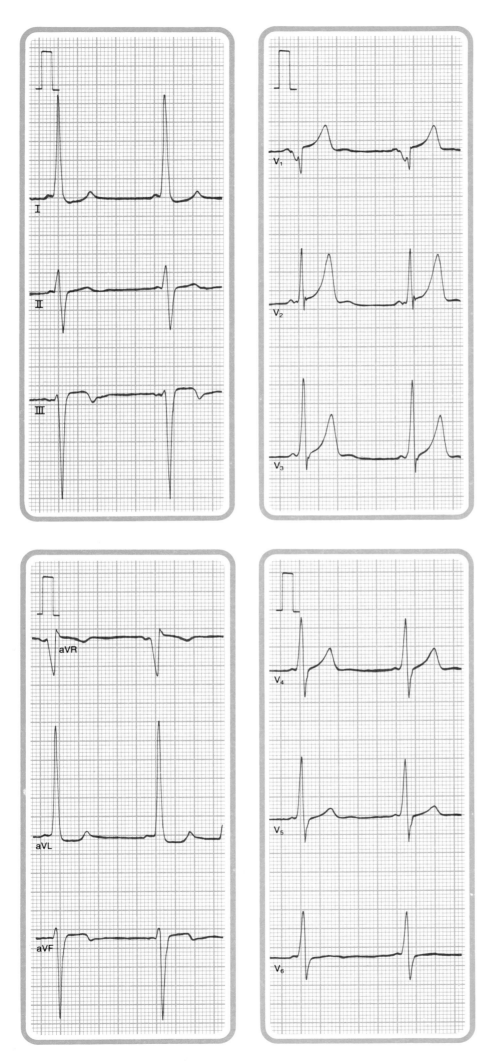

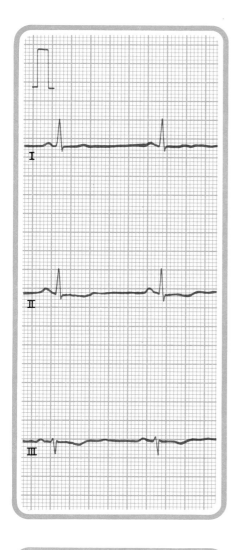

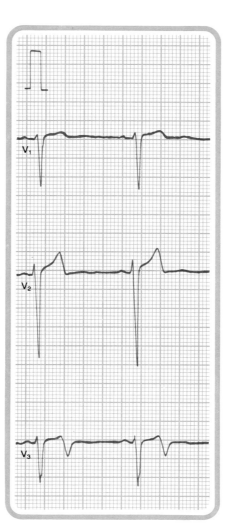

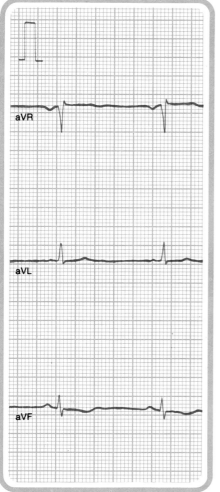

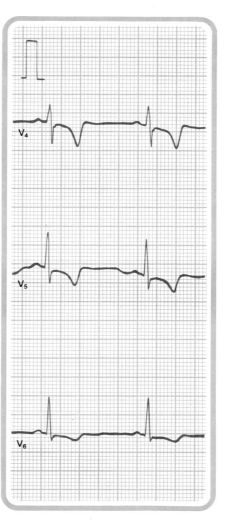

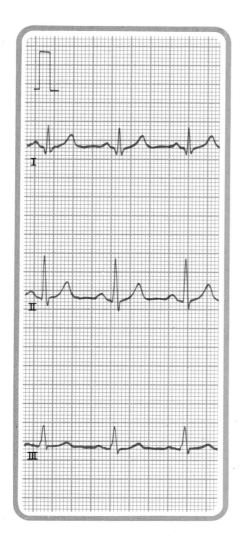

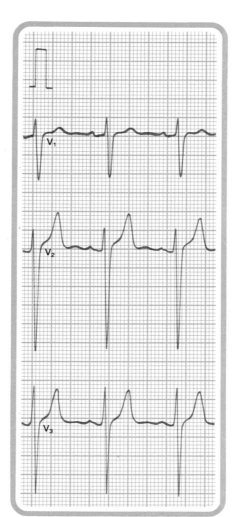

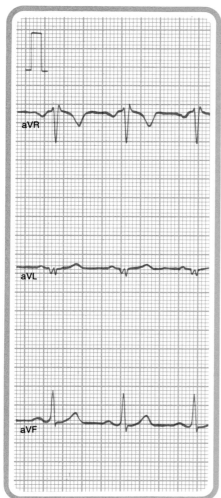

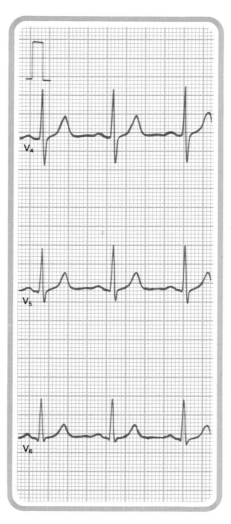

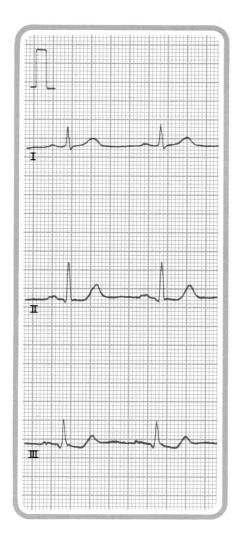

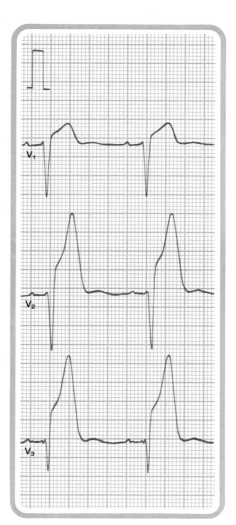

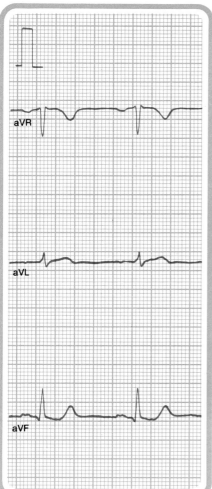

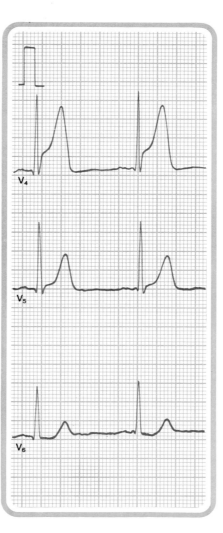

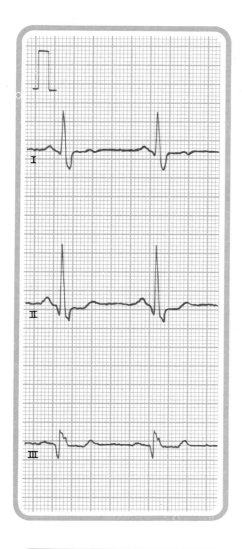

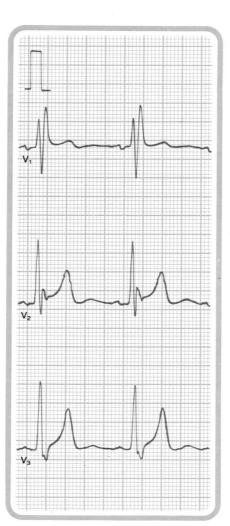

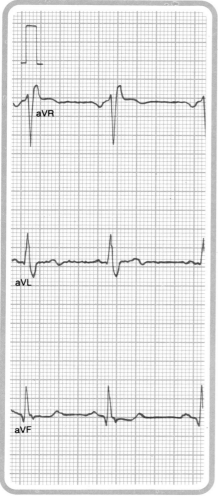

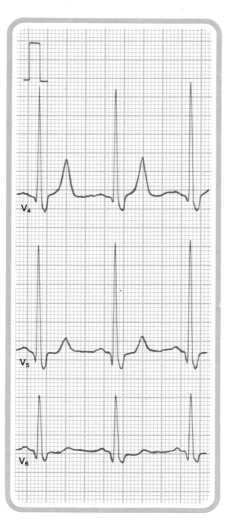

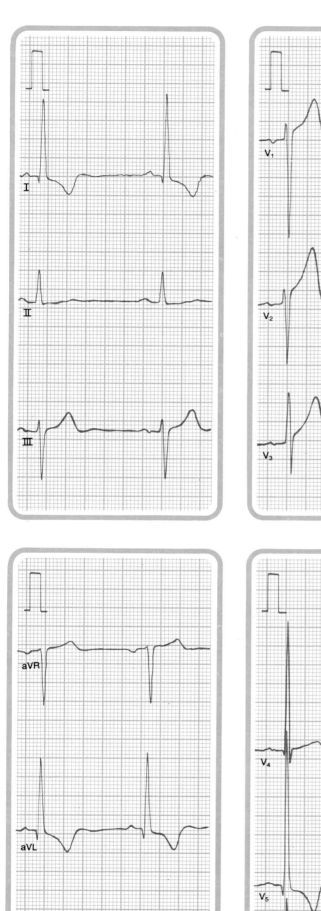

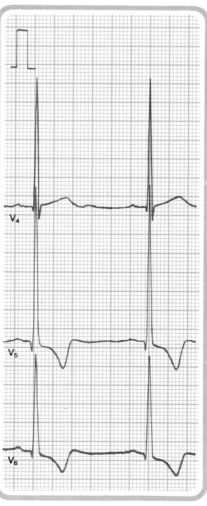

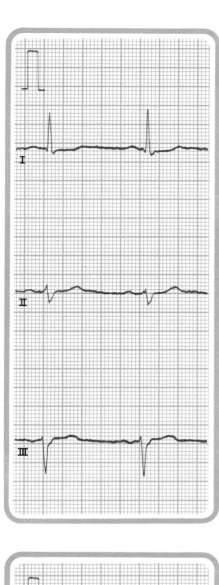
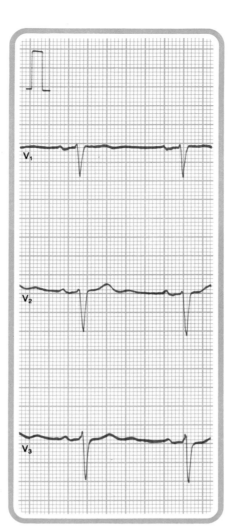
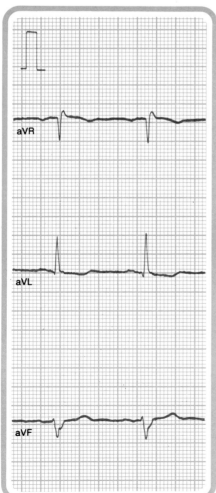
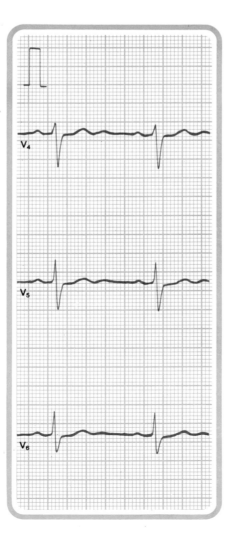

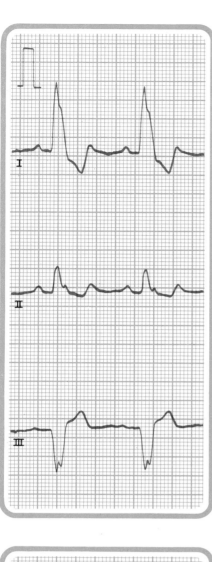

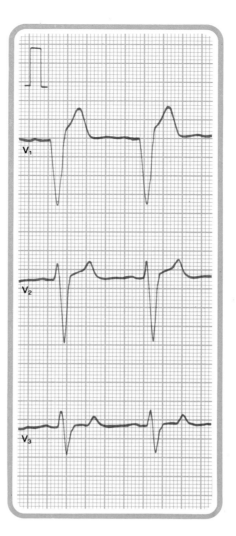

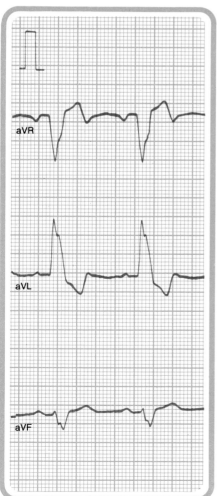

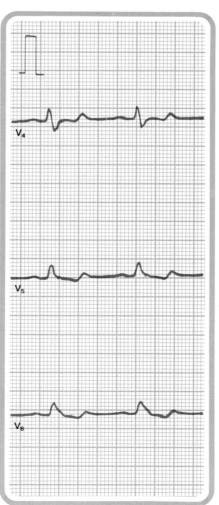

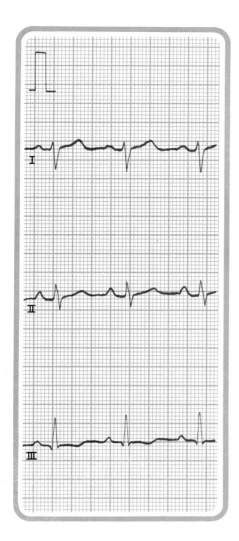

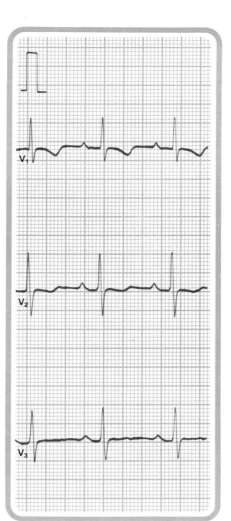

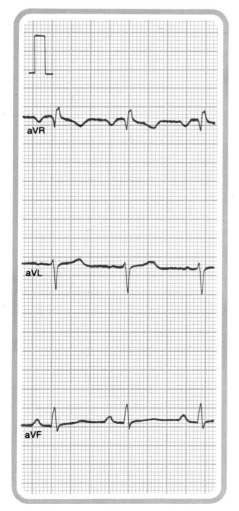

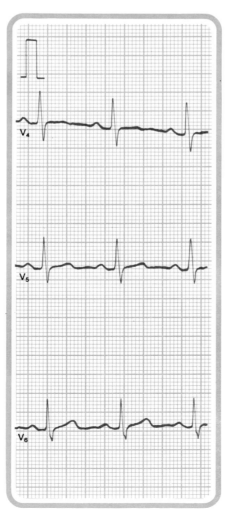

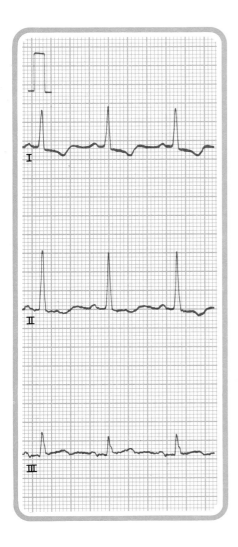

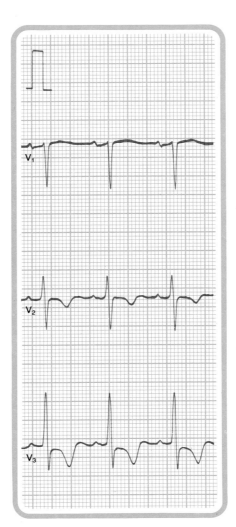

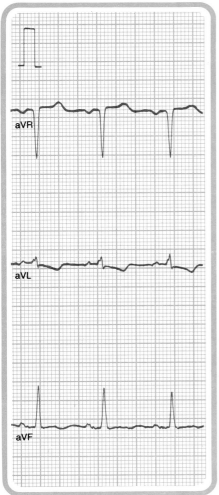

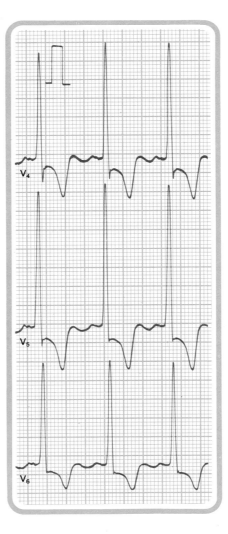

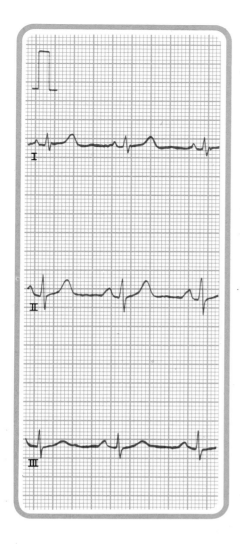

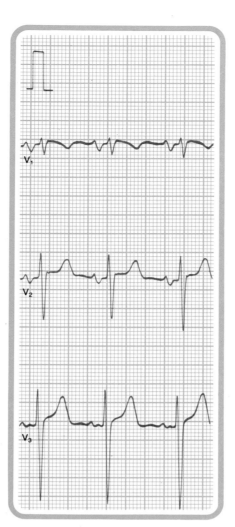

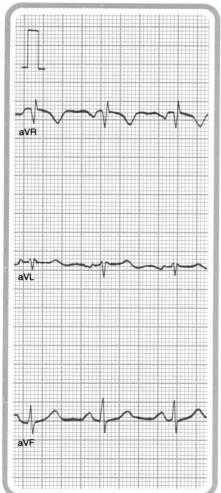

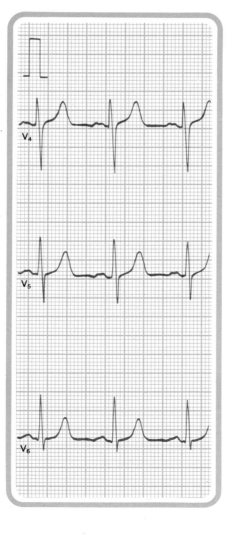

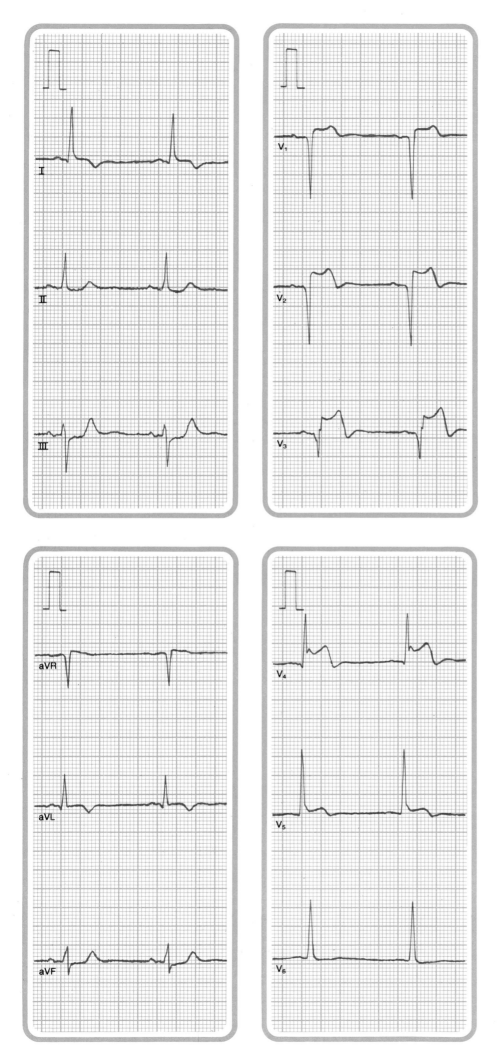

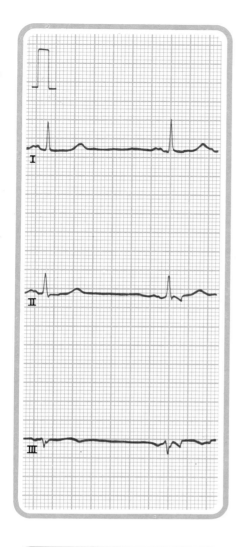

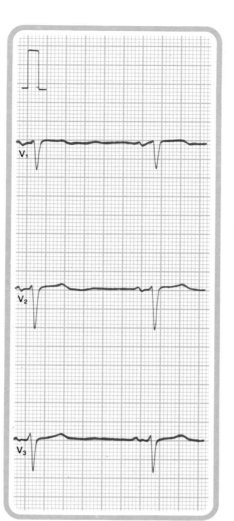

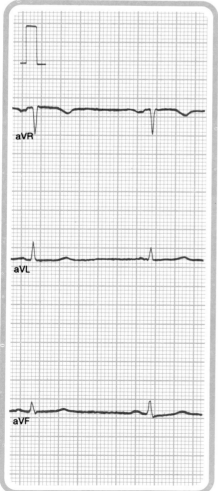

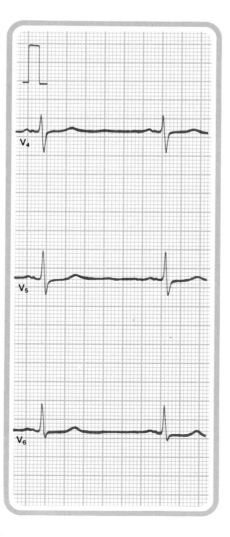

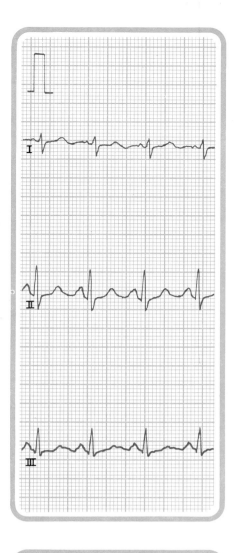

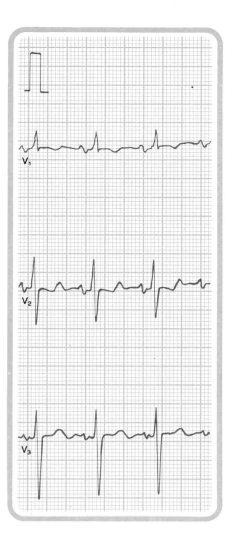

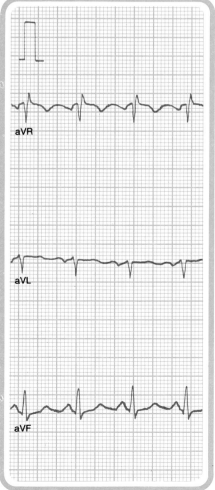

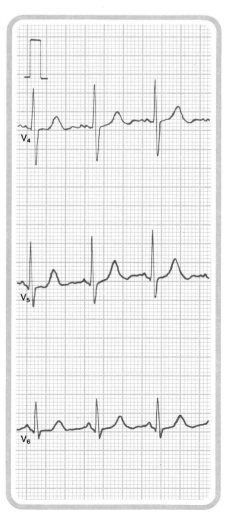

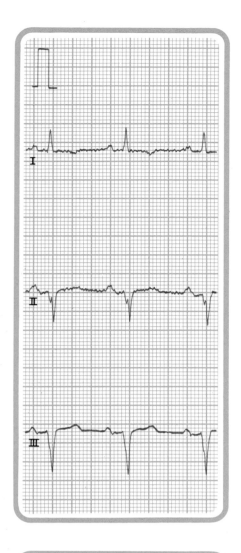

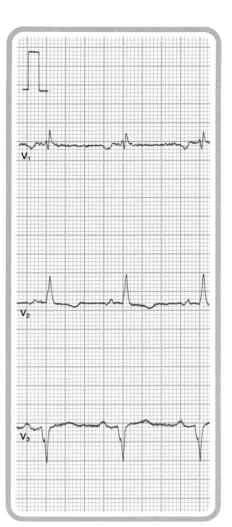

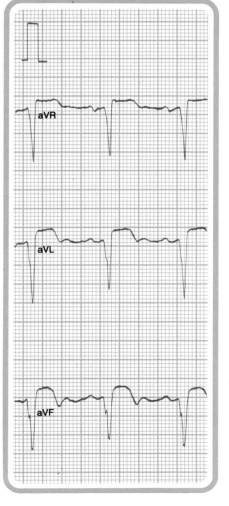

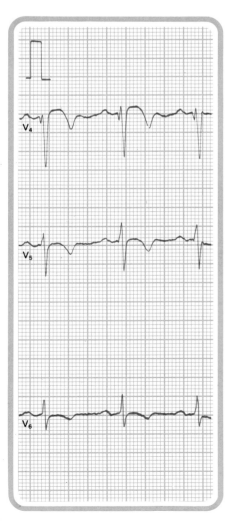

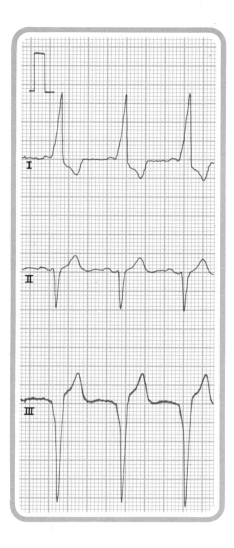

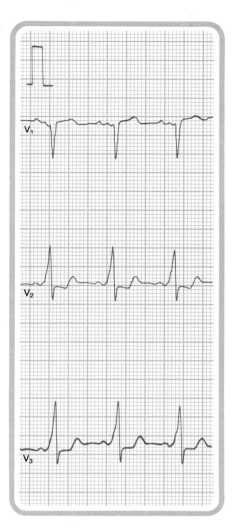

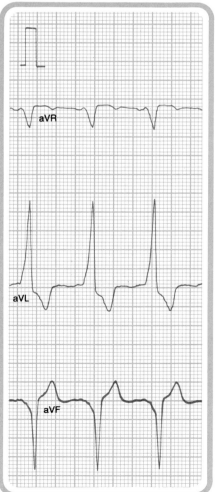

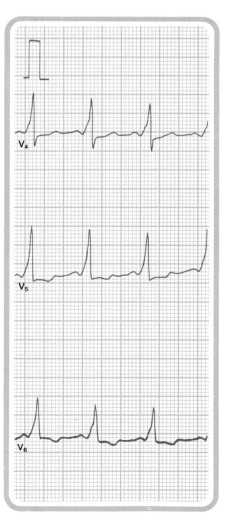

Records 41 to 70

Record 41
Old anteroseptal infarction.
Old inferior infarction.

Record 42
Left ventricular hypertrophy.
Possible left atrial hypertrophy.

Record 43
**Left atrial hypertrophy. Non-specific
S-T, T and U changes – digitalis effect,
hypokalaemia.**
First degree heart block.
Old inferior infarction.

Record 44
Non-specific S-T, T changes.

Record 45
Non-specific S-T, T changes.
**Acute ischaemic S-T segment
depression.**

Record 46
**Recent anterior infarction. Possible
recent inferior ischaemic damage.**

Record 47
Left ventricular hypertrophy.

Record 48
Right bundle branch block.
Sinus tachycardia.

Record 49
Anterior myocardial infarction
(intermediate age).
Old inferior infarction.
Left atrial abnormality.

Record 50
Recent anterior myocardial infarction.
Left anterior hemiblock.

Record 51
**Relatively recent inferior myocardial
infarction.**
Possible anterolateral infarction.

Record 52
Normal (apart from possible left atrial
abnormality). **Technical dextrocardia.**

Record 53
Left bundle branch block.
Abnormal left axis deviation.
Left atrial abnormality.

Record 54
Recent anteroseptal infarction.

Record 55
Ventricular pre-excitation
(WPW type B).

Record 56
Ischaemic S-T, T changes.

Record 57
Normal (Normal Q in aVL).

Record 58
Recent anterior infarction.

Record 59
Right bundle branch block.

Record 60
Left ventricular hypertrophy.
Left atrial hypertrophy.

Record 61
Left anterior hemiblock.
**Non-specific S-T, T and U wave
changes.**
Clockwise cardiac rotation.

Record 62
Left bundle branch block.

Record 63
Right ventricular hypertrophy.
Right atrial hypertrophy.

Record 64
Left ventricular hypertrophy.

Record 65
Left atrial abnormality.

Record 66
**Recent anteroseptal myocardial
infarction.**

Record 67
Myoedema.

Record 68
Right ventricular hypertrophy.
Right atrial hypertrophy.

Record 69
Anterior myocardial infarction
(probable old inferior infarction)
Left axis deviation.

Record 70
Old inferior myocardial infarction.
Non-specific S-T, T changes
(digitalis effect).

Listing of abnormalities in record examples 41–70

Record 41

2. a) V_1 has QS (should have rS).
b) No r wave has developed in V_2 – still QS. These two features indicate anteroseptal infarction.

6. b) The Q wave in aVF is more than one quarter of the height of the ensuing R wave. This indicates an inferior infarction.

ECG diagnosis
Old anteroseptal infarction.
Old inferior infarction.

Record 42

3. c) The R wave in V_5 measures 35 mm (well in excess of the permitted 27 mm).
e) $R_{V_5} + S_{V_5} = 62$ mm (well in excess of the permitted 40 mm).
f) The intrinsic deflection time (well seen in V_6) is 0.05 sec.

4. c) There is T wave inversion in V_5 and V_6.

5. There is S-T segment depression in V_5 and V_6.

7. The frontal plane T wave axis is $-135°$ (the QRS axis is $+15°$ and the angle between the two is therefore abnormal).

8. There is S-T segment depression in Leads I, II and aVL.
These changes indicate left ventricular hypertrophy.

9. The P waves in V_1 have a dominant negative component suggesting a possible left atrial abnormality (probably hypertrophy).

ECG diagnosis
Left ventricular hypertrophy.
Possible left atrial hypertrophy.

Record 43

1. The rhythm is sinus. The P-R interval is abnormally long at 0.26 sec. This indicates the presence of first degree heart block (see Section 3).

4A. The T waves are of low voltage throughout the precordial series.
4B. Prominent (and abnormal) U waves are seen from V_3 to V_6. They are definitely abnormal but are non-specific. They suggest hypokalaemia.

5. There is S-T segment depression from V_3–V_6. These are abnormal but non-specific changes. This patient was actually receiving digitalis and this is probably relevant.

6. The q waves in aVF exceed one quarter of the height of the ensuing R waves. This indicates the presence of inferior infarction.

7A. The frontal plane T axis is indeterminate. Since the frontal plane QRS axis is highly determinate at $0°$, the frontal plane T waves are abnormal.

8. There is S-T segment depression in I, II, aVL and aVF.

9. The P waves are abnormally wide and bifid in II and have a dominant negative component in V_1. These changes indicate the presence of left atrial hypertrophy.

10. It is impossible to assess the Q-T interval since the T waves are of abnormally low voltage and the U waves are prominent.

ECG diagnosis
First degree heart block, left atrial hypertrophy, non-specific S-T, T changes, probable hypokalaemia, possible digitalis effect.

Record 44

4A. c) The T waves are flat in V_3 and of low voltage in V_4. This is a non-specific abnormality.
4B. Prominent U waves are seen in the precordial leads but they are not definitely abnormal.

7. The frontal plane T axis is $+90°$. Since the frontal plane QRS axis is $+30°$, the angle between the two axes is abnormal and the frontal plane T waves are therefore minimally abnormal.
The record shows non-specific (but significant) T wave changes.

ECG diagnosis
Non-specific T wave changes.

Record 45

4A. The T waves are of low voltage from V_3–V_6.

5. There is S-T depression from V_3–V_6. This is of borderline significance in V_3 and V_6, but is definitely abnormal in V_4 and V_5.
The record is frankly abnormal but the changes are non-specific.
(This record was taken from the same patient as Record 44 and within 5 minutes of it. During the taking of Record 44 the patient was asymptomatic. During the recording of Record 45 the patient was complaining of spontaneous anginal pain. The S-T segment depression in the left precordial leads is an example of ischaemic change occurring during spontaneous angina).

ECG diagnosis
Non-specific S-T, T changes occurring in association with chest pain.

Record 46

2. b) The r wave in V_2 is smaller than that in V_1.

3. g) The q wave in V_3 has a depth more than one quarter of the height of the ensuing R wave. This is probably true also in V_4.
These two features indicate the presence of anterior myocardial infarction.

4A. b) There is terminal T wave inversion in V_2.
c) There is T wave inversion from V_2–V_5.

5. There is significant S-T elevation in V_2.

8. There is minimal S-T elevation in III and aVF.
The QRS changes are those of anterior infarction. The S-T and T changes in the precordial leads indicate that the infarct is relatively recent – probably one to four weeks. The S-T segment elevation in III and aVF suggests the possibility of recent inferior ischaemic damage.

ECG diagnosis
Recent anterior infarction. Possible inferior ischaemic damage.

Record 47

2. b) The r wave progression in the precordial leads is not "smooth". There is little or no progression from V_1–V_3 and then a sudden increase. Such appearances can be seen in the presence of an old anteroseptal infarction, but the appearances can also be normal and it is always better to under-interpret (and report) rather than to over-interpret (and report) the electrocardiogram.

3. e) $S_{V_2} + R_{V_5} = 44$ mm.
f) The ventricular activation time is 0.05 sec.
These changes indicate the presence of left ventricular hypertrophy.

9. The P waves are bifid in V_2 or V_3. This suggests possible left atrial hypertrophy, but the criteria for this condition have not actually been fulfilled.

ECG diagnosis
Changes suggestive of left ventricular hypertrophy.

Record 48

1A. The rhythm is sinus. The rate is 107 per min and there is therefore sinus tachycardia.

2. a) V_1 has an rSR′ complex.

3. a) The total QRS duration is 0.14 sec. These changes indicate the presence of right bundle branch block.

4. There is T wave inversion from V_1–V_3 and the T waves are of low voltage in V_4. These are non-specific changes and are likely to be secondary to the QRS abnormality of right bundle branch block.

ECG diagnosis
Right bundle branch block.

Record 49

2. b) The r wave progression is abnormal. The r wave in V_2 is taller than that in V_1 (normal), but the r wave in V_3 is smaller and there is **no** r wave in V_4 (the smaller r wave in V_3 would be acceptable if the r waves in V_4 were normal (page 45)).

3. g) The q waves in V_3, V_4 and V_5 have a depth exceeding one quarter of the height of the ensuing R wave.
These changes indicate the presence of anterior infarction.

2. h) The q waves in V_4 exceed, and those in V_5 equal 0.04 sec in duration. This, too, indicates infarction.

4A. There is T wave inversion in V_5 and V_6. This is a non-specific abnormality. It is likely to be related to ischaemia in the area adjacent to the infarct.

5. There is minimal S-T elevation in V_3 and V_4, suggesting that the anterior infarct is recent.

6. b) The q wave in aVF has a depth exceeding one quarter of the height of the ensuing r wave. This indicates the presence of inferior infarction.

7. No comment of any significance can be made on the T waves in the frontal plane leads since both the frontal plane QRS axis and the frontal plane T axis are indeterminate.

9. There is a dominant negative component to the P wave in V_1 indicating left atrial abnormality. One cannot be sure whether this is related to ischaemia or to hypertrophy.

ECG diagnosis
Old inferior infarction. Left atrial abnormality.

Record 50

2. a) V_1 has no initial r wave. It has a QS complex. V_6 has an RS instead of qR. This is related to the abnormal R wave progression (see below).

b) The r wave progression is grossly abnormal. No r wave appears from V_1–V_4 and the r waves in V_5 and V_6 are smaller than one would expect.

3. a) The total QRS duration is abnormal at 0.14 sec. There is no rSR′ pattern in V_1 to suggest right bundle branch block. There is no initial (septal) q wave in V_6 suggesting the presence of left bundle branch block. However, there is an initial q wave in I and aVL indicating that the septal depolarisation is occurring in the normal direction. This could indicate "through and through" infarction of the interventricular septum with complete left bundle branch block, but this is never a diagnosis one can make with total confidence (page 000). Alternatively the abnormal QRS duration could be indicative of intraventricular block (of the type for which the terms "parietal block" and "peri-infarction block" have been used – see page 000).

b) No r wave exceeds 8 mm. This is due to the presence of anterior infarction – see below.

g) The q waves from V_1–V_4 all have a depth exceeding one quarter of the height of the ensuing R wave. This indicates anterior infarction.

h) The q waves from V_1–V_4 all have a duration exceeding 0.03 sec. This also indicates anterior infarction.

5. There is S-T elevation from V_2–V_5 indicating that the infarction is recent.

6. The frontal plane QRS axis is $-60°$. This indicates an abnormal degree of left axis deviation. There is no evidence of inferior infarction so that the abnormal axis cannot be due to loss of viable myocardium on the inferior wall of the heart. The most likely explanation therefore is block in the anterior division of the left bundle branch system (probably induced by the anterior infarction, though this is speculative).

ECG diagnosis
Recent anterior myocardial infarction. Left anterior hemiblock. Additional intraventricular block (possibly parietal block, possibly LBBB).

Record 51

3. b) No r wave in the precordial leads exceeds 8 mm. This can be due to extracardiac causes reducing the voltage (e.g. obesity, emphysema, pleural effusion), or cardiac causes (e.g. pericardial effusion or anterior myocardial infarction).

6. a) The q wave in aVF exceeds 0.03 sec in duration. This indicates the presence of inferior myocardial infarction.

b) The q waves in aVF have a depth exceeding one quarter of the height of the ensuing r wave. This too indicates inferior infarction.

7. Although the angle between the mean frontal plane QRS and T wave axes is not outside the permitted normal range of $±45°$ (QRS axis = $-15°$, T axis = $-15°$) the T waves in aVF are considered to be abnormal since they are inverted in this lead in association with QRS evidence of infarction in the same lead. These changes suggest that the infarct is relatively recent (i.e. within weeks).

8. There is slight, but significant S-T elevation in aVF and III, suggesting that the inferior infarct is less than a week old.

ECG diagnosis
Relatively recent inferior infarction. Possible anterolateral infarction (on the basis of the low voltage R waves in the left precordial leads).

Record 52

6. a) There are QS complexes in I. It is important to recognise that the P waves are also negative in I. The combination of negative P waves and negative QRS complexes in V_1 is usually due either to technical dextrocardia or to true dextrocardia. Since the form of the QRS complexes in the precordial leads are entirely normal, true dextrocardia can be ruled out.

9. The P waves are bifid in the limb leads. They do not fulfil the criteria for abnormality but raise the possibility of left atrial abnormality.
Apart from the possible left atrial abnormality this is a normal record with technical dextrocardia. (The technician had inadvertently mixed up the right and left arm connections).

The true appearances can be deduced as follows:–

true Lead I = recorded Lead I turned upside down

true Lead II = recorded Lead III

true Lead III = recorded Lead II

true Lead aVR = recorded Lead aVL

true Lead aVL = recorded Lead aVR

true Lead aVF = recorded Lead aVF

true precordial leads = recorded precordial leads

ECG diagnosis
Allowing for the recording error (technical dextrocardia) the record is within normal limits.

Record 53

2. a) V_6 has no initial q.wave. No initial q wave is seen in I or aVL either. This suggests that the interventricular septum is depolarised in an abnormal direction.

b) The r wave progression is less pronounced than usual but not definitely abnormal.

3. a) The total QRS duration is abnormal at 0.16 sec.

The combination of an abnormal QRS duration and absence of the normal septal q wave (in the absence of (i) an rSR' complex in V_1 to indicate right bundle branch block, and (ii) any evidence of ventricular pre-excitation) indicates the presence of left bundle branch block. Further evaluation of the QRS complexes, S-T segments, and T waves (apart from the frontal plane axis) should not therefore be undertaken (unless previous records are available for comparison).

6. d) The frontal plane QRS axis is $-45°$. This is an abnormal degree of left axis deviation. It may indicate defective conduction in the peripheral branches of the anterior division of the left bundle branch system.

9. a) The P wave duration in II is abnormal at 0.14 sec and the P waves are bifid in this lead. This indicates the presence of an abnormality of the left atrium.

c) The P waves are biphasic and have a dominant negative area in V_1. This also indicates an abnormality of the left atrium.

ECG diagnosis
Left atrial abnormality.
Complete left bundle branch block.
Abnormal left axis deviation.

Record 54

2. a) There is no r wave in V_1. It shows a QS complex.

b) The r wave progression from V_1–V_4 is abnormal. No r wave is seen in V_1, V_2 or V_3 and only a small r wave in V_4.

3. g) The depth of the q waves in V_1–V_4 exceeds one quarter of the height of the ensuing r waves indicating anteroseptal infarction.

h) The q waves (actually QS complexes) in V_1, V_2 and V_3 exceed 0.03 sec in duration and are therefore abnormal. The abnormal q waves are indicative of anteroseptal infarction in this case (there is no evidence of left bundle branch block or ventricular pre-excitation).

4A. The precordial T wave cannot really be assessed except in V_6 for in all the other leads the T waves are incorporated in the elevated S-T segment.

5. There is significant S-T elevation in V_1–V_5, indicating that the anterior infarct is recent.

8. There is minimal S-T elevation in I, II and aVF.

9. The P waves are bifid in II. They are not abnormally wide and are therefore not definitely abnormal but they suggest the possibility of left atrial abnormality (e.g. ischaemia or hypertrophy).

ECG diagnosis
Recent anterior infarction.

Record 55

1. The P-R interval is abnormally short at 0.10 sec. This feature, combined with the fact that the total QRS duration is abnormally long (at 0.14 sec), indicates the presence of ventricular pre-excitation.

Because of this finding, the normal criteria cannot be applied to the analysis of the QRS complexes, S-T segments and T waves, and the electro-cardiographic interpretation is best ended at this point, **unless either** a previous record is available for comparison **or** the interpreter is skilled and experienced in electrocardiography.

ECG diagnosis
Ventricular pre-excitation.

Record 56

4A. There is T wave inversion in V_3, V_4 and V_5.

5. There is S-T depression in V_5 and V_6. These are non-specific but definite and highly significant changes. The deep, symmetrical T wave inversion in V_3 is very suggestive of an ischaemic origin.

7. The mean frontal plane T wave axis is indeterminate. The mean frontal plane QRS axis is highly determinate ($+15°$). The T waves in the limb leads are therefore abnormal.

ECG diagnosis
Non-specific S-T, T changes in the limb leads and from V_3–V_6. The appearances in V_3 are suggestive of an ischaemic origin for these changes.

Record 57

6. a) The q waves in aVL exceed 0.03 sec in duration.

b) The q waves in aVL have a depth exceeding one quarter of the height of the ensuing R wave (inevitable – since there are no R waves!).

These changes **can** indicate the presence of anterolateral infarction. However, the mean frontal plane QRS axis in this case is $+75°$ and because of this aVL is a cavity lead and the q waves in aVL are therefore normal.

ECG diagnosis
Within normal limits.

Record 58

2. b) The r wave progression from V_1 to V_3 is abnormal. The r wave in V_2 is smaller than that in V_1, and the r wave in V_3 is smaller still and is actually preceded by a small q wave.

3. g) The q wave in V_3 has a depth exceeding one quarter of the height of the ensuing r wave. Although such a feature can occasionally occur in a normal record in one single precordial lead in the transition zone, it will be most unwise to accept it as normal in this case because of the obvious S-T segment elevation in the precordial series (see below).

The q wave in V_3 is probably indicative of anterior infarction.

5. There is obvious S-T elevation from V_1–V_4, indicative of acute anterior myocardial ischaemic damage.

There is minimal S-T segment depression in V_6 (not actually beyond the limits of normal).

8. There is slight S-T segment depression in II, III and aVF and slight S-T elevation in I and aVL.

The S-T elevation from V_1 to V_4 and in I and aVL is the primary change and the S-T depression in II, III, aVF and V_6 is a reciprocal change.

9. The P waves in II, III and aVF are bifid. This is not a definite abnormality but raises the possibility of left atrial abnormality.

ECG diagnosis
Acute anteroseptal myocardial ischaemic damage.

Record 59

2. a) V_1 has an RSR' complex.

3. a) The total QRS duration is 0.14 sec. The combination of these two findings indicates the presence of right bundle branch block. The right bundle branch block accounts for the presence of the broad, slurred R' wave in V_1 and the broad, slurred S wave from V_3–V_6 and in I and aVL.

ECG diagnosis
Complete right bundle block.

Record 60

3. c) The tallest precordial R wave (V_5) = 41 mm (well in excess of the normal maximum of 27 mm).

e) $R_{V_5} + S_{V_1}$ = 67 mm (well in excess of the normal maximum of 40 mm).

f) The ventricular activation time is abnormal at 0.05 sec.

4A. The T waves are inverted in V_5 and V_6. This is frankly abnormal.

5. There is S-T segment depression in V_5 and V_6. This is frankly abnormal. The S-T depression is asymmetrical and therefore is non-specific. It is not the typical S-T depression of myocardial ischaemia and is likely to be secondary to the QRS abnormalities which are indicative of left ventricular hypertrophy.

6. c) The R wave in aVL measures 20 mm (in excess of the normal maximum).

7. The mean frontal plane T wave axis is $+150°$. The frontal plane QRS axis is $-15°$. The angle between the two is therefore abnormal and the frontal plane T waves are abnormal.

8. There is significant, non-specific S-T depression in I and aVL.

9. The P waves in V_1 have a dominant negative component indicating left atrial abnormality.

ECG diagnosis
Left ventricular hypertrophy with left atrial abnormality (probably hypertrophy).

Record 61

2. a) No initial q wave is seen in V_6. However, there is a q wave in I and aVL and therefore the interventricular septum is being depolarised in the normal direction.

c) The transition zone is further to the left than V_6 (using the definition that the transition zone is reached when a septal q wave develops) or is between V_5 and V_6 (using the definition of the development of a dominant R wave). There is therefore pronounced clockwise cardiac rotation.

3. The tallest R wave in the precordial series (V_6) is only 6 mm. This is abnormally small but this is probably due to the pronounced clockwise rotation.

4A. The precordial T waves in V_5 and V_6 are of low voltage but the voltage is entirely appropriate to the size of the R wave and the T waves are therefore normal.

4B. The U waves are prominent (but not abnormal) in the precordial leads.

6. d) The mean frontal plane QRS axis is abnormal at $-45°$. Since the presence of initial r waves in aVF does not permit an ECG diagnosis of inferior infarction, the abnormal left axis deviation indicates the presence of left anterior hemiblock.

7. The mean frontal plane T axis is $+75°$. The angle between the T and QRS axes is therefore abnormal and the frontal plane T waves are therefore abnormal.

8. There is S-T segment depression in I and aVL.

ECG diagnosis
Left anterior hemiblock, clockwise cardiac rotation, non-specific S-T, T changes in the limb leads.

325

Record 62

2. a) No initial r wave is seen in V_1. No initial q wave is seen in V_6, I or aVL.

3. The total QRS duration is prolonged at 0.18 sec.

In view of the prolongation of the total QRS duration and absence of septal q waves (with no rSR' complex in V_1 to indicate right bundle branch block) and since there is no evidence of ventricular pre-excitation, there is complete left bundle branch block. This precludes any further assessment of the QRS complexes, S-T segments or T waves (except for the assessment of the mean frontal plane QRS axis). If a previous record is available for comparison, or if the interpreter is highly experienced, further interpretation may be possible.

ECG diagnosis
Left bundle branch block.

Record 63

2. a) V_1 has an Rs complex. This is abnormal. It should be an rS complex. Because of this abnormality the r wave progression across the precordial series cannot be normal. There is pronounced clockwise cardiac rotation.

4A. The T waves are iso-electric or minimally inverted in V_3 and V_4 and are of low voltage in V_5.

5. There is S-T depression in V_1 and V_2.

6. The frontal plane QRS axis is $+120°$. This is abnormal.
The combination of a dominant R wave in V_1 with an abnormal degree of right axis deviation indicates right ventricular hypertrophy.

7. The frontal plane T wave axis is $0°$. This is separated from the frontal plane QRS axis by an abnormal angle and therefore the frontal plane T waves are abnormal.

8. There is minimal S-T segment depression in Lead III.

9. b) The P wave height in II is 3 mm. This indicates right atrial hypertrophy.

ECG diagnosis
Right ventricular hypertrophy. Right atrial hypertrophy.

Record 64

2. a) No initial q wave is seen in the left precordial leads or in Lead I or aVL. This can indicate that the interventricular septum is being depolarised in the wrong direction. However, since the total QRS duration is entirely within normal limits, this variation is acceptable. If the QRS duration had been 0.10 or 0.11 sec the ECG diagnosis would have been incomplete left bundle branch block.

3. a) The total QRS duration is within normal limits.

c) The R waves in V_4 and V_5 are abnormally tall (measuring 42 mm in V_5).

f) The ventricular activation time cannot be measured since there is no qR complex in the left precordial leads.

4A. There is T wave inversion from V_2 to V_6.

5. There is S-T segment depression from V_2 to V_6.

7A. The frontal plane T wave axis is $+180°$. Since the frontal plane QRS axis is $+60°$, the angle between the two is abnormal and the frontal plane T waves are abnormal.

8. There is S-T depression in I, II and aVL.
The combination of abnormally tall R waves in the left precordial leads, with S-T segment and T wave changes in the precordial leads and S-T, T changes in the limb leads is indicative of left ventricular hypertrophy. It is surprising that there is no evidence of left atrial hypertrophy.

ECG diagnosis
Left ventricular hypertrophy.

Record 65

6. d) The frontal plane QRS axis is indeterminate, but this is not an abnormality, even though the frontal plane T wave axis is determinate ($+45°$).

9. a) The P wave duration in Lead II is abnormal at 0.13 sec.

c) There is a dominant negative component to the P wave in V_1. These changes indicate left atrial abnormality.

ECG diagnosis
Left atrial abnormality.

Record 66

2. a) No initial r wave is seen in V_1 (or in V_2 or V_3).

3. g) q waves are seen in V_1–V_3 with a duration in excess of 0.03 sec.

h) The q waves in V_1–V_3 have a depth exceeding one quarter of the height of the ensuing R wave.

4A. There is terminal T wave inversion from V_3–V_5 and the T waves are of low voltage in V_6.

5. There is S-T elevation from V_1–V_5. These changes indicate recent anteroseptal infarction.

7. The frontal plane T wave axis is $+120°$. This is at an abnormal angle to the mean frontal plane QRS axis (which is $+15°$). It follows that the T waves are abnormal in the frontal plane leads.

8. There is slight S-T segment elevation in Lead I.

ECG diagnosis
Recent anteroseptal infarction.

Record 67

1. The rhythm is sinus bradycardia.

2. b) No r wave in the precordial series exceeds 8 mm. The precordial R waves are therefore of abnormally low voltage.

4A. The T waves are of low voltage throughout the precordial leads.

9. The P waves are bifid in Lead II and in the precordial leads. This is not a **definite** abnormality, but is sometimes found in left atrial abnormalities.
The overall appearances are abnormal. The combination of sinus bradycardia with low voltage QRS and T waves suggests hypothyroidism.

ECG diagnosis
Sinus bradycardia. Generalised low voltages, suggesting possible hypothyroidism.

Record 68

2. a) V_1 has an Rs complex. This is abnormal. Because of this the R wave progression in the precordial series cannot be normal.

6. d) The mean frontal plane QRS axis is $+105°$.
The combination of a dominant R wave in V_1 with an abnormal degree of right axis deviation indicates the presence of right ventricular hypertrophy.

9. b) The P wave height in II is 3 mm. This is indicative of right atrial hypertrophy.

ECG diagnosis
Right ventricular hypertrophy. Right atrial hypertrophy.

Record 69

2. a) It is not clear whether or not there is a small r wave in V_1 – however –

b) There is no progression of the R wave from V_1–V_4 and this is frankly abnormal.

3. b) No precordial R wave exceeds 8 mm in height.

h) The q wave in V_4 has a height exceeding one quarter of the height of the subsequent R wave.

4A. There is T wave inversion from V_4–V_6.

5. There is S-T segment elevation from V_1–V_4.
These changes indicate the presence of recent anterior infarction. (The main criterion for the diagnosis of infarction in this case is the loss of R wave height from V_1–V_4).

6. a) It is difficult to be sure whether or not there is an initial r wave in Lead II – if not, the QRS complex would be of the QS type and this would be indicative of inferior infarction. However, there is clearly a small r in aVF. In this situation one cannot be confident that there is inferior infarction. It is possible that there has been an inferior infarct and that small r waves have subsequently been generated in place of the initial QS complexes associated with this condition.

d) The frontal plane QRS axis is abnormal at $-60°$.

7A. The frontal plane T wave axis is $+120°$. This is at an abnormal angle to the mean frontal plane QRS axis and the frontal plane T waves are therefore abnormal.

ECG diagnosis
Recent anterior infarction. There is an abnormal degree of left axis deviation. This could be due to old inferior infarction or to left anterior hemiblock. It is not possible with confidence to distinguish between these two possibilities.

Record 70

1. The P-R interval is abnormally short at 0.09 sec. The presence of this feature should lead one to look for the presence of a prolonged QRS duration.

3. (a) The total QRS duration is prolonged at 0.13 sec.
There is slurring of the initial part of the QRS complex. The combination of an abnormally short P-R interval and an abnormally long QRS complex with slurring of the initial part of the QRS complex indicates the presence of ventricular pre-excitation.
Unless a previous record is available for comparison, no further evaluation of the QRS complexes, S-T segments or T waves should be made. (Note, therefore, that the presence of ventricular pre-excitation produces even more severe limitations on ECG interpretation than does the presence of LBBB – for in the presence of the latter condition at least it is justifiable to proceed to the assessment of the frontal plane QRS axis (page 125), whereas this is not so in the case of ventricular pre-excitation). One cannot, therefore, assign any significance to the frontal plane axis (which would otherwise indicate left anterior hemiblock) or to the presence of QS complexes in aVF or V_1 (which would otherwise indicate inferior or anteroseptal infarction).

ECG diagnosis
Ventricular pre-excitation.

Annotated Records from Section 1: Reports

Appropriate reports for the 30 annotated records from Section I (pages 71–101) are given below:-

Record 1

Sinus rhythm. The P-R interval is normal at 0.18 sec. The mean frontal plane QRS axis is +60°. The record is within normal limits.

Record 2

Sinus rhythm. The P-R interval is normal at 0.12 sec. The mean frontal plane QRS axis is +75°. The record is within normal limits. (Note that the q waves which are apparent in aVL, are normal since aVL is, in this case, a cavity lead).

Record 3

Sinus rhythm. The P-R interval is normal at 0.18 sec. The mean frontal plane QRS axis is −15°. **There is a shallow T wave inversion in V_5 and V_6. The angle between the mean frontal plane QRS and T wave axes is abnormal at +135° (the mean frontal plane T wave axis being +120°). There are therefore frankly abnormal T wave changes in the limb leads and in the left precordial leads. These are non-specific abnormalities.** The U waves are prominent but not abnormal in the left precordial leads. (No specific cause can be assigned to the electrocardiographic abnormalities here. Possibilities include myocardial ischaemia and hypokalaemia. It would be unwise to diagnose left ventricular hypertrophy simply on the basis that the R wave height in aVL is minimally above the accepted voltage criteria.)

Record 4

Sinus rhythm. The P-R interval is normal at 0.16 sec. The mean frontal plane QRS axis is +30°. **The precordial QRS complexes just satisfy the voltage criteria for left ventricular hypertrophy. The ventricular activation time is increased at 0.05 sec. These changes are indicative of left ventricular hypertrophy. There is a dominant negative component to the P wave in V_1, indicating left atrial abnormality (quite possibly hypertrophy). There is significant S-T segment elevation in Leads II, III and the foot-lead, and S-T segment depression in Leads I, the left arm-lead and in V_2 and V_3. These changes are indicative of acute inferior myocardial (ischaemic) damage. (The changes in Leads II, III and the foot-lead are primary, those in I, aVL, V_2 and V_3 are secondary.)**

Record 5

Sinus rhythm. The P-R interval is normal at 0.16 sec. The mean frontal plane QRS axis is +45°. **There are unequivocal changes of left ventricular hypertrophy. The precordial voltage criteria for this condition are fulfilled and there are secondary S-T, T changes in leads facing the left ventricle (in this case V_4 to V_6, Leads I, II and aVL). The form of the P waves in V_1 is indicative of left atrial abnormality (probably hypertrophy).**

Record 6

Sinus rhythm. The P-R interval is normal at 0.14 sec. **The mean frontal plane QRS axis is +165° and there is a dominant R wave in V_1. These changes are indicative of right ventricular hypertrophy. The P waves are abnormally tall in the foot-lead (3 mm) indicating right atrial hypertrophy.** (This criterion is normally used in Lead II but can be applied in whichever frontal plane lead is most closely related to the axis of the P wave. This is usually Lead II, but in this case the P wave axis is +75° which is halfway between Leads II and the foot-lead and either of these leads may be chosen). (The other point for comment in this electrocardiogram is the presence of very deep S waves in V_2 and V_3. Deep S waves in the **left** precordial leads are very much part of the pattern of right ventricular hypertrophy, but deep S waves in the **right** precordial leads are not routinely found in this condition. They raise the possibility of additional left ventricular hypertrophy but they are not totally diagnostic).

Record 7

Sinus rhythm. The P-R interval is normal at 0.16 sec. The mean frontal plane QRS axis is −15°. **There is complete left bundle branch block** (the left bundle branch block accounts for the absence of appropriate r wave progression across the precordial leads and for the S-T, T changes in Leads I, aVL and the left precordial leads).

Record 8

Sinus rhythm. The P-R interval is normal at 0.16 sec. **The mean frontal plane QRS axis is −45° indicating an abnormal degree of left axis deviation. There is evidence of an old anteroseptal myocardial infarction** (there is loss of the r waves from V_1–V_3 and inappropriately small r waves from V_4–V_6. It is likely, but not certain, that the abnormal left axis deviation is due to ischaemic damage to the anterior division of the left bundle branch system giving rise to left anterior hemiblock).

Record 9

Sinus rhythm. The P-R interval is normal at 0.20 sec. The mean frontal plane QRS axis is +75°. There is no significant abnormality in the form of the QRS complexes, the S-T segments or the T waves. **There is clear evidence of left atrial hypertrophy in that the P waves in Lead II are broad and bifid and the P waves in V_1 have a dominant negative component.** The combination of left atrial hypertrophy and a mean frontal plane QRS axis towards the right hand end of the normal range in the absence of any other electrocardiographic abnormality suggests the possibility of obstruction at the mitral valve. (This is very commonly due to mitral stenosis and extremely rarely due to the presence of an atrial myxoma).

Record 10

Sinus rhythm. The P-R interval is normal at 0.13 sec. The mean frontal plane QRS axis is +75°. **The form of the QRS complexes in V_1 is borderline abnormal in that the R/S ratio is unity. The form of the P waves in V_1 indicates the presence of left atrial hypertrophy.** A prominent atrial repolarisation wave is seen in the left precordial leads. (The diagnostic criteria for right ventricular hypertrophy are not fulfilled but the presence of an R/S ratio of unity in V_1, together with a mean frontal plane QRS axis, towards the right hand end of the normal range suggests the possibility of minimal right ventricular enlargement). **The P waves in Lead II are also slightly pointed and the possibility of right atrial hypertrophy should be considered although the appearances are not definitive.** The apparent S-T segment depression in the left precordial leads is part of a prominent atrial repolarisation wave which can be seen to begin before the QRS complex. As in Record 9, the most likely clinical accompaniment of such an electrocardiogram is mitral valve obstruction.

Record 11

Sinus rhythm. The P-R interval is normal at 0.12 sec. The mean frontal plane QRS axis is +30°. The record is within normal limits.

Record 12

Sinus rhythm. The P-R interval is normal at 0.20 sec. The mean frontal plane QRS axis is +15°. **There are non-specific S-T, T changes in the limb leads and the left precordial leads.** (The record is frankly abnormal but no specific cause for the abnormality can be assigned. There is no primary abnormality in the QRS complexes and the S-T, T changes are therefore primary. Abnormalities of this type can be found in association with myocardial ischaemia, myocarditis, cardiomyopathy, pericarditis, hypokalaemia and hypothyroidism. The latter is rendered less likely but by absence of a bradycardia.

Record 13

Sinus rhythm. The P-R interval is within normal limits at 0.12 sec. The mean frontal plane QRS axis is +75°. **There is evidence of recent anterior myocardial infarction. (Definitive evidence of infarction appears from V$_1$–V$_4$ and there is also S-T segment elevation in V$_5$ and Lead I.** The q waves in aVL are not necessarily abnormal themselves because the frontal plane QRS axis is +75° and aVL is therefore a cavity lead).

Record 14

Sinus rhythm. The P-R interval is normal at 0.12 sec. The mean frontal plane QRS axis is +45°.
The record is within normal limits. (Note that the T wave inversion in Lead III is not abnormal. The mean frontal plane T wave axis is +15°. The angle between the frontal plane QRS and T wave axes is thus well within the normal range at 30° and it follows that the frontal plane T waves are all within normal limits).

Record 15

Sinus rhythm. The P-R interval is normal at 0.14 sec. The mean frontal plane QRS axis is −15°. **The precordial QRS complexes satisfy the voltage criteria for left ventricular hypertrophy** (note that the precordial leads are half-standardised). **There are non-specific S-T, T changes in the left precordial leads, Leads I, II and aVL. These S-T, T changes are definitely abnormal.** No specific cause for them can be assigned. They may well be secondary to the primary QRS abnormality and thus be part of the picture of left ventricular hypertrophy. However, alternative additional abnormalities may need to be considered as in Record 12.

Record 16

Sinus rhythm. The P-R interval is normal at 0.12 sec. The mean frontal plane QRS axis is 0°. **There is evidence of left ventricular hypertrophy and of inferior myocardial infarction of intermediate age. The precordial QRS complexes satisfy the voltage criteria for left ventricular hypertrophy and the intrinsic deflection time is abnormal. The S-T, T changes in V$_4$, V$_5$ and V$_6$ are probably secondary to the primary QRS abnormality of left ventricular hypertrophy.** The form of the QRS complexes in V$_4$ could be indicative of a localised anterior infarction (since there is appreciable reduction in the r wave compared with that seen in V$_3$ and that seen in V$_5$), but it would be unwise to make a confident diagnosis of this since the r wave can occasionally be inappropriately small in a single lead in the precordial series in the transition zone (page 45). **There is definitive q wave evidence of infarction in aVF where the q waves are abnormally deep and abnormally broad. The T wave inversion in Leads II, III and aVF is probably part of the pattern of inferior infarction. If so it indicates that the infarct is of intermediate age.** It is not a very recent infarction since there is no residual S-T segment elevation. However, one cannot be sure that the T wave changes in the inferior limb leads are related to the infarction. They could also be related to the left ventricular hypertrophy.

Record 17

Sinus rhythm. The P-R interval is normal at 0.16 sec. **The mean frontal plane QRS axis is −45°. This is an abnormal degree of left axis deviation.** The deviation is probably due to left anterior hemiblock. **There is evidence of old anteroseptal myocardial infarction. Small initial r waves are seen in V$_1$ but the r wave is smaller or absent in V$_2$, and V$_3$ shows q waves. The QRS configuration in V$_1$, V$_2$ and V$_3$ therefore unequivocally represents an anteroseptal infarction** (the total QRS duration being within the normal range). The abnormal degree of left axis deviation occurring in the absence of QRS evidence of inferior myocardial infarction indicates the presence of left anterior hemiblock. There is minimal S-T segment depression in V$_6$ but one cannot be sure of the significance of this since the baseline is not truly horizontal.

Record 18

Sinus rhythm. The P-R interval is normal at 0.15 sec. The mean frontal plane QRS axis is +15°. **There is evidence of left ventricular hypertrophy with counterclockwise cardiac rotation (the precordial QRS complexes satisfy the voltage criteria for left ventricular hypertrophy and the ventricular activation time is prolonged. There are non-specific S-T, T changes from V$_3$–V$_6$.** These are almost certainly secondary to the primary QRS abnormality. The transition zone is between V$_2$ and V$_3$, indicating pronounced counterclockwise cardiac rotation. **There are non-specific S-T, T changes also in the limb leads.** These too are almost certainly secondary to the primary QRS abnormality).

Record 19

Sinus rhythm. The P-R interval is normal at 0.16 sec. The mean frontal plane QRS axis is +45°. The record is within normal limits.

Record 20

Sinus rhythm. The P-R interval is normal at 0.15 sec. The mean frontal plane QRS axis is +15°. The record is within normal limits.

Record 21

Sinus rhythm. The P-R interval is normal at 0.19 sec. The mean frontal plane QRS axis is +30°. **There is evidence of left ventricular hypertrophy and left atrial hypertrophy. (The S-T, T changes in the left precordial leads and in the limb leads are almost certainly secondary to the primary QRS abnormality).**

Record 22

Sinus rhythm. The P-R interval is normal at 0.16 sec. The mean frontal plane QRS axis is indeterminate. The complexes in all these leads are of low voltage and **no precordial R wave satisfies the minimum voltage criterion of 8 mm. This is a non-specific feature, but raises the possibility of anterior infarction. The q wave in aVF is abnormal and indicates the presence of an old inferior infarction.** (The abnormally low r wave voltage across the precordial leads could be due to obesity or emphysema. Hypothyroidism should also be considered, but this is relatively unlikely in view of the lack of sinus bradycardia).

The generalised low voltage of the T waves is not of any separate significance for the T waves are bound to be of low voltage since the QRS complexes are of low voltage. The significance of the low voltage in the precordial leads can only be assessed by secondary interpretation. It is conceivable that there has been extensive loss of R wave voltage as a result of previous infarction, but in the presence of obesity or emphysema it would be most unwise to make such a deduction. The q waves in aVF, which are easily missed, are indicative of inferior infarction. This is perhaps best seen in the third QRS complex in aVF.

Record 23

Sinus rhythm. The P-R interval is normal at 0.16 sec. The mean frontal plane QRS axis is +75°. **There is complete right bundle branch block** (the "splintering" of the QRS complexes in V_2, V_3 and V_4 is simply part of the right bundle branch block).

Record 24

Sinus rhythm. The P-R interval is normal at 0.14 sec. The mean frontal plane QRS axis is +15°. The record is within normal limits. (The q wave in aVL is at the upper end of the normal range, but is not definitely abnormal).

Record 25

Sinus rhythm. The P-R interval is normal at 0.12 sec. The mean frontal plane QRS axis is +15°.

There is evidence of an old anterior myocardial infarction. (There are QS complexes in V_1 and V_2, abnormally deep and wide q waves with very small r waves in V_3, and abnormally deep and wide q waves in V_4. There are non-specific S-T, T changes throughout the precordial leads. These are almost certainly secondary to the primary QRS abnormality. Non-specific S-T, T changes are also seen in these limb leads).

Record 26

Sinus rhythm. The P-R interval is normal at 0.13 sec. The mean frontal plane QRS axis is −30°.

There is evidence of inferior myocardial infarction of intermediate age. Non-specific S-T, T changes are seen in the left precordial leads suggesting apical extension of the ischaemic or infarcted zone (inferior myocardial infarction is not infrequently associated with ischaemic changes in the left precordial leads, the area of infarction or ischaemia being referred to either as "apical" or "inferolateral". There is no definitive evidence of lateral myocardial infarction in this case although the R waves are rather lower in voltage in the left precordial leads than one would expect).

Record 27

Sinus rhythm. The P-R interval is normal at 0.19 sec. The mean frontal plane QRS axis is +45°.

There are non-specific S-T, T changes in the left precordial leads and in the limb leads. (There is no abnormality in the form of the QRS complexes. The non-specific S-T, T changes are therefore primary). As usual therefore, it is not possible to assign a specific cause for the abnormality.

Record 28

Sinus rhythm. The P-R interval is normal at 0.14 sec. The mean frontal plane QRS axis is −15°.

There is complete left bundle branch block. (Note that the QS complexes in the inferior limb leads do not signify inferior myocardial infarction since there is left bundle branch block. In the same way, the absence of r wave progression in V_1–V_3 does not signify myocardial infarction. Both these features are part of the left bundle branch block pattern).

Record 29

Sinus rhythm. The P-R interval is normal at 0.20 sec. **The mean frontal plane QRS axis is +120°. There is evidence of right ventricular hypertrophy** (the dominant r wave in V_1 together with the abnormal degree of right axis deviation indicates right ventricular hypertrophy. **The pronounced clockwise cardiac rotation is simply part of the pattern of right ventricular hypertrophy as are the S-T, T changes which are present in this record from V_1–V_4.** Prominent U waves are seen in V_3 and V_4 but these are not definitely abnormal).

Record 30

Sinus rhythm. The P-R interval is normal at 0.17 sec. The mean frontal plane QRS axis is +45°.

The record is within the normal limits although the QRS complexes in V_1 and V_2 could be consistent with an old anteroseptal infarction (the r wave progression from V_1–V_3 is not typically normal and there is no doubt that it is possible that there is an old anteroseptal infarction. However, appearances of this type are sometimes seen in normal records and as a general rule it is best to under-report rather than to over-report the electrocardiogram. It must be remembered that not only may **this** pattern be associated with an anteroseptal infarction, so may a completely normal electrocardiogram!).

Epilogue

Every effort has been made, in the writing of this text, to encourage the development of confidence in electrocardiographic interpretation on the part of the reader. It is, nevertheless, essential also to remember that the electrocardiogram has severe limitations as a diagnostic tool. It provides information about depolarisation and about repolarisation of myocardium. Information about disease in the coronary arteries is not directly provided by the electrocardiogram, though it may often be inferred if the electrocardiogram is abnormal. A normal electrocardiogram in no way excludes significant stenosing atheroma of the coronary arteries. The following two cases illustrate this.

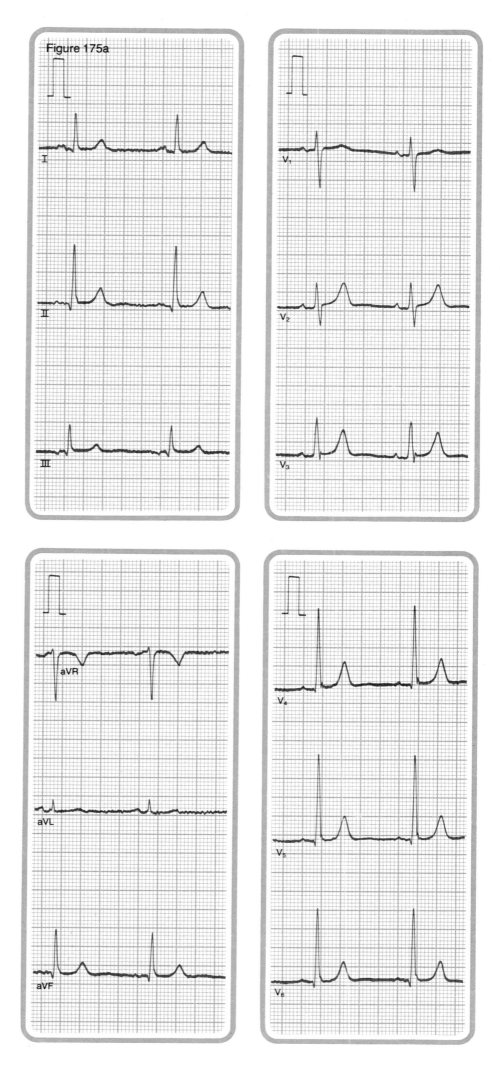

Figure 175a

331

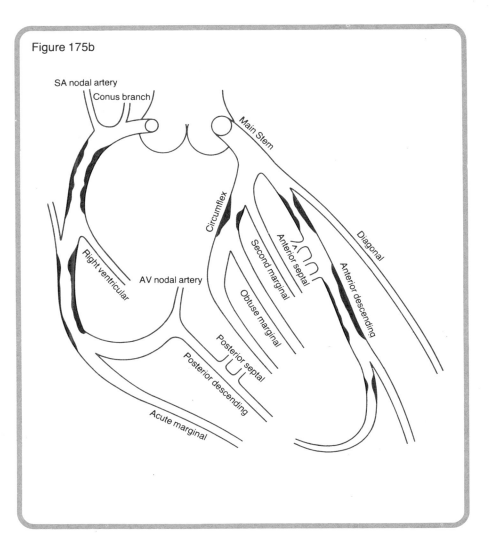

Figure 175b

Case 1

J.R. A 54-year-old lady with an unequivocal story of angina pectoris. The electrocardiogram is shown in Figure 175a. This ECG would be reported as follows:-
"Sinus rhythm. The mean frontal plane QRS axis is +45°. The record is within normal limits".

Figure 175b shows the coronary angiographic appearances in this patient. There is evidence of severe, stenosing atheroma in the anterior descending and circumflex branches of the left coronary artery, and in the main right coronary artery.

This patient thus has involvement of all three major coronary arteries without any electrocardiographic abnormality whatsoever.

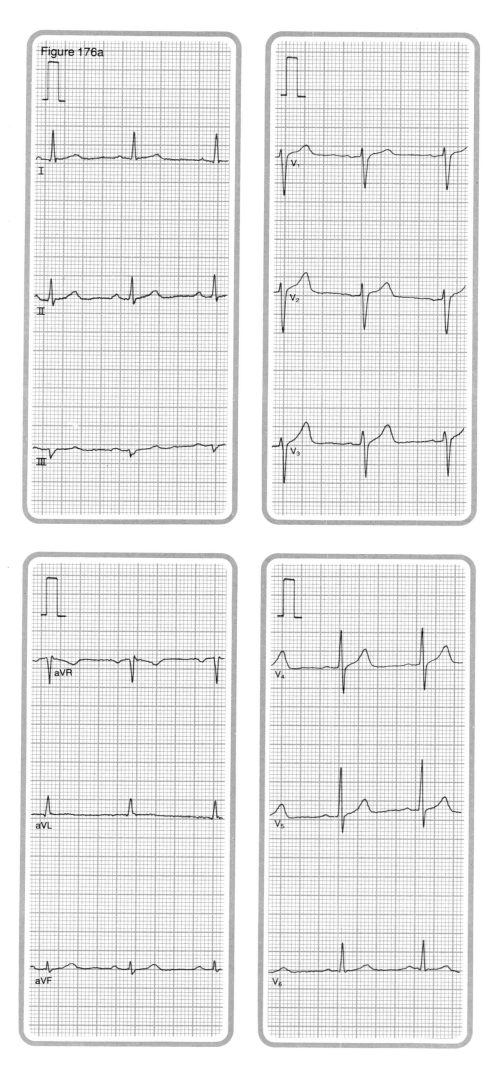

Figure 176a

I
II
III

aVR
aVL
aVF

V₁
V₂
V₃

V₄
V₅
V₆

333

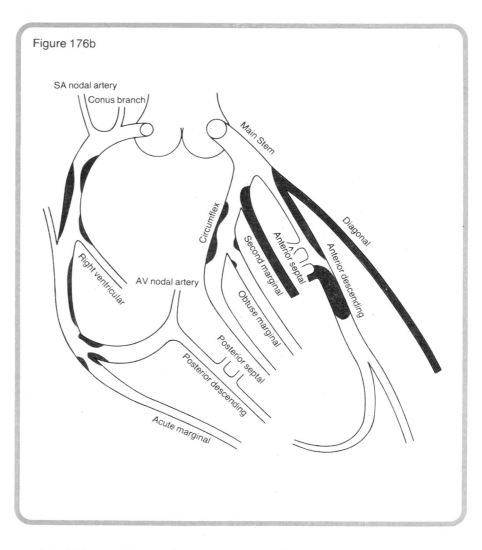

Figure 176b

SA nodal artery

Conus branch

Main Stem

Circumflex

Diagonal

Second marginal

Anterior septal

Anterior descending

Right ventricular

AV nodal artery

Obtuse marginal

Posterior septal

Posterior descending

Acute marginal

Case 2

A.A. A 50-year-old man with severe, disabling angina pectoris and repeated hospital admissions with episodes of chest pain. The electrocardiogram is shown in Figures 176a. This electrocardiogram would be interpreted as follows:-

"Sinus rhythm. The mean frontal plane QRS axis is +15°. The record is within normal limits".

Figure 176b shows the coronary angiographic appearances in this patient. There is very extensive disease in the right coronary artery, there is complete occlusion of the diagonal branch of the left coronary artery and of the distal part of the anterior descending branch of the left coronary artery. There is complete occlusion of the second marginal branch of the circumflex coronary artery and significant narrowing in the main circumflex artery itself. In addition, this patient had actually already received four coronary saphenous by-pass grafts, two of which were completely blocked, one of which was severely narrowed and one of which was working normally.

It is hoped that these two cases will provide a cautionary tale sufficient to discourage anyone from believing that a normal electro-cardiogram in any way excludes significant disease in the coronary arteries.